Physical Examination, History Taking & Health Assessment Test Bank

1500+ Test Bank Questions with Rationales

Nursing Spring

What's in this test bank?

This test bank is a comprehensive all-inclusive reviewer on patient health assessment, particularly physical examination, and history-taking, reflecting the latest standards and technology in this field.

This compilation stores more than 1500 questions categorized into 27 chapters. All items were developed based on numerous references for patient assessment.

The questions are held to the highest standards and include the latest updates on physical examination and history-taking concepts. They have undergone extensive checking and testing so that they closely reflect those in real exams.

The items are a combination of multiple choice and SATA (select all that applies) types. The questions are compiled per body system and includes the assessments of children, pregnant women and older adults.

The rationales serve as a concise reviewer for the most pertinent information in the subject matter. And as a bonus, it comes with a chapter dedicated to strategies in physical examination!

Who can use this test bank?

The questions in this test bank are designed for students taking up a course on patient health assessment, especially in nursing. It also serves as an invaluable reviewer and practice material for those who would sit for the NCLEX or the US nursing board exams.

Who developed the practice questions?

The questions in this test bank were developed by experts who have taken the examinations themselves and have extensively applied the concepts discussed therein throughout their careers. The team consists of educators and clinical instructors who are trained in honing the critical thinking skills of test-takers. These experts have utilized the question development standards as mandated by the NCSBN (National Council for State Boards of Nursing).

What are the benefits of using this test bank?

Listening to lectures and watching live demos inside the classroom help to grasp concepts on health assessment but are never enough to pass the course or the NCLEX.

Students and Board examinees need to practice answering a lot of NCLEX-style questions to familiarize themselves with the subject as well as the test-taking techniques, both of which lead to mastery and confidence.

 This set of tests is a sort of dry-run before the real exam, and is, therefore, indispensable.

Table of Contents

Introduction to Health Assessment

Questions

1. A nurse admits a client with a chief complaint of pain in the right lower quadrant of the abdomen. She understands that to obtain objective data, she has to
   a. Ask about the patient's last meal
   b. Put the client on NPO
   c. Perform a physical examination
   d. Ask the patient what could have triggered the pain

2. To which of the following patient should a focused physical examination be more appropriate?
   a. A 56-year old male with a 4-inch laceration on the arm, coherent and responsive.
   b. A 2-year old girl with low grade fever and a rash
   c. A 25-year-old male asking for a medical certificate for employment purposes
   d. A 76-year-old female having 5 loose stools since the day before

3. The nurse is preparing the patient for physical examination. Which of the following events need improvement on the part of the nurse?
   a. Nurse enters the room with the client and goes out to gather supplies
   b. Nurse adjusts the light to accommodate the examination accordingly
   c. Nurse asks the client for consent and positions the client comfortably on the examining table
   d. Nurse begins checking the general appearance and then takes the vital signs

4. A 52-year old female client presents to the clinic for the first time with a chief complaint of weight loss and extreme fatigue. The nurse assesses the client accordingly. As the nurse examines the breasts, the nurse palpates an immovable 3-inch mass on the left breast and some dimpling of the skin. The client states, "I've noticed this lump for some time now but didn't really mind it. What do you think it is?" Which of the following is the most appropriate nursing response?
   a. "I am not certain, but it can be breast cancer. Don't be alarmed. The doctor will order some tests to be   sure."
   b. "Don't worry about it now. We'll know tomorrow."
   c. "Let's stay positive. It can be nothing, you know."
   d. "It's a 3-inch mass. We will have to finish our examination and the doctor will have to perform some more tests on you."

5. The nurse prepares a female client for a genito-urinary examination and helps her assume a lithotomy position. Which of the following nursing actions warrants further evaluation?
   a. The nurse secures the drapes around the examining table
   b. The nurse uses a warmed speculum to assess the genitalia
   c. The nurse puts on sterile gloves before touching the client's genitalia
   d. The nurse politely leaves the room after examination.

6. During a focused physical examination, the patient suspected of cholelithiasis asks to urinate. What is the most appropriate nursing response?

    a. Offer a hospital gown and assist the client to the toilet
    b. Offer a urinal and leave the room
    c. Politely ask the client to 'hold it'
    d. Explain to the client briefly why he needs to lie still

7. The nurse is preparing to examine the patient's eye. Which of the following equipment/instrument is not necessary?
    a. A snellen chart
    b. Opthalmoscope
    c. Pen light
    d. Stadiometer

8. During abdominal examination, which of the following is the right sequence in performing assessment?
    a. Auscultation, inspection, percussion, palpation
    b. Inspection, auscultation, percussion, palpation
    c. Palpation, Percussion, Inspection, auscultation
    d. Inspection, palpation, percussion, auscultation

9. A nurse plans to inspect the patient's spine. To what position will the nurse assist the client to assume?
    a. Semi-Fowler's position
    b. A neutral position while sitting or standing, and the client's back fully exposed to the nurse
    c. Prone position with the upper extremities drawn to the sides, and the client's back fully exposed to the nurse
    d. In a standing position assuming a 'military stance'

10. A 65-year old male has been admitted for a possible blood transfusion. Which of the following client information is most pertinent to obtain during history taking?
    a. Socioeconomic status
    b. Marital status
    c. Spiritual and cultural beliefs
    d. Vaccination history

11. The nurse is preparing to measure the blood pressure of a morbidly obese adult client. Which of the following is the correct nursing action?
    a. The nurse obtains a standard adult cuff size and wraps it around the client's forearm
    b. The nurse prepares to use the bell of the stethoscope to auscultate for the pulse
    c. The nurse obtains a thigh cuff and wraps it around the client's forearm
    d. The nurse does none of the above and asks the physician to do the measurement

12. It is a method of tapping body parts with the tips of the fingers to help determine the size,

consistency, and borders of body organs, or the presence or absence of fluid in body cavities.
a. Palpation
b. Auscultation
c. Inspection
d. Percussion

13. The nurse hears the client says "My mother has diabetes. My dad died of cancer." The nurse is sure to document this part of health history under
a. Adult illnesses
b. Childhood illnesses
c. Past medical condition
d. Family history

14. A 66-year-old male client accompanied by his wife is seen in the clinic because he failed to recognize his son. When asked about the present year, the answered, "I'm sure it's 1975." Which of the following is the best action the nurse should take with regards to history taking?
a. Proceed to obtain information from the wife
b. Ask about his health condition around 1975
c. Let the client rest for 30 minutes and proceed to ask information from the client
d. Ask the client if he has experienced memory loss before

15. When obtaining a patient's history, the nurse performs which of the following?
a. Gathers data about the patient's chief complaint
b. Palpates the patient's abdomen
c. Auscultates for the patient's heart sounds
d. Documents vital signs

16. The following are the purposes of a nursing health assessment EXCEPT:
a. To help establish a medical diagnosis
b. To determine the patient's need for health teaching
c. To help identify risk factors
d. To help develop a nursing care plan

17. A 55-year old male client has undergone a coronary angioplasty a week before and comes to the clinic for a scheduled visit. Which type of assessment would the nurse most appropriately perform?
a. A comprehensive health history
b. An emergency history
c. Problem oriented assessment
d. Follow-up history

18. A 19-year old soccer player was admitted with a laceration to the arm and is bleeding profusely.

Which type of history/assessment is best to perform?
a. A comprehensive health history
b. An emergency history
c. Problem oriented assessment
d. Follow-up history

19. This section of the history is a complete, clear, and chronologic account of the problems prompting the patient to seek care.
a. Past History
b. Health Patterns
c. Chief Complaint(s)
d. History of Present Illness (HPI)

20. Which of the following set of questions can be used to assess for risk factors?
a. Have you had your MMR shots? How many DTaP shots did you receive in all?
b. Do you use or have you ever used marijuana, cocaine, heroin, or other recreational drugs? How much alcohol do you drink per sitting and per week?
c. Has anyone in your family been diagnosed with hypertension? Cancer?
d. What types of tests were done on you and when?

21. Which of the following statement about health is TRUE?
a. Health is primarily referring to the physical wellbeing of a person.
b. Health is all about the absence of disease.
c. Health is achieved by just eating the right kind of food.
d. Health is living to one's potential and is the sum of facets that make up the individual.

22. A mother of three recently learned that she lost her job. Although she was saddened by the news, she regarded her circumstance as an opportunity to look for a higher-paying job. Which facet of the mother's health is reflected in this situation?
a. Physical health
b. Emotional health
c. Cultural influences
d. Developmental level

23. Which of the following describes the development facet of an individual's health?
a. Absence of disease
b. The surroundings are favorable to promote and maintain health
c. Able to find solutions to both common and complex everyday problems
d. Presence of supportive family and friends

24. Which of the following is NOT an indicator of a successful health maintenance?
a. Able to adapt

   b. Preserving the facets
   c. Able to align the facets
   d. Adhering strictly to set standards for oneself

25. Which of the following comprise a nursing health assessment? Select all that apply.
   a. A comprehensive health history
   b. A systems review
   c. A complete physical examination
   d. A neurobiological assessment

26. Which of the following is TRUE about a nursing health assessment?
   a. It focuses primarily on the review of systems
   b. It is a systematic way of collecting patient data to develop the most appropriate and effective plan of care
   c. It primarily involves interviewing the patient to seek pertinent health information
   d. The patient need not participate in the data collection

27. Which of the following are parts of the nursing process? Select all that apply.
   a. Developing a medical diagnosis
   b. Determining a patient's health status, risk factors, and need for teaching
   c. Extrapolating the patient's health data
   d. Prioritizing the findings
   e. Formulating and implementing the plan of care

28. Which of the following goals does Healthy People 2020 hope to achieve overall?
   a. Perform health teaching
   b. Correct misconceptions about health
   c. Eradicate chronic diseases
   d. Increase quality of life

29. Which of the following directly achieves the goal of cultivating an awareness that will eliminate health disparities under Healthy People 2020?
   a. Planning for health promotion
   b. Health education
   c. Participating in research
   d. Creating policies for implementation

30. Which of the following questions assesses the reason for the patient's visit to the clinic or hospital?
   a. "Who do you talk to when you have questions about your health?"
   b. "What are the reasons for your previous hospitalizations?"
   c. "What do you do when you feel sick?"
   d. "Tell me why you are here today."

31. Which of the following nurse actions will elicit the patient's verbal response to the nurse's assessment?
    a. Measuring the patient's blood pressure
    b. Observing the patient's facial expression
    c. Asking the patient what medications he is taking
    d. Checking the patient's body movements

32. Which of the following reflects the role of the nurse in keeping the community healthy? Select all that apply.
    a. Contributing to the creation of public policies on health
    b. Using the nursing process to alleviate the pain of the patient in the emergency room
    c. Assessing family dynamics
    d. Providing feedback that will be useful in making decisions for community health

33. Which of the following statements is TRUE?
    a. The nurses' initial role in health assessment is the implementation of a health care plan
    b. Nurses provide holistic care.
    c. The nurses' observations and attention to details primarily happen in the initial stage of care provision.
    d. Culture and the environment have very little influence on a patient's health.

34. Which of the following patients will need a comprehensive assessment?
    a. A 30-year-old mother of two who is asking for a contraceptive
    b. A 66-year old man presenting with chest pain in the emergency room
    c. A 2-year old boy with a greenstick arm fracture
    d. A 48-year old woman complaining of weakness and malaise for several months' now

35. On which of the following patients will the nurse need to perform a comprehensive assessment?
    a. A patient who was stabilized in the emergency room after being treated for high blood sugar for the first time
    b. A patient bleeding in the arm after a vehicular accident
    c. A patient for a return check-up
    d. A hospice patient who is asking for a change of medication

36. Which of the following patients would need a focused assessment?
    a. A post-surgical patient who returned to the clinic for wound cleaning
    b. A jobseeker who is for checkup, fulfilling an HR requirement
    c. A middle-aged man complaining of vague abdominal pain for the last six months
    d. A 5-year-old who is underweight despite being given proper diet

37. Which of the following can be a source of data when collecting the health information of a patient? Select all that apply.
    a. Past medical records
    b. The patient himself
    c. The patient's neighbors
    d. The patient's family
    e. The patient's social media status

38. Which of the following nurse actions will help the patient make decisions regarding their health? Select all that apply.
    a. Provide health teaching
    b. Ask for the patient's input
    c. Encourage the patient to choose the nurse's personal recommendations
    d. Encourage the patient to ask their friends with a similar health conditions on what to do
    e. Answer the patient's questions regarding health using the latest clinical evidence

39. A new patient who has a blood pressure reading of 160/100 has just been given an antihypertensive medication. Which of the following actions reflects the ability of the nurse to make timely assessments?
    a. Prepare the patient for an emergency procedure
    b. Measure the patient's blood pressure again after 30 minutes.
    c. Perform a comprehensive assessment while waiting for the medication to take effect
    d. Tell the patient to refrain from eating fatty foods for the next two weeks

40. Which of the following reflects the nurse's ability to recognize the patient's spiritual needs?
    a. Making the patient elaborate on the ways they handle stress
    b. Asking the patient about their relationship with their children
    c. Referring a clergy from the patient's religious affiliation when the patient so requests
    d. Asking the patient to tell more about the days they feel sad

41. Which of the following nursing actions reflects the nurse's ability to recognize a patient's social needs during a comprehensive assessment?
    a. The nurse asks the patient what they usually do when they get stressed
    b. The nurse observes a 1-year-old baby walk
    c. The nurse asks the patient how many times in a week they experience headaches
    d. The nurse refers the patient to a support group

42. Which of the following statements about making assessments is INCORRECT?
    a. Sufficient time is needed to make a thorough and detailed assessment.
    b. Making assessments using the '7 facets' is a major responsibility of the nurse.
    c. Nurses must identify what is needed by the patient on a monthly basis.
    d. Accurate history taking and physical examination are the foundations of nursing practice.

43. Which strategies are aligned with Healthy People 2020? Select all that apply.
    a. Reducing the length of hospitalization
    b. Health promotion
    c. Disease prevention
    d. Eradication of cancer
    e. Finding a cure for AIDS

44. The Healthy People agenda provides guidelines for healthy living for how many years?
    a. 3 years
    b. 5 years
    c. 10 years
    d. 20 years

45. Which of the following will help determine the type of assessment that needs to be completed in a given situation?
    a. The patient's age
    b. The patient's current situation and condition
    c. The patient's preference
    d. The nurse's preference

ANSWERS

1. C

    In performing a physical examination, the nurse obtains objective data. Asking information from the client is gathering subjective data. Putting the client on NPO is not part of assessment but of intervention

2. A

    The 56-year old male with a 4-inch laceration on the arm, coherent and responsive will benefit from a focused assessment because his wound needs to be treated immediately.

3. A

    A patient who is to undergo physical examination is most likely anxious and should never be left alone in the examining room. The nurse gathers supplies first before entering the room with the client.

4. D

    The nurse is not allowed to assume a medical diagnosis however overwhelming the evidence gets. The nurse may tell the client an objective data in a matter-of-fact way. It is non-therapeutic to give false reassurances.

5. D

    The nurse never leaves the client by herself to get out of lithotomy position. The nurse first assists the client to get down from the examining table and helps her get dressed.

6. A

    The comfort of the client is a priority during an examination. If the client is without an emergent condition, the nurse assists the client put on a gown if necessary and escorts the client to the toilet. A urinal is not necessary and denying the client the request is unethical.

7. D

    A stadiometer is used to measure height

8. B

    When assessing the abdomen, it is best to do percussion and palpation after auscultation because these maneuvers can affect bowel motility that can consequently alter abdominal sounds

9. B

    To assess the spine, the nurse asks the client to assume a neutral position while sitting or standing, and the client's back fully exposed to the nurse. All other positions will not help determine misalignment or assess curvature.

10. C

Some religions and culture forbid blood transfusion. It is important to assess beliefs to appropriately establish care.

11. C

Using the correct cuff size is pertinent to obtain the most accurate blood pressure measurement. For morbidly obese clients whose arm circumference is more than 46 cm, the thigh cuff is most appropriate to use.

12. D

Percussion is the method of tapping body parts with the tips of the fingers to help determine the size, consistency, and borders of body organs, or the presence or absence of fluid in body cavities. Palpation is the method of feeling with the fingers or hands during a physical examination. Auscultation is listening to sounds within the body either directly or through a stethoscope or other instrument. Inspection is careful viewing of a body part without touching.

13. D

Family history provides information on age and health, or age and cause of death, of siblings, parents, and grandparents. It also contains data on presence or absence of specific illnesses in the family, such as diabetes and cancer.

14. A

A disoriented client is not a reliable source for a comprehensive history. In cases such as these, the wife becomes the most reliable source of information. The nurse documents that information was sourced out from the client's wife.

15. A

Chief complaint is a direct statement of the client of why he is seeking medical attention. B, C and D are part of the physical examination.

16. D

The purposes of a nursing health assessment are to determine the patient's need for health teaching, to help identify risk factors and to help develop a nursing care plan. The medical diagnosis is established by the doctor upon confirmation by a specific or a series of diagnostic procedures

17. D

The follow-up history is a form of a focused assessment. The patient comes back to the clinic on a scheduled visit to have a problem or treatment plan evaluated. This type of assessment can also be used by a nurse upon endorsement of another nurse from earlier shift or from another department. This assessment helps evaluate the outcomes of the plan of care.

18. B

    The emergency history is best to perform in this situation because the data collection is focused on the patient's emergent problem and the nurse begins to assess ABC's, Airway, Breathing and Circulation followed by the affected body part.

19. D

    History of Present Illness (HPI) is a narrative that should also include the onset of the problem, the perceived precipitating factors, its manifestations, and any treatments. The HPI should reveal the patient's responses to the symptoms and the effect the illness has had on his daily life.

20. B

    Asking the client on his use of alcohol, tobacco and illicit drugs as well as presence of environmental hazards assesses risk factors.

21. D

    Health is a state wherein a person is living their potential and not merely referring to the absence of disease. It is the summation of all facets of an individual, and not just the physical. There are seven facets that make up health, and these are physical health, emotional health, social well-being, development, and cultural, spiritual and environmental influences.

22. B

    Emotional health refers to having a positive outlook in life and being able to channel emotions in a healthy manner.

23. C

    A healthy individual has a developmental level that is appropriate for their age. The developmental facet of health describes how a person thinks, provide solutions to problems and perform decision-making.

24. D

    Signs of successful health maintenance include being able to adapt without compromising the facets of health and also being able to harmoniously align the facets that make up an individual's health.

25. A , C

    A nursing health assessment is comprised of a comprehensive health history and a complete physical examination.

26. B

    A nursing health assessment is a systematic way of gathering pertinent health information from the patient. The data is to be used to develop a plan of care that is most appropriate and effective for the patient.

27. B, C, D, E

The nursing process involves determining the status of the patient's health and identifying risk factors for health conditions as well as their need for teaching, extrapolating the patient's health data, prioritizing the findings and formulating and implementing the plan of care.

28. D

Healthy People 2020 is an agenda in the US wherein the health issues, and risk factors of health conditions are identified. The overall goal of Healthy People 2020 is to improve the quality of life by promoting healthy lifestyle, providing teaching to the people to eliminate health disparities, and preventing diseases.

29. B

Healthy People 2020 hopes to create awareness to eliminate health disparities. To do this, the nurse performs health education to disseminate the right information regarding health issues and conditions.

30. D

Part of the nursing assessment is determining the patient's views on health and what they want to happen during their visit to the clinic or hospital. The nurse may ask the patient to elaborate on the reason for their visit, and what they expect to accomplish during their visit.

31. C

Verbal responses are what the patient tells the nurse. Nonverbal responses are observable actions that the patient shows in response to the nurses' assessments.

32. A, D

The provision of health by nurses goes beyond the individual patient. The nurse may contribute to the promotion and maintenance of community health by helping out in the creation of policies on health, and by providing relevant feedback that would positively influence decision-makers in nurturing the community. Other options refer to care given to individuals and families as patients.

33. B

Nurses provide holistic care to patients. During health assessments, their first responsibility is to collect patient information. Throughout the entire care process, nurses continuously observe and pay attention to details and even nuances. Patients are influenced by many things, such as culture, the environment, and their spiritual beliefs, among others.

34. D

Patients who present with new complaints or problems will need a comprehensive assessment. Emergency situations will necessitate an urgent assessment.

35. A

The nurse needs to perform a comprehensive assessment on patients who were treated for an acute condition but are presently stable.

36. A

A focused assessment is the type of assessment that is done on patients who had already undergone a comprehensive examination and are currently being seen for a return checkup.

37. A, B, D

The best sources of information regarding a patient's health are the patient himself, his family, and his past medical records. The inputs of the patient's neighbors are not reliable unless they are directly involved in the patient's care.

38. A, B, E

Patients must be active participants in their own care. To help them in decision-making, it is best to seek the patient's input. The nurse must also provide them with information using the latest clinical evidence so that they are properly guided in all aspects of decision-making. The nurse must not influence them with their personal biases and must also refrain from encouraging the patient to seek information from unreliable sources.

39. B

During the course of patient care, the nurse must be able to determine the need for reassessments so that the nursing care plan could be updated appropriately. Taking the patient's blood pressure the second time means that the nurse is to make timely assessments.

40. C

A nurse should be able to recognize the patient's spiritual needs during an assessment. A sign of knowing a patient's spiritual needs is referring a clergy who can meet the patient's spiritual needs.

41. D

The nurse shows the ability to recognize the patient's social needs when they refer them to support groups. Socialization with the other group members will benefit the patient.

42. C

The nurse should make assessments and identify the patient's needs on a daily basis. All other options are correct statements.

43. B, C

Healthy people 2020 aims to improve the quality of life by developing health promotion and disease prevention strategies aimed at changing people's lifestyle. It also intends to increase awareness through appropriate health teachings.

44. C

The Healthy people agenda have goals and objectives that aim to improve the health of Americans, targeting 10-year increments.

45. B

When determining which type of assessment is needed, the nurse must first look into the patient's current situation. Focused assessments are appropriate to use during emergencies as well as in follow-up visits when detailed assessments have been previously performed. However, when a patient presents a new problem that is still undiagnosed, a comprehensive assessment is indicated.

Critical Thinking and Evidence Based Assessment

Questions

1. Collecting health promotion data is an important part of evidence-based assessment. Which of the following does NOT describe evidence-based data collection?
   a. It allows for customization of information regarding risk reduction and health promotion information
   b. It encourages existing positive behaviors
   c. It reflects best clinical evidence
   d. It is a process of drawing conclusions to make a diagnosis

2. Lana is a 15-year old girl who was admitted due to uncontrolled vomiting and diarrhea. The nurse performed history taking and physical examination. Which of the following is TRUE about the information Lana told the nurse?
   a. It comprises subjective data
   b. It comprises objective data
   c. It forms the client's database
   d. It is part of history taking and may be unreliable

3. The nurse is caring for a client who has been admitted due to possible meningococcemia. She collects subjective and objective data, and looks for cues. She then makes a diagnostic hypothesis, and then proceeded to re-examine the client and evaluate her data. The nurse demonstrated which skill?
   a. Data management
   b. Diagnostic reasoning
   c. Data collection
   d. Diagnostic examination

4. The nurse is analyzing health data, and identifying a diagnosis for a client with arteriosclerosis. In the process, she re-examines the client's BP because her last reading shows that the blood pressure has not changed after taking an antihypertensive medication. Which of the following did the nurse just demonstrated?
   a. Initial data collection
   b. Clustering data
   c. Organizing data
   d. Data validation

5. A novice nurse is reviewing her concepts on standards of practice in nursing prior to her first nursing duty. Which of the following is NOT TRUE about standards of practice in nursing?
   a. It was previously called the nursing process
   b. It has six phases namely assessment, diagnosis, outcome identification, planning, implementation, and evaluation
   c. It is a step-by-step process wherein a step is a pre-requisite to the next and should not overlap

6. The nurse recognizes the importance of critical thinking in the attainment of positive patient outcome. Which of the following correctly demonstrates critical thinking?
    a. The client's baseline blood pressure reading while on antihypertensive medication maintenance is 130/90. Her current BP reading is 120/80 and the nurse administers her PRN meds for hypertension
    b. The client has just been given a sedative and requests to use the restroom. The client has no mobility restrictions, and the nurse allows her to use the restroom.
    c. A client presents to the emergency department with fever and vesicular rashes all over his body. The nurse isolates the client and makes further assessments.
    d. A teenage client requests for pain medication but is seen laughing at a friend's joke. The nurse withholds the pain medication because she concludes with her assessment that the client may not be in real pain.

7. Critical thinking is an important part of nursing education and practice. Which of the following is TRUE about critical thinking?
    a. It entails thinking outside the box
    b. It focuses on the mastery of pathophysiology
    c. It is a linear approach to finding solutions to a problem
    d. It involves making assumptions with the data gathered

8. An obese client is being seen in the clinic for his annual check-up. The client has no health complaints. The nurse focuses her questions on the client's lifestyle and diet without further assessments and laboratory tests. What is the nurse demonstrating in her assessment?
    a. Diagnostic reasoning
    b. Making assumptions
    c. Validating data
    d. Critical thinking

9. Several clients are being seen by the nurse. One female client diagnosed with Guillain- Barre is becoming agitated and is complaining of having less air to breath. Another client is complaining of colicky abdominal pain which was unrelieved by defecation and antacids. A female client with Reynaud's disease needs instructions on her antihypertensive medication. Which of the clients is considered first priority?
    a. The client with Guillain-barre
    b. The client with abdominal pain
    c. The client with Reynaud's disease
    d. Both the client with abdominal pain and Reynaud's disease

10. Several clients are being seen by the nurse. One client diagnosed with Guillain- Barre is becoming agitated and is complaining of having less air to breath. Another client is complaining of colicky abdominal pain that was unrelieved by defecation and antacids. A female client with Reynaud's disease needs instructions on her antihypertensive medication. Which of the clients has second-

level priority problem?
   a.   The client with Guillain-barreThe client with abdominal pain
   b.   The client with Reynaud's disease
   c.   Both the client with abdominal pain and Reynaud's disease

11. Several clients are being seen by the nurse. One client diagnosed with Guillain- Barre is becoming agitated and is complaining of having less air to breath. Another client is complaining of colicky abdominal pain which was unrelieved by defecation and antacids. A female client needs instructions on her antihypertensive medication. Which of the clients is having third level priority problem?
   a.   The client with Guillain-barre
   b.   The client with abdominal pain
   c.   The client with Reynaud's disease
   d.   Both the client with abdominal pain and Reynaud's disease

12. Professional nurses on duty should demonstrate evidence-based practice. Which of the following correctly describes evidence-based practice?
   a.   It is a multilinear approach to practice
   b.   It primarily takes into account nurse's experience and expertise
   c.   It emphasizes the use of evidence that lead to positive health outcomes
   d.   It does not take into account client preferences

13. There are numerous barriers to evidence-based practice. Which of the following is considered a barrier?
   a.   Nurses lack research skills
   b.   Institution have financial challenges to enforce evidence-based practice
   c.   Most research are unreliable
   d.   Research database are digitalized

14. The nurse is doing evidence-based assessment to create a complete database of a client suspected of having diabetes. Which of the following is included in the complete (total health) database?
   a.   Detailed history taking and a thorough physical examination
   b.   Client's perception of illness
   c.   Client's own management of illness
   d.   All of the above

15. A post-cholecystectomy client has been discharged. During his first clinic visit after surgery, the nurse makes an evidence-based assessment. The results of her assessment is called
   a.   Complete database
   b.   Follow-up database
   c.   Problem-centered database
   d.   Emergency database

16. A post-tracheostomy client who has been discharged a month ago comes to the clinic unscheduled and asks for help cleaning his tracheostomy. Which of the following database is the most appropriate for the nurse to complete?
    a. Complete database
    b. Follow-up database
    c. Problem-centered database
    d. Emergency database

17. A dazed client with a bleeding arm laceration sustained from a minor vehicular accident is accompanied by police officers to the clinic. The client is manifesting signs and symptoms of extreme alcohol intoxication. The nurse assesses ABC's, vital signs and level of consciousness, and asks the client when his last drink was. The nurse more appropriately needs to establish which database?
    a. Problem-centered database
    b. Emergency database
    c. Complete database
    d. Follow-up database

18. Health promotion and disease prevention are the primary emphasis of health care delivery to augment illness, injury and death. Which of the following is a correct distinction of Health promotion from disease prevention?
    a. Health promotion is deciding to start, maintain or improve healthy lifestyle while disease prevention is stopping or reducing unhealthy lifestyle and habits
    b. Disease prevention is deciding to start or maintain healthy lifestyle while health promotion is stopping or reducing unhealthy lifestyle and habits
    c. Disease prevention focuses on teachings and assisting the client to make healthier choices while health promotion deals with efforts to quit smoking, to moderate alcohol intake and to stop drug use.
    d. Health promotion and disease prevention increases morbidity cases

19. A 55-year old woman comes to the clinic for her scheduled check-up. Which of the following measures of health promotion and disease prevention is the LEAST appropriate?
    a. Screening history for dietary intake, physical activity, substance abuse,
    b. Chemoprophylaxis of folic acid to prevent having children with neural tube defects
    c. Physical examination for height and weight, BP, and screening for cervical cancer and HIV
    d. Counseling for fall prevention
    e. Screening for depression

20. According to the U.S. Census Bureau, by the middle of this present century, 50% of US population will comprise of people of different cultures, race and ethnicity. Which of the following factors are challenges of cultural diversity?
    a. People from different culture interpret disease differently

b. Health care providers incorporate a culture's unique beliefs and practices
c. There are efforts to uphold cultural health rights
d. Health care providers obtain education, training and practices in a variety of settings

21. Mrs. M, a client with right sided heart failure, is seen in the Outpatient Department with a primary complaint of sudden weight gain. During history taking, the nurse is heard asking the client these questions: "Do your shoes feel tighter than usual? Was there a need to let out your belt?" The nurse is assessing the client for:
    a. Sodium imbalance
    b. Edema
    c. Kidney disease
    d. Dysrhythmias

22. The nurse is seen in a depressed community collecting sputum specimens from the residents. The specimens are to be sent to the laboratory for tuberculosis screening. This is an example of what level of prevention?
    a. Primary level of prevention
    b. Secondary level of prevention
    c. Tertiary level of prevention
    d. Fourth level of prevention

23. A client presents to the clinic for the first time with chief complaint of difficulty moving his arms and legs. During history taking, which of the following is NOT an appropriate question by the nurse?
    a. "Do any of your parents have diabetes?"
    b. "Do you smoke?"
    c. "Do you have diplopia?
    d. "How many are you at home?"

24. The nurse is assessing Mr. V for a possible sexually transmitted disease. In taking the client's health history, the nurse is careful to include the following pertinent questions except:
    a. "Do you experience unusual discharge from or sores in your penis?"
    b. "How many sexual partners have you had in the last 6 months?"
    c. "Do you have sex with men, women or both?
    d. "Why did it take you this long to come for a check-up?"

25. A 5-year old girl is brought to the clinic by her mom for a possible fracture of the arm. The girl has bruises in various stages of healing and is trying to stifle her cry. Which of the following is an appropriate nursing action?
    a. The nurse politely asks the mother to leave the room and interviews the child alone.
    b. The nurse asks the mother to stay with her child to comfort her and asks the client, "How did you get hurt?"

c.   The nurse promptly endorses the care of the child to the afternoon shift nurse after the end of her shift.

d.   The nurse documents the incident as "an accident that she fell off the bed"

26.   A 36-year old female who is openly pro-abortion is to be assessed by a nurse who is against the procedure. Which of the following is an appropriate nursing action?
a.   Respectfully decline to interview the client
b.   Perform self-reflection pre-interview to prevent biases and assumptions from affecting assessment
c.   Rely mostly on objective data to avoid confrontation with patient
d.   Ask to perform health teaching on why abortion is against human rights

27.   Which of the following statement by the nurse is NOT therapeutic and reflect the need for further evaluation?
a.   "What brings you to the clinic today?"
b.   "How does your illness affect your daily life?"
c.   "You must feel sorry for yourself. You don't have to be."
d.   "By 'brain fog' do you mean you get confused and don't know what to do?"

28.   It is the phase of the interview process wherein the end of the client interview is determined.
a.   Pre-interview
b.   Introduction
c.   Working phase
d.   Termination phase

29.   During history taking, the client tells the nurse, "I didn't even have a wink last night." The nurse replied, "Do you mean you had trouble sleeping last night?" This is an example of which communication technique?
a.   Summarizing
b.   Clarification
c.   Focusing
d.   Paraphrasing

30.   A 23-year old female is accompanied by her parents to the clinic after she has not eaten anything for three days. She had recently broken-up with her fiancé. She refuses to speak with the nurse and holds back tears. Which of the following is an appropriate nursing response?
a.   The nurse holds the client's hands and says, "Everything's gonna be all right."
b.   The nurse says, "You must be hungry. I'll go and get you something to eat." and went to get the client food.
c.   The nurse gently pats the client on the arm and says, "I'll sit with you."
d.   The nurse asks the client, "would you like some privacy?"

31. A 54-year old male has otosclerosis and is hard on hearing on his left ear. The nurse is to make initial interview. Which is the most appropriate nursing response?
    a. Try to talk in a louder voice and speak slowly
    b. Sit slightly to the right of the client and speak clearly in a normal tone and rate while facing the client
    c. Exaggerate lip movement because people hard on hearing read lips
    d. Take a board and write words that the client cannot hear.

32. A 15-year old girl of Asian descent is talking in a very soft tone of voice with the nurse and refrains from having eye contact. When asked a direct question, she replies either "Yes, mam" or "No, mam." The nurse understands that
    a. The girl is being rude and sarcastic
    b. The girl is shy
    c. The girl is showing respect
    d. The girl is disinterested in being interviewed.

33. The following are components of the comprehensive health history EXCEPT:
    a. Chief complaint
    b. Health Patterns
    c. Review of Systems
    d. Ordered diagnostic exams

34. Establishing rapport with the client happens in which phase of interview?
    a. Pre-interview
    b. Introduction
    c. Working
    d. Termination

35. The nurse understands that there are 7 attributes of a symptom. Which attribute is the nurse referring to when she asks the client "Is there anything that makes it better or worse?"
    a. Onset
    b. Duration
    c. Associated Manifestations
    d. Relieving/Exacerbating Factors

36. When assessing risk factors during history taking, the nurse understands that the CAGE questionnaire is used to gather data about
    a. Alcohol use
    b. Drug abuse
    c. Tobacco use
    d. Environmental hazards

37. A senior nurse is seen assessing a 45-year old client. The student nurse hears the senior nurse ask the client for the presence of jaundice, heartburn or hemorrhoids. The student nurse understands that the senior nurse is doing a review of which system?
    a. Cardiovascular
    b. Gastrointestinal
    c. Musculoskeletal
    d. Nervous

38. A 66-year old male patient is newly diagnosed with colon cancer and tells the nurse, "I don't think any treatment will work on me now." The best nursing response is
    a. "Can you tell me why you think no treatment will work on you now?
    b. "I will refer you to an experienced therapist."
    c. "Don't lose hope. Let's talk to your doctor about your options"
    d. "It's better that you know than not knowing what's wrong with you".

39. A nurse is assessing a 4-year old boy who is suspected of overdosing with his medication for fever. The nurse wants to verify the possible time of ingestion. Which of the following is the most appropriate response?
    a. "Did you take this medication before or after lunch?"
    b. "What time do you think you took this medication"
    c. "Where is the hand of the clock pointing when you took the medication?"
    d. "Why did you take all the medication?"

40. A 3-year old girl is seen in the clinic by the nurse. She is obviously in pain and in distress. The nurse wants to assess her level of pain. Which of the following is the most appropriate nursing action?
    a. Ask the client to scale her pain having 1 as the least pain, and 10 the worst pain.
    b. Show her pictures of faces having different levels of pain and have her point out which face most likely resembles her pain
    c. Ask her to describe her pain in her own way
    d. Ask her to squeeze your hand and instruct her to squeeze tighter for more pain

41. What are nursing assessments for?
    a. To create organizational policies
    b. To develop nursing care plans
    c. To determine a medical diagnosis
    d. To carry out physicians' orders

42. The nurse starts their physical examination using the head-to-toe procedure. Which step of the nursing process is physical examination a part of?
    a. Assessment
    b. Diagnosis
    c. Planning and implementation

d. Evaluation

43. The nurse has gathered enough patient data during the assessment phase of the nursing process and is now analyzing the available information to make hypotheses as to the patient's problem. Which of the following is the nurse demonstrating?
    a. Skills in data collation
    b. Proper etiquette
    c. Proper evaluation
    d. Clinical reasoning

44. Using the nursing process, what should the nurse do next after defining the patient's problem?
    a. Ask the patient if their condition has improved
    b. Evaluate the patient's progress
    c. Develop a nursing care plan
    d. Implement the plan

45. Which of the following is an objective information?
    a. Dizziness
    b. HR = 54
    c. Headache
    d. Malaise

46. A 55-year-old male patient tells then nurse that he feels weak most of the time ever since his wife died a year ago. According to the patient, he had been hospitalized twice for having pneumonia. During the physical examination, the nurse took his height and weight measurements. Which of the following set of patient information is subjective?
    a. Age, gender, height and weight measurements
    b. Patient feels weak most of the time, the reason for the previous hospitalizations
    c. Patient feels weak most of the time, the reason for previous hospitalization, height, and weight
    d. Age, gender, patient feels weak most of the time

47. A nurse is interviewing a patient regarding their chest pain. The nurse asks the patient when the pain began. According to the OLD CART technique of interviewing, which of the following detail about the pain does the nurse want to know?
    a. Characteristic symptoms
    b. Location
    c. Onset
    d. Associated manifestation

48. Several nurses are listening to the patient as the patient provides details about their abdominal pain, which is their primary complaint. Which of the following interview questions aims to know the associated manifestation of the abdominal pain?

a. "Could you describe the pain you are feeling? Is it colicky?"
b. "What else do you feel or notice when you experience the pain in your belly?"
c. "What time of day is the pain worst?"
d. "Is the pain continuous?"

49. A patient is being seen in the outpatient department because of tingling sensations in the hands and feet. The patient tells the nurse that the tingling is already felt upon waking up in the morning and it persists most of the day. The tingling is accompanied by decreased sensation to the affected areas. The patient said they tried using a hot compress to relieve the symptom but to no avail. The tingling sensation has been going on for days and that was the reason they sought medical attention. Which of the following details of the patient's account refers to relieving factors?
a. The pain is already felt upon waking up in the morning and persists most of the day
b. The tingling is accompanied by decreased sensation to the affected areas
c. The patient tried using hot compress to relieve the sensation
d. The tingling sensation has been going on for days

50. Which of the following statement about the nursing process is INCORRECT?
a. It is methodical
b. It is a broad systematic framework
c. The steps do not overlap
d. It addresses the human responses and needs of each patient

51. Which of the following components of the nursing process refers to the clinical judgment made after analyzing patient information obtained through physical examination and history-taking?
a. Assessment
b. Diagnosis
c. Planning
d. Implementation

52. A 55-year old male patient presents to the emergency room with headache, weakness, and difficulty breathing. The nurse took his vital signs. After the physician's examination, it was determined that the patient has hypertension. An anti-hypertensive medication was consequently prescribed. The nurse duly administered the medication, and after 30 minutes, the nurse measured the patient's blood pressure again. Which part of the nursing process is the nurse performing when she measured the patient's blood pressure the second time?
a. Assessment
b. Diagnosis
c. Implementation
d. Evaluation

53. Which of the following are types of reasoning for clinical problem-solving? Select all that apply.
a. Learning from experience

b. Pattern recognition
c. Development of schemas
d. Positive responses
e. Application of relevant and basic clinical science

54. A nurse is assessing a patient and makes a record of her findings. The nurse documents the following signs and symptoms under the same category: a sore throat, inflamed tonsils, white patches are seen on the tonsils, low-grade fever. Which of the following process did the nurse demonstrate?
    a. Identifying abnormal findings
    b. Clustering the findings
    c. Interpreting the findings
    d. Testing the hypothesis

55. A patient is being seen in the emergency department. The patient presented with maculopapular reddish rash, high-grade fever, and malaise. The patient recalls being in the same room with another person who has had measles a few days back. The nurse is interpreting the findings. Which of the following is the probable nature/cause of the patient's manifestations?
    a. Traumatic
    b. Nutritional
    c. Toxic
    d. Infectious

56. Nursing diagnoses are made after the identification, clustering, and interpretation of findings. Typically, nursing diagnoses are written as statements of the patient's response to a health condition. Which of the following is the most common basis for these diagnoses? Select all that apply.
    a. Changes in the patient's life
    b. Altered processes
    c. Changes in the patient's decision-making after receiving information
    d. Changes in the patient's condition after interventions were made
    e. Specific causes

57. A nurse is asking about the patient's immunization status, the health screenings that they have undergone, and the learning sessions that they have taken to keep themselves healthy and disease-free. Which of the following category of history-taking is the nurse gathering data for?
    a. Prevention of disease progression
    b. Rehabilitation
    c. Health maintenance
    d. Cure for a disease

58. Which of the following describes the proper way of developing a care plan?
    a. The nurse must ask for the patient's input
    b. The care plan must not be modified once it has been completed
    c. A new development or a change in the patient's condition necessitates that the old plan be discarded, and a new plan be created
    d. The plan should be developed according to the assessment findings which have been identified

59. Which of the following is an ideal short-term goal?
    a. The patient would be free of cancer in three months
    b. After two days of antibiotic treatment, the infection will be resolved
    c. After health teaching, the patient would be able to demonstrate proper deep breathing technique 3x a day.
    d. After a month, the patient will lose 1/3 of her current body weight

60. Which of the following ways of documentation is best to use when writing about the patient's family history, particularly for tracing genetic disorders?
    a. A detailed narrative
    b. The use of direct quotes
    c. A diagram
    d. A chart

61. A staff nurse examines the patient's HEENT (Head, Eyes, Ears, Nose, Throat) and the result of their assessment is written as PERRLA. The novice nurse should know that PERRLA stands for:
    a. Pupils are equally round and reactive to light and accommodation
    b. Pupils are even, radiant and reactive to light acquisition
    c. Pupils are evidently responding to reasonable light and accommodation
    d. Pupils are evidently refractive and reactive to light ambiance

62. After assessing the musculoskeletal system of the patient, the nurse writes down 'FROM in hands, wrists, elbows, shoulders, spine, hips, knees, and ankles' in the patient's records. The student nurse interprets this finding as:
    a. A symptom of a disease process
    b. A sign of a disease process
    c. A kind of a disease process
    d. Normal findings

63. Which of the following techniques ensures the quality of the patient data gathered?
    a. Asking the patient closed-ended question only
    b. Giving the patient suggestions to build up a hypothesis
    c. Applying the principles of data analysis to the patient's information
    d. Rectifying data collection mistakes at a later time

64. Which of the following are the characteristics of a proper progress note?
    a. It should include all the assessment findings from the initial examination
    b. It should be clear and sufficiently detailed
    c. It must be easy to follow
    d. It should reflect the nurse's clinical reasoning
    e. It should follow the SOAP format: Subjective, Objective, Apprehensions, and Pains.

65. Which is the correct interpretation of the following example of a principle of test selection "The specificity of CK-MB in patients with possible myocardial infarction is > 90%'?
    a. More than 90% of patients with myocardial infarction will have falsely elevated CK-MB.
    b. Only less 10% of patients with myocardial infarction will have elevated CK-MB
    c. Of 100 patients without myocardial infarction <10% will have a normal CK-MB; in >90% the CK-MB will be falsely elevated.
    d. Of 100 patients without myocardial infarction >90% will have a normal CK-MB; in <10% the CK-MB will be falsely elevated.

ANSWERS

1. D
    Collecting health promotion data allows risk reduction and health promotion information to be personalized while encouraging positive behaviors that already exist. It should reflect the best clinical evidence. The process of drawing conclusions to make a diagnosis is called diagnostic reasoning.

2. B
    All information that the client says about her health comprises subjective data and is part of history-taking. All assessment parameters that the nurse gathers through physical examination are objective data. Subjective and objective data, client records and laboratory results comprise the client's database.

3. B
    Diagnostic reasoning is the analysis of data followed by making a conclusion to identify a diagnosis. It involves looking at available cues, making a hypothesis, gathering more data in relation to the hypothesis, subjecting the hypothesis to evaluation with the newly gathered data, and arriving at a final diagnosis.

4. D
    Validation of data is looking for gaps and missing pieces to make sure that initial data gathered are accurate. It is an essential critical thinking skill.

5. C
    Standards of practice in nursing is a process repeatedly used in the proper care of clients. It allows nurses to perform any of the phases simultaneously to address the varying needs of the client.

6. C
    Critical thinking is needed to make an appropriate diagnostic reasoning and a sound clinical judgment. Isolation of a client on the first sign of a communicable disease demonstrates critical thinking.

7. A
    Critical thinking entails thinking outside the box. It goes beyond mastery of pathophysiology and involves multidimensional thinking. It avoids making assumptions.

8. B
    In this situation, the nurse is assuming that the client's obesity is due to unhealthy lifestyle and diet. Evidence-based assessment means conducting history-taking and physical examination and considering pathology also as a cause of the client's obesity.

9. A

    The client with Guillain-Barre is exhibiting ascending paralysis most likely affecting her lungs. Her difficulty breathing is a first-level priority problem because it can lead to a life-threatening situation. First-level priority problems involve air, breathing, circulation and vital signs problems.

10. B

    The client complaining of colicky abdominal pain that was unrelieved by defecation and antacids has a second-level priority problem. Second-level priority problems are next in urgency status and they mean further client deterioration.

11. C

    A female client with Reynaud's disease who needs instructions on her antihypertensive medication is having third level priority problems. Problems in this level usually are related to knowledge deficit, coping, mobility and rest.

12. C

    Evidence-based practice uses a systematic approach to care and emphasizes primarily the use of evidence that lead to positive health outcomes. The nurse's assessment findings, experience and expertise and client preferences are also taken into account.

13. A

    Lack of nursing research skills, lack of time to do research, and lack of confidence to implement change are some of the barriers to evidence-based practice.

14. D

    A complete database includes data from a detailed history taking, and a thorough physical examination. It also includes client's responses to health problems such as perception of illness, and attempts to manage illness.

15. B

    A follow-up database comprises of data obtained at regular intervals to monitor for changes, improvements and coping strategies to follow-up on health problems.

16. C

    A problem-centered database is of smaller scope than the complete database. It focuses on a particular problem that in this situation is lack of skill in tracheostomy care. At this point, the hospital must have already obtained the complete database and some follow-up database.

17. B

    An emergency database should be established when there is immediate threat to life or if there is a possibility of rapid client deterioration. It entails focused assessment done in a rapid accurate manner while doing life-saving measures concurrently.

18. A

   Health promotion is deciding to start, maintain or improve healthy lifestyle while disease prevention is stopping or reducing unhealthy lifestyle and habits such as smoking, alcohol and drug use. Health promotion and disease prevention lead to decreased morbidity and mortality.

19. B

   Chemoprophylaxis of folic acid to prevent having children with neural tube defects is the least appropriate at this time because she is not within childbearing age anymore.

20. A

   The main challenge of cultural diversity is that people from different cultures have varying interpretation of and approach to diseases, therefore, the need to gather accurate culturally sensitive data is important.

21. B

   Asking the patient if the client felt usual shoes or belts tighten is assessing the client for fluid retention or edema in terms that the client can answer accurately. Although fluid retention can be caused by sodium imbalance, kidney disease or dysrhythmias, asking those questions does not confirm the direct cause.

22. B

   Screening for and treatment of diseases is under the secondary level of prevention. Primary level of prevention involves lifestyle change and the development of healthy habits. Tertiary level of prevention deals with rehabilitation and maximizing function after disability. Fourth level of prevention is yet to be defined.

23. C

   During history taking, it is inappropriate to use medical terms that the client may not be able to understand. It is important to ask questions in a matter-of-fact way without being judgmental and in a manner that the patient can comprehend.

24. D

   "Why" questions are inappropriate and judgmental and will not elicit any information that will help in client assessment.

25. A

   In a suspected case of abuse, it is important to ask the client to be interviewed alone to prevent the possible abuser from intimidating the client. This strategy can also help in acquiring more accurate data from the client. All possible cases of abuse should be reported to the nursing supervisor and consequently to the authorities immediately. Client response should be documented as direct quotes.

26. B

Self-reflection before meeting the client is important prior to interview to prevent biases and assumptions from affecting assessment. It is also a way of being respectful of individual differences. There is no need to decline the task of interviewing the client. C and D are both inappropriate.

27. C

This statement is assuming on the client's feelings and offers false reassurance. Both are non-therapeutic.

28. A

Determining when the interview should end is done during the pre-interview when goals are being set. This is to inform the client the approximate time the interview would finish. The termination phase is a time for summarizing the patient's problems and reviewing the plan of care, and allowing the client to ask questions pertaining to his care or illness.

29. D

Paraphrasing is repeating client's statements in similar words. Summarizing is stating the main points of the client. Seeking clarification makes the client's overall meaning more understandable. Focusing helps recognize an emotion behind words.

30. C

In this response, the nurse conveys her presence without being intrusive. (A) is giving false reassurance while B and D are inappropriate responses because the nurse suggests to leave the patient in distress.

31. B

If a patient has a unilateral hearing loss or deficit, the nurse sits on the hearing side and speaks at normal volume and rate. The nurse also avoids covering her mouth or looking down at papers. Sign languages, questionnaires or a communication board are appropriate for those with complete hearing loss apart from speaking in a normal tone and rate.

32. C

Women, especially young girls from Asia, usually refrain from maintaining eye contact and they speak softly as a sign of respect.

33. D

The comprehensive health history is composed of Chief Complaint(s), History of Present Illness, Past History, Family History, Review of Systems, and Health Patterns.

34. B

In the introduction phase, the nurse meets the client for the first time and establishes rapport. Together they identify objectives for the interview.

35. D

   To assess factors that relieve or exacerbate a symptom, the nurse asks what makes the symptom better or worse

36. A

   The CAGE Questionnaire is an easily validated tool to screen for alcohol use. It questions about Cutting down, Annoyance if criticized, Guilty feelings, and Eye-openers.

37. B

   In assessing the gastrointestinal system the nurse may ask about trouble swallowing, heartburn, appetite, nausea, bowel movements, stool color and size, change in bowel habits, pain with defecation, rectal bleeding, black or tarry stools, hemorrhoids, constipation, diarrhea, abdominal pain, food intolerance, excessive belching or passing of gas, jaundice, liver, or gallbladder trouble and/or hepatitis

38. A

   This response is most therapeutic because it allows the client to further verbalize feelings. It is always inappropriate to "pass the buck" when a patient states a concern. C is offering false reassurance although after interview, the nurse may help the client seek physician's advice for options. D is a non-therapeutic response.

39. A

   Preschoolers are most likely still confused about their concept of time. The nurse must ask if the event happened before or after a particular routine such as meals to get more accurate information.

40. B

   Young children do not have a clear concept of numbers, more so of scaling. It is best to show them pictures of faces in various levels of pain to which they can relate to easily.

41. B

   The goal of nursing health assessments is to develop an individualized plan of care for each patient.

42. A

   During the assessment phase of the nursing process, the nurse gathers data through history-taking and physical examination. Assessment is the first step of the nursing process.

43. D

   The nurse is demonstrating clinical reasoning when the nurse gathers, collates, and analyzes patient's data and then make hypotheses of the patient's current health condition.

44. C

   During the nursing process, the nurse develops the nursing care plan after defining the patient's problem and making nursing diagnoses.

45. B

   Objective data are those that the nurse has observed or measured themselves. Examples of objective information are the patient's vital signs, such as the heart rate.

46. B

   Subjective data are information that the patient provides the nurse. In the case scenario, the subjective data are the patient's feeling of weakness, and the reason for their hospitalization.

47. C

   Onset refers to the time that a sign or symptom began. When a patient tells the nurse a new complaint, the nurse must ask details, such as when the symptom was first felt.

48. B

   Associated manifestations refer to the other signs or symptoms that the patient notices appearing with the primary complaint, which in this case is the abdominal pain. The associated manifestation is nausea.

49. C

   Relieving factors are any attempts that the patient has sought to alleviate the symptom. In this case, the patient tried applying a hot compress to the area to relieve the tingling sensation. The relieving factor is the hot compress.

50. C

   The nursing process is a broad systematic framework that addresses the human responses and needs of the patients. It is a methodical problem-solving approach that starts with assessment. The assessment is followed by diagnosis, planning, implementation, and evaluation. Although the steps happen in this order, in many cases, the nurse can simultaneously do the steps to address different client problems.

51. B

   The nursing diagnosis is the clinical judgment made regarding the patient's response to their health condition. It is the basis from which the nurse selects interventions to address the patient's health concerns.

52. D

   Evaluation is done after implementing the care plan. It aims to determine if the goals of improving the patient's condition have been achieved. In the scenario, the nurse measures the patient's blood pressure after administering the anti-hypertensive medication to determine if the medication was successful in lowering the patient's blood pressure.

53. B, C, E

In clinical problem-solving, clinicians such as nurses use three types of reasoning. One such reasoning is pattern recognition wherein nurses recognize and compare cues they had previously observed in the same patient or in a different patient with a similar condition. Another type of reasoning is the development of schemas. It is a case-based reasoning that relies on previous successful problem-solving, which eventually lead to the acquisition of generalized knowledge. The application of relevant and basic clinical science, on the other hand, is the use of knowledge gained from the nursing education to address patient needs.

54. B

During the clustering of findings, the nurse analyzes the abnormal findings and then looks for clues that suggest the interrelatedness of the manifestations. The nurse then documents the findings in groups to make the interpretation of data more meaningful and accurate.

55. D

Even with minimal clinical knowledge, the novice nurse must be able to interpret the patient's manifestations using scientific reasoning. A patient presenting with fever, rash and malaise would most probably have a disease process which is infectious in nature. In this case, the nurse learns to interpret her findings.

56. A, B, D

Nursing diagnoses are made after assessing the patient and making a hypothesis of the patient's health problems. They are statements that are based on the changes in the patient's life, or about altered processes and specific causes of a health condition.

57. C

Health maintenance is an important category that reflects a common patient problem. To gather data on health maintenance practices, the nurse asks about the patient's immunization status, the health screenings that they have undergone, any health teachings that they have received, and other practices that they do to be healthy.

58. A

When making a nursing care plan, the nurse must seek the input of the patient. The patient must be an active participant in its development and must be given choices whereby possible. The patient must agree to the plan before its implementation. The plan can be modified as needed in accordance with the patient's responses to treatments. There is no need to create an entirely new plan, but all updates must be properly documented. The plan should be developed from the diagnoses, and not from the assessment findings.

59. C

A short-term goal is an aim that the nurse, together with the patient plan to accomplish within the immediate period after a particular intervention. An example of a short-term goal is being able to properly demonstrate and apply a skill that the patient has learned within that day. When setting goals, the nurse must remember that they should be timely and realistic.

60. C

A diagram is best to use when documenting family history for tracing genetic disorders. A histogram would clearly show relationships, the diseases that afflict both sides, and their statuses, whether they are living or already deceased.

61. A

PERRLA means Pupils are Equally Round and Reactive to Light and Accommodation. The nurse documents PERRLA in the patient's records to indicate that the patient has a normal pupillary reaction during the assessment of the patient's eyes.

62. D

FROM of the joints such as the hands, wrists, elbows, shoulders, spine, hips, knees, and ankles means that these joints have Full Range Of Motion, an expected and normal finding in the assessment of the musculoskeletal system.

63. C

From assessments to developing a nursing care plan and documenting, the nurse must ensure the quality of patient data. To ensure quality, the nurse must ask open-ended questions to allow the patient to elaborate. The 'OLD CART' mnemonic can help the nurse to elicit more significant information from the patient. The nurse can also apply the principles of data analysis to the patient information, and then immediately rectify any mistakes identified in the data collection and interpretation.

64. B, C, D

A progress note is a documentation of the patient's clinical status, and it sites any improvements or decline. It should be of the same standard as the first assessment. It should reflect the nurse's clinical reasoning and must also be clear and easy to understand, with sufficient details. Progress notes usually follow the format SOAP, which stands for Subjective, Objective, Assessment, and Planning.

65. D

Specificity identifies the proportion of people who test negative in a group of people known to be without a given disease, or the proportion of people who are true negatives compared with the total number of people without the disease. 'The specificity of CK-MB in patients with possible myocardial infarction is > 90%' means that of 100 patients without myocardial infarction >90% will have a normal CK-MB and in <10%, the CK-MB will be falsely elevated.

Cultural Competence and Spiritual Assessment

Questions
1. The United States is becoming more of a nation of diverse culture. Which factor contributes to cultural diversity in the US?
    a. Medical tourism
    b. Decreased acceptance of lifestyle choices that are out of the norm
    c. Globalization
    d. Racial discrimination

2. When caring for a client of a different culture, understanding cultural diversity is important. What is the key to understanding diversity of culture in the practice of nursing?
    a. Some knowledge of different health practices of various cultures
    b. Being assertive of evidence-based practice
    c. Self-awareness and knowledge of one's own culture
    d. Prioritization of client's health beliefs and practices over established protocols and guidelines

3. The nurse wants to be aware of poverty issues when providing care for a multicultural set of clients. Which of the following ethnic and racial group has the LEAST poverty rate?
    a. Alaska natives
    b. Non-Hispanic whites
    c. African Americans
    d. Hispanics

4. The nurse should understand that the largest percentage of immigrants presently coming to the US come from
    a. Asia
    b. Mexico
    c. Latin America
    d. Europe

5. Of all factors considered to be 'determinants of health', which has the greatest influence on health?
    a. Quality of neighborhood
    b. Culture
    c. Genetics
    d. Poverty

6. Health disparities exist in our society. This means that certain health problems are particularly high in a given 'vulnerable population.' Which racial/ethnic group has the highest cases of the following: gonorrhea, congenital syphilis, AIDS, nonfatal firearm-related injuries, new cases of tuberculosis, homicides, and drug-induced deaths?
    a. Asians
    b. African Americans
    c. Hispanics

    d. Alaskan Natives.

7. The National Standards for Culturally and Linguistically Appropriate Services in Health Care determines standards designed to help meet the health needs of immigrants. Which detail of the first standard refers to a set of behaviors, attitude, and policies related to language and culture that enables effective multicultural care?
    a. Respectful care
    b. Effective care
    c. Cultural and linguistic competence
    d. Critical thinking

8. Religion has a big impact on how a person reacts to and thinks about health and illness. Which of the following indicates positive religious coping?
    a. A person feels a strong connection to God or a supreme being
    b. There is constant struggle to do good to others
    c. Illness is viewed as a form of punishment
    d. Recovery from illness depends totally on God

9. A nurse is caring for a client who appears melancholic. When interviewed by the nurse, she states that she has problems of the heart. The nurse clarifies if she meant she was sad. Her reply in broken English was, "I don't know. I don't know what sad means in our language." To which cultural group does the client most probably belong?
    a. Mediterranean
    b. Chinese
    c. Ugandan
    d. Mexican American

10. The nurse is reviewing her concepts on cultural diversity to further improve her competency. Which of the following characterize the biomedical theory of illness causation?
    a. The body can be understood by reducing it to smaller components, such as understanding bodily systems or a particular organ.
    b. Health exists when there is perfect balance of all factors of health in an individual
    c. Human life is only a part of the big universe
    d. Foods are transformed into yin and yang energy after being metabolized

11. A Filipino client is a professed Christian Baptist. He firmly believes that evil spirits have caused his undiagnosed abdominal pain. This is an example of which causation of illness?
    a. Biomedical
    b. Naturalistic
    c. Magicoreligious
    d. Hot and cold theory

12. A female client is experiencing dystocia and insists on seeing a braucher who has the right potion to help progress her labor. To which cultural/ethnic/racial group does the client belong?
    a. European
    b. Amish
    c. Hispanics
    d. Blacks

13. An American Indian client scheduled for an operation requests blessings from their medicine woman. The nurse is correct when she requests visitation from the
    a. Curandero
    b. Espiritista
    c. Acupuncturist
    d. Shaman

14. The nurse knows that understanding culture is pertinent to nursing practice. Which of the following is a characteristic of culture?
    a. It is naturally learnt from birth through the learning of language, and through experiencing the life of which a person is born to
    b. It is having a unique experience, lifestyle and point of view that are shared with the ethnic group to which the person belongs
    c. Its adaptation is primarily dependent on the environment, natural resources, and technology
    d. It persists to influence the cultural group for long periods of time with no or little change

15. Choi is a Korean national who immigrated to the US eight years ago. He was once a conservative teenager who wore checkered shirts and slacks. After three years, he is seen wearing what kids his age also wear. He also has picked up some expressions that he hears from his peers. When he is home, he speaks Korean, and still enjoys home-cooked Korean meals. What correctly describes this situation?
    a. Establishing ethnic identity
    b. Acculturation
    c. Assimilation
    d. Biculturalism

16. Sarai is a 5-year girl of Mediterranean race who has come to the US with her family. She tells her mother that she is having a hard time talking and playing with friends, and she refuses to go to school. What is Sarai most likely experiencing?
    a. Assimilation
    b. Biculturalism
    c. Multiculturalism
    d. Acculturative stress

17. Nurse Kaye has been a health nurse in a community whose residents are mostly Muslims. When one of her clients died, she was careful not to touch the body. She also notified the family immediately. Being in that community for ten years, she has understood their culture, and has attended to her patients' needs. Her clients have expressed their satisfaction of her service. What did Nurse Kaye demonstrated?
    a. Cultural sensitivity
    b. Cultural awareness
    c. Cultural competence
    d. Cultural assimilation

18. A client of African culture is being seen by the nurse. Which of the following would the nurse allow the client to take for health restoration that will reflect culturally competent provision of care?
    a. Ginseng
    b. Asafoetida, herbs and roots
    c. Swamp root and Olbas
    d. Manzanilla

19. Which of the following groups believes that disharmony with nature can have negative effects on health?
    a. Native Americans
    b. Asians
    c. Hispanics
    d. Europeans

20. A patient is for surgery and the nurse requests that the client remove his bracelet. The client refused and said that the bracelet is an amulet against the Mano Negro. To which ethnic/racial group does the client most probably belong?
    a. European
    b. African
    c. Spanish
    d. American Indian

21. Which of the following is true of a cultural assessment? Select all that apply.
    a. It looks into the patient's social and personal details
    b. It primarily aims to establish short-term and long-term goals
    c. It is systematic
    d. It is comprehensive
    e. It aims to gather data about the patient's health beliefs, values, and practices

22. Which of the following is the primary cause of a growing culturally diverse population?
    a. Rapid improvements in technology
    b. Increasing number of religions
    c. Global migration
    d. Increasing number of communication modes

23. Which of the following is NOT true about culture?
    a. It is about patterns of behavior that are socially transmitted
    b. It is a set of the products of human work and thought that is common to a population
    c. It is a system of shared ideas, rules and meanings
    d. It is a manner of dividing people into groups based on various sets of physical attributes

24. A male Caucasian patient walks in an emergency department because of sudden blurred vision. He believes that the new medication he had been taking since a few days before is causing the blurry vision. He is Roman Catholic and lives with a roommate. Which of the following is the information about the patient's race?
    a. The belief that the new medication he took caused the health problem
    b. Caucasian
    c. Roman Catholic
    d. Lives with a roommate

25. Which of the following identify themselves with the culture of their group?
    a. Muslims
    b. Mexican
    c. White
    d. Africans

26. Which of the following goals of Healthy People 2020 targets health equity for all regardless of cultural background?
    a. Achieve high-quality and long life free of diseases that could be prevented
    b. Eliminate health disparities
    c. Create healthy social and physical environments
    d. Promote quality of life

27. Which of the following are the characteristics of the care and services that would be provided to patients in accordance with the principal standards in the National CLAS Standards? Select all that apply.
    a. Special
    b. Just
    c. Effective
    d. Honest
    e. Equitable

28. Which of the following nurses demonstrates cultural competence?
    a. The nurse who starts an IV line on the patient's non-dominant hand
    b. The nurse who allows a religious relic to be held by a Roman Catholic patient
    c. The nurse who puts on a colorful coat when talking to a 2-year-old patient
    d. The nurse who voiced an opinion to the doctor

29. Which of the following can help make a nurse culturally competent?
    a. Genuinely seeking cultural encounters
    b. Requesting a different assignment when dealing with Asian patients
    c. Starting an IV line in an African American teen
    d. Providing information to a Muslim couple

30. Which of the following strategy should be used to analyze situations to develop cultural awareness?
    a. Theoretical framework
    b. Statistical analysis
    c. Stereotyped thinking
    d. Reflective thinking

31. Which of the following nurses demonstrates cultural humility?
    a. The nurse who approaches a patient with respect
    b. The nurse who non-judgmentally interacts with the parents of a 5-year-old girl who just underwent female circumcision
    c. The nurse who greeted a patient 'Happy birthday'
    d. The nurse who gave health teaching to a childless couple

32. A nurse shows that she prefers interacting with a patient who is neatly dressed and looking very professional than with the patient who is wearing black lipstick and short skirts. Which of the following does the nurse reflect?
    a. Stereotype
    b. Prejudice
    c. Bias
    d. Insensitivity

33. A nurse begins to provide health teachings regarding proper dieting to an obese male patient. The patient has not undergone any assessments to determine the cause of his obesity. Which of the following did the nurse reflect?
    a. Stereotype
    b. Dishonesty
    c. Prejudice
    d. Incompetence

34. A nurse is telling a male patient that he should get a job, because he is the father, and that having a job is expected of him as the head of the family. Which of the following did the nurse demonstrate?
    a. Bias
    b. Incompetence
    c. Stereotype
    d. Prejudice

35. Which of the following questions can be used for self-reflection to become culturally competent?
    a. Should I do volunteer jobs at the nearest home care facility?
    b. Do I know how to ask for the services of an interpreter should the need arise?
    c. Do I keep my patient's information confidential at all times?
    d. Am I being honest to my patient?

36. Which of the following dimensions of cultural humility refers to identifying one's own biases?
    a. Self-awareness
    b. Respectful communication
    c. Competent care
    d. Collaborative partnerships

37. A nurse has asked for the services of a certified interpreter to be able to develop a nursing care plan with the patient. Which dimension of cultural humility did the nurse demonstrate?
    a. Competent care
    b. Collaborative partnerships
    c. Self-awareness
    d. Respectful communication

38. A patient has recently died, and the nurse sees the patient's wife crying. The nurse says, "This is a difficult situation for you. It is ok to cry." Which of the following components of the RESPECT model did the nurse exemplify?
    a. Rapport
    b. Empathy
    c. Support
    d. Partnership

39. Which of the following shows Support to the patient according to the RESPECT model?
    a. Using verbal clarification techniques
    b. Conveying one's presence and availability when help is needed
    c. Respecting cultural practices
    d. Avoiding making assumptions

40. Which of the following situations describes a culturally bound syndrome?
    a. The nurse is telling an African American patient their right as a patient
    b. The husband of a Korean patient tells the nurse his wife is experiencing Hwabyung
    c. The nurse asks a teen patient what a 'bling' is
    d. The nurse asks for Kosher diet for a Jewish patient

41. A patient who believes that there is a God who is all good suddenly lost his wife to murder. The nurse must prepare to care for a patient with:
    a. Religious affiliation
    b. Somatization disorder
    c. Culturally-bound syndrome
    d. Spiritual distress

42. Which of the following is an example of a developmental loss?
    a. Retirement
    b. Loss of the ability to have a child due to advanced age
    c. Death of a child
    d. Being fired from work

43. Which of the following patient responses signal spiritual distress?
    a. "Why do I have cancer?"
    b. "What caused my disease?"
    c. "Who should I talk to regarding my diagnosis?"
    d. "I would like the tests to be repeated."

44. A nurse is making a spiritual assessment and is asking a patient if they have any unmet hopes and dreams. What type of loss does the nurse want to determine?
    a. Loss of self
    b. Loss of other people
    c. Concrete losses
    d. Abstract losses

45. Which of the following questions assesses for the patient's source of hope and strength?
    a. "Are there any religious practices that are important to you?"
    b. "Who helps the most when you are afraid?"
    c. "Has being sick changed anything in your faith?"
    d. "Do you believe in a God?"

ANSWERS

1. C
    Immigration and globalization are the major factors that contribute to cultural diversity in the US.

2. C
    Self-awareness and knowledge of one's own culture is the key to understanding the diversity of culture in nursing practice because one's own culture and beliefs can influence the nurse's own practices, behavior and coping mechanisms.

3. B
    The national average of poverty rate is least for non-Hispanic whites at 13% while Alaska natives, African Americans and Hispanics have the greatest poverty rates.

4. C
    The current wave of immigrants mostly comes from Latin America, followed by Asia.

5. D
    Among the determinants of health, poverty exerts the greatest influence on health. This is according to results of evidence-based research.

6. B
    African Americans have the largest health disparities in relation to cases of gonorrhea, congenital syphilis, AIDS, nonfatal firearm-related injuries, new cases of tuberculosis, homicides, and drug-induced deaths.

7. C
    Cultural and linguistic competence refers to a set of behaviors, attitude, and policies related to language and culture that enables effective multicultural care.

8. A
    Signs of positive religious coping are a strong connection to God or a supreme being, a strong connection towards others, and having a peaceful and kind outlook in life.

9. B
    The Chinese have no local term equivalent to 'sad', and to express themselves, they usually refer to their melancholic feelings as problems of the heart.

10. A
    The biomedical theory of illness causation states that the body can be understood by reducing it to smaller components, such as understanding bodily systems or a particular organ. Another concept that pertains to the biomedical theory of illness causation is the germ theory, wherein

bacteria, viruses, fungi and other microorganisms cause illness.

11. C

Magicoreligious theory of illness causation states that supernatural forces, such as black and white magic, good and evil spirits, angels and demons, voodoo and witchcraft, cause health and illness.

12. B

A brauche is the Amish' traditional healing practice and a braucher is the healer. A braucher prepares tonics, potions and herbs to treat different ailments and diseases.

13. D

The American Indian healer or medicine person is referred to as the Shaman.

14. A

Culture is naturally learnt from birth through the learning of language, and through experiencing the life of which a person is born to. It is having commonness that is shared by the group. Its adaptation is related to the environment, natural resources, and technology but it does not rely primarily on them. Culture is also non-stagnant and undergoes constant change.

15. D

Biculturalism is picking up from the culture of the majority while maintaining one's original culture in his own ethnicity.

16. D

Acculturative stress refers to the difficulties that a person of a different culture is experiencing in adjusting and adapting to a new culture.

17. C

A nurse is culturally competent when she demonstrates understanding the total context of a culture including factors that cause stress, social factors, and similarities and difference in culture.

18. B

Patients with African culture believe that Asafoetida, herbs and roots would restore health.

19. A

Native Americans and Africans believe that disharmony with nature can have negative effects on health.

20. C

People with Spanish heritage believe that the amulet bracelet will protect them from the Mano Negro, the evil one.

21. C, D, E

Cultural assessment is an important part of nursing care. It is a systematic and comprehensive process that aims to gather data about the patient's health beliefs, values, and practices. The patient may be an individual, a family, a group or community.

22. C

Increasing global migration has made the US population more culturally diverse. Cultural diversity has posed a big challenge to providers who have beliefs and practices that are very different from their patients.

23. D

Culture is the collection of all patterns of behavior, arts, beliefs, values, customs, way of life and all the products of human work and thought put together that a group of people uses to view the world and make decisions. It is a system of viewpoints and meanings.

24. B

Race refers to a concept of differentiating people according to various sets of physical attributes that are usually related to ancestry. Caucasian, Asian, and African are examples of a race.

25. A

Some people identify themselves with the culture of their groups, such as those belonging to a particular age group or religion.

26. B

Healthy People 2020 aims to eliminate disparities among ethnic and cultural groups in the US by providing quality care that is responsive to diverse cultural backgrounds.

27. C, E

The Principal Standard of the National CLAS Standards is: "Provide effective, equitable, understandable, and respectful quality care and services that are responsive to diverse cultural health beliefs and practices, preferred languages, health literacy, and other communication needs". (source)

28. B

Cultural competence is the ability to understand and respect people across cultures. A culturally competent nurse is able to communicate and interact with patients who have set of beliefs and practices different from their own. An example is allowing religious items that do not pose any health risks in the patient's room.

29. A

Nurses become culturally competent by actively seeking cultural encounters and information. They can also do this by becoming sensitive to cultural needs, and by being aware of cultural diversity.

30. D

To analyze actions and events, and develop cultural awareness, the nurse needs to use reflective thinking. The nurse can do this by identifying their own biases and prejudices about other cultures.

31. B

Cultural humility is the practice of humility while doing self-reflection and self-critique in the care of patients with a different cultural background.

32. C

Bias is a preference or a tendency to give impartial judgment to a person or group with a different culture. In the case scenario, the nurse showed preference to the patient who is well-groomed over the other patient who is not.

33. C

Prejudice is a negative reaction toward a person or situation without any factual basis. In the case scenario, the nurse has a prejudice that the patient became obese due to overeating.

34. C

A stereotype is a fixed, often overgeneralized view of a particular group of people. In this case, the nurse has a stereotype that the patient, as the father, has to be the head of the family and the parent who has to have a job.

35. B

Self-reflection is an important part of being culturally competent. To do self-reflection, the nurse may ask themselves several questions on how they would pursue competence when dealing with people with different set of beliefs and practices. An example of the questions to ask oneself is "Do I know how to ask for the services of an interpreter should the need arise?"

36. A

To practice cultural humility, the nurse must be able to identify their own biases. This process of learning personal biases is called self-awareness.

37. B

To practice cultural humility, the nurse must build collaborative partnerships, which is all about having the nurse-patient relationship built on respect and having mutually agreeable plans.

38. B

One way of showing respect to the patient is by demonstrating empathy. Empathy can be exemplified by acknowledging and legitimizing the feelings of the patient.

39. B

In the Support component of the RESPECT model, nurses are encouraged to convey their presence and their availability to the patient in their times of need.

40. B

A culturally-bound syndrome is a recognized disease among people of a cultural group. In this case scenario, Hwabyung is recognized by Koreans as a malady that is caused by anger and depression.

41. D

Spiritual distress is experienced when one loses their ability to find meaning in life through their relationship with others or a supreme being. A cause of spiritual distress is a loss of a significant other.

42. B

Developmental losses are experienced as part of the natural developmental process, such as aging.

43. A

Nurses must be alert for patient responses that signal spiritual distress. When patients ask why they have acquired a certain disease, or when they tell the nurse that they are at a loss on what to do, they are experiencing spiritual distress.

44. D

Abstract losses are those that cannot be measured or observed because they had not been visible. Examples of abstract losses are the loss of dreams, hopes, and childhood, among others.

45. B

When the nurse assesses a patient's source of hope and strength, the nurse may ask the patient who helps them when they are in distress or in need. The nurse may also ask what kind of help is available to them and who the most important person is to them.

Interviewing and Health History

Questions

1. A client interview or history-taking is likened to a contract between the nurse and the client. Prior to the process, the details of what the client needs and expects, and what the nurse can offer are clearly communicated. Which of the following is the LEAST important/ inappropriate to establish?
    a. Purpose of the interview
    b. Duration of the interview
    c. Cost of the interview
    d. List of persons who will not be given the client's information

2. Ana is a nurse in the medical-surgical ward who was temporary reassigned to the geriatric medical ward. She finds it difficult caring for older clients because she "just couldn't get them." Ana is having a challenge on which internal factor of communication?
    a. Liking others
    b. Empathy
    c. The ability to listen
    d. Self-awareness

3. An experienced nurse is mentoring a novice nurse on how to improve communication. Included in her instructions is a control of external factors that can affect communication. Which of the following is an example of an external factor?
    a. Knowing oneself
    b. Use of technology
    c. Conducting the interview within curtained partitions
    d. Feeling with the patient

4. A nurse is to perform an interview. Which of the following functional use of space is appropriate?
    a. Putting a 3-ft distance between nurse and the client
    b. Putting a 4-ft distance between nurse and the client
    c. Putting a 6-ft distance between nurse and the client
    d. Putting a 7-ft distance between nurse and the client

5. A clinical instructor is acting as a preceptor of several novice nurses. Which of the following demonstrates that additional teachings are needed?
    a. The nurse speaks with a moderate tone of voice when standing by the bedside of a bedridden client
    b. The nurse positions both chairs at 90-degree angle
    c. The nurse takes a chair and sits by the bedside of a client who is lying supine
    d. The nurse discourages the use of a hospital gown and conducts the interview while the client is still in his own clothes

6. The nurse is conducting a health history and wants to know the number of cigarette sticks the client smokes per day. What kind of communication strategy is most appropriate?
    a. Asking an open-ended question
    b. Asking a closed-ended question
    c. Eliciting feelings
    d. Conveying empathy

7. The nurse is conducting an interview. The client confides to the nurse, "I am worried about being able to provide for the baby since I don't have a steady job," to which the nurse replies, "You are worried you cannot provide for your child." The nurse is using which communication technique?
    a. Facilitation
    b. Reflection
    c. Empathy
    d. Clarification

8. While the nurse is talking with the client, the client states, "I cannot tell my husband about my cancer diagnosis" and the nurse replies, "Could it be because you are worried of how he will react to your news?" This demonstrates what communication technique?
    a. Clarification
    b. Interpretation
    c. Explanation
    d. Summary

9. A conversation is going on between the nurse and the client. The nurse asks the client, "You mentioned that you were in a foster home since age 12. But now you are saying "mom". Did you mean your foster mom?" The client says, "Yes, my foster mom." This is an example of
    a. Clarification
    b. Interpretation
    c. Confrontation
    d. Explanation

10. The nurse is conducting a client interview. The client states, "I don't know what to do. First, my mom got sick. Then my husband left me. Now my teenage daughter is pregnant. I am so at a loss! In fact I did not even have a wink last night." Which of the following nurse response conveys empathy?
    a. "It must be difficult for you."
    b. "You feel you have had many stressors."
    c. "By saying you didn't have a wink last night, did you mean not having enough sleep?"
    d. "You seem distressed."

11. The nurse takes the client to a private room to conduct an interview. The client asked the nurse, "Which contraceptive do you think is best for me?" The nurse replies, "I think it would be best if you use the pill. Most of the people I know who use it were successful without experiencing drastic side effects." Which type of non-productive verbal response did the nurse exhibited?
    a. False reassurance
    b. Giving one's own opinion/personal advice
    c. Emphasis on authority
    d. Distancing

12. The nurse visited the bedside of a client with cancer scheduled for an operation. The client states, "I don't know what's gonna happen to me after the surgery." Which of the following response by the nurse is therapeutic?
    a. "Let me call the doctor so you can discuss your concerns better."
    b. "I will have my duty on your scheduled surgery. I will take care of you."
    c. "Don't worry, be positive and everything will be all better."
    d. "You seem distressed. I will recommend that the doctor prescribe you a medication to help you out."

13. A novice nurse is heard conversing with the client who is for cholecystectomy. In which of the following response should the preceptor provide additional instructions to the novice nurse?
    a. "Let me show you the room where you will recover after surgery."
    b. "I will be the nurse on duty on the day of your surgery."
    c. "The doctor will remove the gallbladder."
    d. "You seem anxious."

14. The nurse is asking the client several questions. Which of the following questions the nurse asked is considered biased or leading?
    a. "Have you had a bowel movement today?"
    b. "Do you keep a record of your medications?"
    c. "Are you sexually active?
    d. "You don't smoke, right?"

15. The nurse is asking the client about family life. On several questions pertaining to this topic, the client rarely makes eye contact and responds only after a long pause or a sigh. The client also uses monotonous, slow, soft voice. What feeling or demeanor is the client conveying?
    a. Anxiety
    b. Dishonesty
    c. Sarcasm
    d. Depression

16. The nurse is about to interview a 5-year old girl and her companions, a man and a woman. Which of the following gestures is appropriate and fosters right communication?
    a. The nurse puts on a colorful top over her uniform

b. The nurse addresses the man and the woman as "mom" and "dad"

c. The nurse focuses her questions on the child to get more direct information

d. The nurse uses grandiose and exaggerated gestures to encourage imagination

17. The nurse asks for some information from a Mediterranean client who was accompanied by her teenage daughter. The nurse guided them in a partitioned room and positioned them 5 feet from her on an angled position. The client has little understanding of English and the nurse have asked the help of her daughter to translate for her. She speaks in a normal tone of voice and takes notes from time to time. Which of the following actions of the nurse reflects the need for further teaching?
    a. Guiding them in a partitioned room
    b. Positioning them 5 feet from her at an angled position
    c. Taking notes from time to time
    d. Asking the daughter's help to act as an interpreter

18. A client who is hearing impaired comes to the clinic. The nurse asks the client for information. Which of the following actions needs to be improved?
    a. The nurse speaks in a loud voice and pronounces words so that lip movement becomes obvious
    b. The nurse speaks slowly in a moderate tone of voice.
    c. The nurse faces the client so that there is adequate lighting on the nurse's face.
    d. The nurse verifies client responses such as a nod or a yes.

19. There are several nurses on the floor conducting interviews with their clients. Who of the nurses performed an INCORRECT technique in doing the interview?
    a. The nurse who says to the client high on methamphetamine, "Please stop fidgeting. I need to know your marital status. Are you married?"
    b. The nurse whose client became tearful when the nurse asked, "Do you have any children?"
    c. The nurse who asked "What is your name?" to a person who was just brought in after a vehicular accident and who is with a large gaping wound to the stomach
    d. The nurse who asked the help of an in-house interpreter when her Chinese client had difficulty communicating with the nurse

20. The nurse has asked the service of an interpreter to communicate with a Jewish patient. The nurse is trying to explain what an MRI is. The nurse explains sentence by sentence that, "The MRI is a test that produces images using sound waves. You will need to lie down under a big machine that produces loud sounds. It does not hurt. It will be done tomorrow at noon. It will take about 30-40 minutes. You should not wear anything with metal. I know you feel a bit under the weather, but I will accompany you to the MRI room." Which sentence needs to be restated by the nurse?
    a. The MRI is a test that produces images using sound waves.
    b. You will need to lie down under a big machine that produces loud sounds.
    c. You should not wear anything with metal.

d. I know you feel a bit under the weather, but I will accompany you to the MRI room.

21. A male client is admitted due to a large laceration to the arm after having an accident at home. Which of the following is the least appropriate to ask?
    a. Diet
    b. Allergies
    c. Name and address
    d. Contact person

22. The nurse is taking the health history of the client to establish a database before client admission. Which of the following does NOT reflect a correct nursing action?
    a. The nurse writes on the area 'reason for seeking care': severe migraine for 5 hours since morning
    b. The nurse notes person who provided information: Mr. John Cruz, interpreter for Ms. Ady Castillo from Spain
    c. The nurse collects information in this sequence: biographic data, reason for seeking care, present health or history of present illness, past history, medication reconciliation
    d. The nurse asks information on activities of daily living after review of systems

23. Several nurses have documented the pain that their client is experiencing. Which of the following record entries should be clarified?
    a. Head pain, bitemporal, throbbing felt since yesterday, unrelieved by acetaminophen
    b. Stomach pain of moderate intensity felt since yesterday and relieved by food.
    c. Substernal chest pain that is like a squeezing sensation, felt at 10am, relieved after one sublingual nitroglycerin
    d. Pain of the joints of the hands and wrists, of moderate intensity, usually felt early in the morning, unrelieved by acetaminophen

24. When assessing the client's pain, the nurse must include details to help describe the pain. Which of the following describes setting?
    a. Right upper quadrant abdominal pain
    b. Dull ache
    c. Felt after eating fatty, oily foods
    d. Unrelieved by defecation

25. The nurse gathered information by interviewing the client. The nurse proceeded to collate the data. Which of the following does not belong to the cluster of data?
    a. Heart failure secondary to myocardial infarction
    b. Rheumatoid arthritis, adult onset
    c. Croup
    d. Diabetes type II

26. A female client's obstetrical record reads: Grav 4, Term 3, Preterm 1, Ab 0, Living 3. Which of the following is a correct interpretation of this data?
    a. The client has been pregnant 4x, and three children were delivered alive at full term, while one was born a stillborn. She has no abnormal child. Only three of the children are currently alive
    b. The client has four children, and three children were delivered at full term, while one child was born premature. Only three of the children are currently alive
    c. The client has been pregnant 4x, and three children were delivered at full term, while one child was born premature. Only three of the children are currently alive; there was no abortion
    d. The client has four children, and three children were delivered at full term, while one child was born premature. Only three of the children survived at birth; no abortion

27. A 26-year old client's immunization status is reviewed. Which of the following entries on vaccination record should the nurse verify?
    a. Pneumococcal
    b. Td/Tdap
    c. Varicella
    d. Zoster

28. The nurse is conducting a systems review with the patient. Which of the following assesses health promotion for the mouth and throat?
    a. Do you have any pain in your mouth?
    b. Do your gums bleed when you brush your teeth?
    c. How often do you visit your dentist?
    d. How often do you get tonsillitis?

29. The nurse wants to assess the sexual health of the client. Which of the following questions is INAPPROPRIATE to ask the client?
    a. Are you sexually active?
    b. How satisfied are you about the aspects of sex?
    c. Do you use any contraception?
    d. What are your routines prior to sex?

30. A client is brought to the clinic because of an alcohol-related accident. In establishing database for the client, the nurse wants to screen the client for excessive alcohol intake. Which of the following is an INAPPROPRIATE question to ask the client when using the CAGE questionnaire?
    a. Have you ever thought of cutting down your alcohol intake?
    b. Have you been ambivalent about drinking?
    c. Do you feel guilty when you drink?
    d. Do you take a drink before or after breakfast?

31. The home health nurse is creating a complete database for a client prior to admission to a facility. The nurse asks, "How do you view your situation now? What are your health goals?" What is the nurse trying to assess?
    a. Personal habits
    b. Perception of health
    c. Cognition
    d. Preferences

32. The nurse is assessing the child for possible allergies. The nurse mentions several causes of food allergies. Which of the following is a rare cause of food allergy?
    a. Egg
    b. Dairy
    c. Seafood
    d. Grapes

33. A psychosocial review of symptoms for adolescents is used to foster communication with the young people. The HEEADSSS method of conducting an interview focuses on the assessment of several parameters. Which of the following parameters is not under the HEEADSSS assessment?
    a. Home
    b. Education and entertainment
    c. Eating
    d. Sexuality

34. The HEEADSSS method has color-coded questions that will help identify the importance of the questions asked. Which color represents the most essential to ask?
    a. Red
    b. Blue
    c. Green
    d. Yellow

35. The HEEADSSS method has color-coded questions that will help identify the importance of the questions asked. Which color represents additional important questions to ask if there is adequate time?
    a. Red
    b. Blue
    c. Green
    d. Yellow

36. The nurse is assessing the sleep pattern of a teenage boy. What is the correct response by the nurse when the boy asks how many hours he must sleep at night?
    a. 6 hours
    b. 7 hours

   c. 8 hours

   d. 9 hours

37. The nurse is using the HEEADSSS method in conducting an interview. Which of the following is an example of a red question?
   a. Have there been any recent changes in your weight?
   b. Have you ever been suspended in school?
   c. Do you feel as if you belong in your school?
   d. Are you crying more than usual?

38. A nurse is asking a series of questions to a mother of three. "Does your child easily adapt to new situations?" "How does your daughter handle problems?" "Did she ever seek counseling?" Which parameter do these questions assess?
   a. Personal habits
   b. Interpersonal relationships
   c. Coping and stress management
   d. Family cohesion

39. A nurse is conducting a review of systems. Which system is the nurse assessing if she asks about presence of palpitations, coldness of extremities, cyanosis and murmurs that the client knows about?
   a. Hematologic system
   b. Cardiovascular system
   c. Neurologic system
   d. Hematologic system

40. A nurse is conducting an interview of a divorced woman who is the mother of a child recently diagnosed with leukemia. Which of the following questions by the nurse needs to be restated?
   a. "What is the name of your husband?"
   b. "What is your daughter's favorite food?"
   c. "Did you notice any bruises?"
   d. "Does she tire easily?"

41. The nurse is interviewing a 55-year old patient. During the course of the interview, the client states, "I have pain in my abdomen about 2 hours after eating at a fast food restaurant". To get a more focused assessment of her primary concern, the nurse uses the OLD CART pneumonic, which stands for:
   a. Onset, Latency, Duration, Common symptoms, Associated manifestations, Relieving factors, Treatments
   b. Onset, Location, Duration, Common symptoms, Associated manifestations, Risk factors, Treatments
   c. Onset, Location, Duration, Characteristic symptoms, Associated manifestations, Relieving

factors, Treatments
   d. Overview, Latency, Duration, Characteristic symptoms, Associated manifestations,
       exacerbating factors, Treatments

42. A 31-year old mother of 3 seeks medical help to address her frequent headaches. The nurse hears
    her say that when she has episodes, she tries taking a nap, having her eyes checked and reducing
    the bright lights. She said these actions offered only brief relief. Using the OLD CART pneumonic,
    under which category should you document the patient's statement?
    a. Characteristic symptoms
    b. Associated manifestations
    c. Relieving factors
    d. Treatments

43. The nursing process is a broad and systematic framework that provides a methodical base or
    structure which is applicable to the practice of nursing. Which of the following is NOT true of the
    nursing process
    a. It aims to validate the signs and symptoms that the nurse has gathered to come up with a
        sound medical diagnosis
    b. It is a problem-solving strategy used to address human responses and the needs of an
        individual, a family or a community
    c. It is used as a tool in developing standards of nursing practice
    d. It focuses on the patient and is customized to meet client needs

44. Making hypotheses about the nature of the patient's problem is a crucial part of clinical reasoning.
    The nurse understands that she needs to consult clinical literature primarily for which reason?
    a. To develop a plan that is agreeable to the patient
    b. To make sound, evidenced-based decisions on how to establish care
    c. To be able to create an individualized nursing care plan
    d. To expand the nurse's knowledge

45. The following are correct about formulating the nursing care plan EXCEPT:
    a. Gather subjective and objective data from the client and check previous medical records as
        part of the assessment process.
    b. Establish nursing diagnoses, and prioritize according to level of importance
    c. Finalize plans and meet with the client to start with the interventions immediately
    d. During the evaluation part, check against your plan if goals have been met and revise as
        needed

46. A 46-year old male comes to the clinic for the first time and started narrating his story. The client
    tells the nurse, "I get nasty headaches in the mornings, sometimes I feel it in my nape. I tried taking
    Tylenol, I get some relief, but the pain just comes back again. I'm scared, you know, my mom and
    granny died of heart attack. You think I have a brain cancer or something?" What is the correct

documentation for the above?
a. Chief complaint: The client experiences headaches usually in the mornings and feels pain in the nape
b. Relieving factors: takes Tylenol
c. Adult Illnesses: heart attack
d. Chief Complaint: "I get headaches in the mornings, sometimes I feel it in my nape"

47. It is one of the principles of test selection and use. It indicates how well repeated measurements of the same relatively stable phenomenon will give the same result and is also known as precision.
a. Reliability
b. Validity
c. Specificity
d. Sensitivity

48. The nurse knows that a rectal thermometer will provide more accurate measurement of body temperature than an axillary thermometer. This means that the temperature taken by rectal thermometer is more _____ than that of an axillary thermometer.
a. Reliable
b. Valid
c. Specific
d. Sensitive

49. The nurse understands that the specificity of C-reactive protein in people with bacterial infections is 94%. The nurse knows that
a. of 100 patients without bacterial infections, 94% will have a normal C-reactive protein and the remaining in 6% will have false positive CRP results
b. of 100 patients with bacterial infections, 94% will have a normal C-reactive protein and the remaining in 6% will have false positive CRP results
c. of 100 patients without bacterial infections, 94% will have a normal C-reactive protein and the remaining in 6% will have false negative CRP results
d. of 100 patients without bacterial infections, 94% will have a decreased C-reactive protein and the remaining in 6% will have false positive CRP results

50. The nurse is developing a plan of care for a client who had recently undergone an abdominal surgery. One of your diagnoses read: Ineffective breathing pattern due to pain on the surgical site. Which of the following is not an appropriate intervention to address the problem?
a. Encourage deep breathing exercises especially during the peak effect of his pain medication
b. Administer pain meds on time
c. Clean the surgical site with hydrogen peroxide solution using aseptic technique
d. Provide health teaching on the importance of deep breathing on healing

51. A community nurse is seeing an elderly woman with hypertension and develops her nursing plan of care. One of your priority diagnoses is knowledge deficit. Which of the following is an appropriate long term goal?
    a. To be able to identify 2 out of 4 possible causes of hypertension after health teaching
    b. To lower blood pressure within normal of her age in the next 2 weeks.
    c. To be able to reduce sodium intake by eliminating table salt and other condiments during meals.
    d. To be able to identify 4 out of 5 lifestyle changes needed to lower BP and the strategies for such after 4 weekly home visits.

52. What is the body mass index of a 22-year old male who stands 5'9" tall and weighs 176 lbs?
    a. 35
    b. 26
    c. 29
    d. 31

53. The nurse is developing her nursing care plan for a client diagnosed with emphysema and made the following nursing diagnoses: knowledge deficit due to misinformation on the cause of cigarette smoking, impaired gas exchange due to accumulation of secretion, ineffective breathing pattern due to hyper aerated barrel chest, pain of the newly created tracheostomy. She knows that she should list them in order of which priority?
    a. knowledge deficit due to misinformation on the cause of cigarette smoking, impaired gas exchange due to accumulation of secretion, ineffective breathing pattern due to hyper aerated barrel chest, pain of the newly created tracheostomy
    b. Ineffective breathing pattern due to hyper aerated barrel chest, pain of the newly created tracheostomy, impaired gas exchange due to accumulation of secretion, knowledge deficit due to misinformation on the cause of cigarette smoking
    c. pain of the newly created tracheostomy, impaired gas exchange due to accumulation of secretion, ineffective breathing pattern due to hyper aerated barrel chest,knowledge deficit due to misinformation on the cause of cigarette smoking
    d. impaired gas exchange due to accumulation of secretions, ineffective breathing pattern due to hyper aerated barrel chest, pain of the newly created tracheostomy, knowledge deficit due to misinformation on the cause of cigarette smoking

54. It is the phase in the nursing process where the nurse jots down strategies on how to address the client's problems. In this stage, the nurse and the patient establishes long and short term goals.
    a. Assessment
    b. Diagnosis
    c. Planning
    d. Intervention

55. The nurse is developing a plan of care for a client and understands that one of the following is true
    a. The nurse categorizes the plans according to assessment findings
    b. The nurse can evaluate and do interventions simultaneously
    c. After evaluation, the nursing process ends
    d. The patient plays an active role in the planning phase only

56. A 50 year old woman who is active in church seeks medical attention when her abdominal pain cannot be relieved by her self-medication. She is suspected of having peptic ulcer. The client states that the pain is worse after meals. She says that on a scale of 1-10, her pain is a 9. She is forced to avoid food because eating causes pain. She also reports passing of black stools. She takes an antacid to relieve pain until just recently the medication offered no relief to her anymore. She frequently eats instant noodles because she says it is easier on her stomach. She drinks about 5 cups of brewed coffee a day. Her past medical record shows that she previously weighed 65kg. Current weight is now 57kg. Her vital signs are all within normal. She believes she has a form of cancer as God's punishment to her for her sins and accepts her symptoms wholeheartedly. Which of the following is NOT an appropriate nursing diagnosis?
    a. Pain, acute (abdominal) related to irritation and lesion of gastric mucosa
    b. Imbalanced Nutrition, Less Than Body Requirements related to pain
    c. Knowledge Deficit: the prevention and treatment of symptoms
    d. Anxiety, chronic, related to the nature of the disease and long-term management.

57. The following are data gathered from assessment: RR: 20, shallow breathing, PR: 90, bounding pulse, BP 150/100, heart rate regularly irregular, pain on surgical site (chest), tobacco use since age 18, use of hash occasionally, alcohol 1 glass 2x a day, Tylenol for headaches, anxiety due to disease progression. Which of the following is a correct clustering of problems?
    a. Tylenol for headaches, anxiety due to disease progression
    b. tobacco use since age 18, use of hash occasionally, alcohol 1 glass 2x a day, Tylenol for headaches
    c. VS: RR: 20, PR: 90, BP 150/100; pulse bounding, heart rate regularly irregular
    d. Pain on surgical site (chest), Tylenol for headaches, anxiety due to disease progression

58. A nurse is talking to a 70 year old client. Which of the following is an appropriate response during the introduction phase of the interview?
    a. "Good morning grandma! How are you feeling today?"
    b. "How are you feeling dear? It's a pleasure to meet you."
    c. "My name is Sarah. How are you?"
    d. "Good morning Mrs. White. I'm Sarah. How do you want me to address you?"

59. A client who had just undergone explore laparotomy is transferred to the recovery room. His wife asks to see his charts. What is the best nursing response?
    a. Politely decline request and explain that she needs to wait until her husband wakes

because he will be the one to give the consent
b. Give the wife the chart
c. Ask permission from the nursing supervisor before handing the chart to the wife.
d. Request an order from the doctor to release the information to the wife.

60. The nurse is writing an expected outcome statement that is quantifiable. Which of the following is an example of such outcome?
a. Verbalization of new knowledge gained after health teaching
b. A decrease in the level of pain from in 6 hours.
c. Enumeration of 5 out of 6 reasons why hand washing is important
d. Ability to move legs within 24hours

61. Which of the following is an example of self-reflection?
a. Determining one's biases before caring for patients who underwent abortion
b. Voicing out one's clinical reasoning to advocate for the patient
c. Reviewing one's skill in handling patients in traction
d. Taking time to listen to the patient's story

62. In what phase of the interview process should the nurse review her clinical behavior and appearance?
a. Pre-interview phase
b. Introduction phase
c. Working phase
d. Termination phase

63. Which of the following is a correct way of adjusting the environment for conducting the interview?
a. Conduct the interview in the waiting area or along the hallway
b. Ask for the patient's permission to draw the curtains and then close the curtains
c. Speak softly to the patient when the interview happens within hearing distance of others
d. Ensure that the room is very cool to use

64. Which of the following interviewing techniques is INCORRECT?
a. Taking notes using short phrases and dates
b. Maintaining eye contact
c. Taking notes when the patient tells a sensitive issue
d. Asking the patient to tell their story while directly facing the patient

65. A student nurse is to interview an adult patient for the first time. Which of the following nurse response indicate the proper way of greeting the patient for the first time?
a. "Hi, Sandra. My name is Kate. I am a nurse."
b. "Hi, Mrs. Downey. How are you? I am nurse Kate."
c. "Nurse Kate here. You are Sandra, right? Nice morning, isn't it?"

d. "Hi there! How are you? I am here to conduct an interview."

66. Which of the following greetings can depersonalize and demean the patient, and should, therefore, be avoided?
    a. "Hello, Mr. Stone. I am Eva, your nurse for this shift."
    b. "Nice to meet you, Ms. Holloway."
    c. "How are we feeling this morning, George?"
    d. "Hello, dear. How are you this morning?"

67. Which of the following interview techniques is inappropriate and should be avoided?
    a. Moving aside table and chairs that are in the way
    b. Using the patient's intimate space for interviewing
    c. Sitting at eye level with the patient
    d. Putting the patient at ease with small talk

68. Which of the following response is best to use to invite the patient to elaborate more on their primary complaint?
    a. "What type of headache are you experiencing?"
    b. "Do you have any idea as to what caused your headache?"
    c. "Is your headache related to stress?"
    d. "Tell me more about your headache."

69. A nurse is assessing a patient. During the interview, the patient did not provide enough details of their complaint even if they have given the chance to elaborate, so the nurse explores their perspective on their illness. Which of the following questions is best to ask to determine the patient's perspective on illness?
    a. "How has your headache affected you?"
    b. "When does your headache usually occur?"
    c. "How long does your headache usually last?"
    d. "Did you get relief from over-the-counter medications?"

70. Which of the following interview questions is non-therapeutic?
    a. "You said you were feeling blue. What did you mean?"
    b. "Does anyone in your family have or had cancer, tuberculosis, diabetes, or hypertension, and are they still living?"
    c. "Do you feel the tingling sensation at night?"
    d. "How did the pain affected you?"

71. A nurse is conducting an interview to assess an elderly female patient in a home care. When the nurse asked the patient who she lived with, she said she has lived like a hermit all her life. The nurse responded, "What exactly did you mean by living like a hermit all your life?" What type of

therapeutic communication technique did the nurse use?
a. Reflection
b. Clarification
c. Validation
d. Summarizing

72. A nurse is interviewing a patient who was raped two weeks ago. During the assessment, the patient started crying. In response, the nurse says, "a person who has been traumatized can still feel the pain even after weeks have passed." What type of therapeutic communication technique did the nurse use in this situation?
a. Reassurance
b. Transition
c. Validation
d. Summarizing

73. A patient is anxious about her surgery which is scheduled later that day. Which of the following nurse response is NOT therapeutic?
a. "Don't worry. Everything will be fine."
b. "I will be the nurse who will take care of you while you are in the recovery room."
c. "Do you have any concerns about your surgery?"
d. "The surgical team will do its best to make the surgery successful."

74. Which of the following are ways to empower patients? Select all that apply.
a. Conveying interest in the patient's personal affairs
b. Asking for the patient's perspective
c. Avoiding listening to emotional content
d. Revealing the limits of your knowledge
e. Limiting the patient's participation in the planning stage

75. Which of the following responses uses the therapeutic communication technique of proper transitioning?
a. "What did you mean by having a fair share of bad days?"
b. "Now we are done with the interview. I will examine you next. I will give you a few minutes to put on this hospital gown."
c. "You said you started having those headaches four months ago and has since been having them most days of the week for almost the entire day. You also noticed watery discharge from your nose, and that you could not do much work on those days, is that right?"
d. "Is there anything else would you like to tell me?"

76. Which of the following should the nurse do if they encounter a silent patient? Select all that apply.
a. Continue being attentive
b. Encourage the patient to continue and elaborate more

   c. Ask a series of short-answer questions

   d. Say, "You seem quiet. Have I done something to offend you?"

   e. Shorten the interview process

77. During the interview of a confusing patient, what should the nurse do if they suspect a psychiatric disorder?

   a. Continue the interview process and take notes of understandable answers

   b. Stop the interview and refer the patient to a psychologist immediately

   c. Do not gather a detailed history and shift to a mental status exam

   d. Restrain the patient

78. Which of the following is best for the nurse to do if their patient has impaired capacity?

   a. Keep the interview short and simple

   b. Look for the patient's lawyer

   c. Find a surrogate informant

   d. Be quick when interviewing a family member

79. Which type of therapeutic communication technique would be most helpful when interviewing a talkative patient?

   a. Summarizing

   b. Transitioning

   c. Validating

   d. Reflecting

80. Which of the following is NOT therapeutic when dealing with a crying patient?

   a. Give the patient the permission to cry

   b. Say, "It is good to express your feelings."

   c. Offer a tissue and give the patient time to recover.

   d. Leave the patient and come back after the patient has regained their composure

81. Which of the following refers to a document by which the patient makes provision for health care decisions when the time comes that they will be incapable of making those decisions?

   a. Health care proxy

   b. DNR

   c. Advance directives

   d. Durable Power of Attorney.

82. Which of the following is INCORRECT when using interpreters?

   a. The nurse must interact with the patient and not the interpreter

   b. Let the patient know that every conversation will be interpreted for them

   c. Choose interpreters that are close to the patient, such as a relative or a friend, to advocate for the patient

    d.   Use simple language and short sentences

83. Which of the following is NOT appropriate when interviewing a patient with impaired hearing?
    a.   Face the patient directly and use good lighting
    b.   Eliminate background noise
    c.   Speak loudly and exaggerate mouth movements to make lip reading easier
    d.   If the patient has glasses, let them wear it

84. Which of the following patients will benefit most from Augmentative and Alternative Communication (AAC)?
    a.   A patient with impaired hearing
    b.   A patient with impaired vision
    c.   A patient with severe cognitive disabilities
    d.   A talkative patient

85. A ma le patient tells the nurse that he has something important to say but the nurse should promise first to keep the matter confidential between just the two of them. Which response by the nurse is most therapeutic?
    a.   "You can trust me to keep it secret, but you have to tell me first."
    b.   "I cannot make such a promise. There are pieces of information that I may need to share with the appropriate people."
    c.   "We took an oath to keep patient information confidential at all times."
    d.   "I promise not to tell anyone."

86. An elderly patient is to be admitted to a long-term care facility. Which of the following types of history is most appropriate to gather?
    a.   A comprehensive health assessment
    b.   A focused or problem-oriented assessment
    c.   A follow-up history
    d.   An emergency history

87. A patient who is recovering from an abdominal surgery sustained a wound that shows signs of infection. Which of the following types of history is most appropriate to gather?
    a.   A follow-up history
    b.   An emergency history
    c.   A comprehensive health assessment
    d.   A focused or problem-oriented assessment

88. The afternoon-shift nurse is asking a patient if they had a bowel movement since the nurse from the morning shift has noted that the patient has not defecated for three days now. The afternoon-shift nurse proceeded to ask about the details of the patient's constipation problem. Which type of history did the afternoon-shift nurse gathered?

a. A focused or problem-oriented assessment
b. A follow-up history
c. An emergency history
d. A comprehensive health assessment

89. Which of the following is TRUE of comprehensive assessments?
a. It is appropriate for patients returning for a follow-up
b. It is appropriate when assessing more signs and symptoms of a particular complaint
c. It evaluates a particular body system only
d. It helps identify or rule out the causes related to patient complaint

90. On which of the following patients would the nurse need to obtain an emergency history?
a. A patient who comes to the ER complaining of chest pain
b. A patient who is seen in the clinic for the first time
c. A patient who complains of easy fatigability in the last few months
d. A patient with a primary complaint of a recurring headache and night sweats

91. Which of the following is a subjective information?
a. Dizziness
b. HR = 54
c. BP = 120/70
d. BMI = 20

92. Which of the following is part of the Identifying data component of the adult health history?
a. Chief complaint
b. Source of history
c. Childhood illnesses
d. Past hospitalizations

93. Which of the following component of the adult health history pertains to the patient's symptoms or concerns that prompted them to seek medical attention?
a. Past history
b. Reliability
c. Chief complaint/s
d. Present illness

94. Which of the following reflects the correct way of documenting a patient's chief complaint?
a. Morning headache, bitemporal
b. "I think the patient has a migraine."
c. "My head hurts, especially in the morning, and I feel like throwing up every time."
d. Headache usually felt in the morning, unrelieved by acetaminophen

95. Which of the following are attributes of a symptom that the nurse should include in their assessment of the patient's present illness? Select all that apply.
    a. Location
    b. Quality
    c. Past experience of the symptom
    d. Reason for hospitalization
    e. The setting in which the symptom occurs

96. The nurse is asking a male patient about his present medications, supplements, and his intake of non-prescription drugs. The nurse would document their findings under which category of the adult health history?
    a. Personal and social history
    b. Review of systems
    c. Chief complaint
    d. Present illness

97. Which of the following should the nurse document under the category health maintenance? Select all that apply.
    a. Cause of death of parents and relatives
    b. Immunization status
    c. Use of herbal medicines
    d. Screening tests
    e. Past surgeries

98. The nurse is asking the patient if they are using hearing aids. Which body system is the nurse reviewing?
    a. General
    b. Respiratory
    c. HEENT
    d. Peripheral vascular

99. Which of the following symptom is under the review of the hematologic system?
    a. Anemia
    b. Joint stiffness
    c. Depression
    d. Heat intolerance

100. Which of the following types of documentation is the best to use to identify disease patterns within the family quickly?
    a. Bulleted form
    b. Narrative
    c. Genogram

d. Chart

101. A nurse is interviewing a patient and is using the CAGE questionnaire to get information from the patient. Which information is the nurse obtaining when the CAGE questionnaire is used?
    a. Drinking problem
    b. Abuse
    c. Mental problem
    d. Cognitive disabilities

102. A patient answers yes to three of the CAGE questions. Which question is appropriate to ask next?
    a. "Have you ever experience blackouts or accidents after drinking?"
    b. "Which type of drink do you take?"
    c. "How much alcoholic drink are you having in a day?"
    d. "Which type of alcohol do you usually drink?"

103. The nurse is asking about the immunization status of an elderly patient. Which of the following vaccines are routinely given ONLY to older people aged 60 years old and above?
    a. Varicella
    b. Meningococcal
    c. Singles
    d. Hib

104. The nurse is asking a 50-year-old female patient if she has knowledge of her mother ever taking DES or Diethylstilbestrol while pregnant with her. The nurse is asking this question because DES is linked to the development of:
    a. Breast cancer
    b. Vaginal or cervical carcinoma
    c. Lymphoma
    d. Bone carcinoma

105. Which of the following is appropriate to ask the patient if the nurse is to assess the patient's self-perception or self-concept?
    a. "What time do you usually retire?"
    b. "How do you feel about your ability to handle frustration?"
    c. "What is your source of strength and hope?"
    d. "Please describe your leisure activities."

106. The nurse is asking the patient who they live with and who supports their family's need. The nurse also asked the patient if they feel safe. Which of the following topics on personal/social history is the nurse assessing?
    a. Coping-stress-tolerance

b. Role-relationship
c. Self-perception-self-concept
d. Value-belief

107. Which of the following should the nurse remember when broaching sensitive topics? Select all that apply.
a. Respectfully explain to the patient your disapproval for negative sexual behaviors
b. Deny your discomfort asking sensitive questions and proceed with the interview
c. Do not be judgmental
d. Explain the need for knowing certain information
e. If the patient feels uncomfortable with the questions, skip the questions and ask them at a later time

108. A nurse is gathering data about a patient's sexual history. Which of the following questions is NOT appropriate to ask?
a. "Are you sexually active?"
b. "Do you have sex with men, women or both?"
c. "To know about your risk factors for reproductive diseases, I need to ask you about your sexual health and practices.
d. "How many sexual partners have you had in the last six months?"

109. Which of the following questions could the nurse ask a female patient to assess the sensitive topic of possible violence in the family?
a. "Is there any time in your relationship that you feel unsafe or afraid?"
b. "Is there a history of violence in your family?"
c. "Do you feel like crying at times?"
d. "Have you been hospitalized because of accidents?"

110. In the course of an interview, the nurse begins to suspect that the patient has been abused. Which of the following are signs that abuse may be happening to a patient? Select all that apply.
a. The patient is an elderly
b. A person living with the patient has an alcohol or drug problem
c. The patient's companion does not leave the room and answers for the patient even if the patient is capable of answering for themselves
d. The patient seems disinterested in interacting with the nurse
e. The patient is overly eager to get all the information from the assessment

ANSWERS

1. D
    Prior to the interview, the nurse discusses the purpose, duration, and cost if applicable, to the client.

2. A
    To be happy and successful in the nursing profession, specifically in communicating with clients, families and other health professionals, there should be an innate and genuine liking of other people.

3. C
    Ensuring privacy by choosing the right place for interview is one of the external factors of communication. Other external factors are controlling the physical environment and avoiding interruptions.

4. B
    The most appropriate distance between the nurse and the client should be 4-5 feet. Conducting the interview closer than 4 feet invades personal space and can cause anxiety, while being farther away conveys indifference.

5. A
    Client interview should be conducted wherein the visual message of the communication must be conveyed. Standing over a patient communicates a hurried demeanor. The nurse should be at eye level with the client. Asking the client to change into a hospital gown emphasizes hierarchy and power difference and makes the client feel exposed.

6. B
    Asking a closed-ended question is most appropriate in this situation because it elicits specific information. The nurse can ask directly, "How many sticks of cigarettes do you smoke per day?"

7. B
    Reflection conveys that the nurse understands the client's story. It entails repetition of some words of the client.

8. B
    Interpretation is the strategy of trying to link contents of what the client is saying and implying causation. It relies on inference.

9. A
    Clarification entails asking for more explanation of an ambiguous statement.

10. A

Empathy is feeling 'with' the client and not 'like' the client. The nurse tries to identify the feeling and allows the client to express it.

11. B

In professional nursing practice, giving unsolicited advice or one's own opinion that will influence the client's choice is non-therapeutic. The nurse should explain the advantages and disadvantages of options, and support the client through the decision –making process but she should not incorporate her own personal opinion on the matter.

12. B

One of the ten traps of interviewing is giving false reassurances. False reassurances trivialize the client's concerns and feelings and create a barrier in communication. Therapeutic reassurance can be conveyed by telling the client that as a nurse, you care about her by ensuring your service and presence.

13. C

Distancing is using language that puts distance between a threat to health and the self. An example is using "the" instead of 'your' or 'my' when pertaining to client's body parts. The therapeutic response should be "The doctor will remove your gallbladder."

14. D

A biased or leading question asks that the client choose the 'better' or the 'good' choice. It is non-therapeutic. In this case, the nurse seems to imply that the good choice to answer is, "No, I don't smoke."

15. D

People who are depressed rarely make eye contact. They respond only after a long pause or a sigh, with some reluctance or hesitancy. If they respond, their voice is usually, slow, monotonous and sometimes, barely audible.

16. A

The white uniforms that nurses wear can elicit fear and anxiety in a young child. Putting on a colorful coat or top makes the interview more casual. The nurse must not assume that the man and the woman who brought her to seek medical consult are her parents. The nurse should direct most of her questions on the primary caregiver if the child's age is 6 years old and below.

17. D

Using an "ad hoc" interpreter (a non-professional interpreter who is usually a relative or a friend) is convenient. However, it is not recommended because the client's confidentiality may be breached, and because the ad hoc interpreter may not have enough knowledge on medical terminology to carry out the task with reliability.

18. A

When dealing with a hearing-impaired client, it is not appropriate to speak in a loud voice or to exaggerate lip movements. The nurse should use a normal tone of voice, being careful that the face of the nurse is visible to the client. The nurse may also use pantomime for deaf people.

19. A

A client who is high on amphetamine may have inappropriate behaviors. Asking the client to stop fidgeting is confrontational and is non-therapeutic. All options reflect correct techniques in interviewing.

20. D

When explaining about a medical procedure, it is best to get an interpreter who knows about medical procedures. The procedure should be explained using simple language. The nurse should provide details such as description, body parts to be examined, the schedule and duration of the test. The nurse, however, must not use idioms, such as "feel a bit under the weather".

21. A

During an emergency case, it is appropriate to conduct a focused interview. In this situation that the client is bleeding due to a laceration, there may be a need for surgery. Important biographical information are necessary as well as allergies that may be significant in a surgical procedure. Diet is the least important information to ask the client at this time.

22. A

The reason for seeking care should be written in direct quotes and should not contain a medical diagnosis even if the diagnosis has been pre-established. If the nurse asked for the services of an interpreter, the name of the interpreter should be indicated. The correct sequence of the interview is as follows: 1. Biographic data, 2. Reason for seeking care, 3. Present health or history of present illness, 4. Past history, 5. Medication reconciliation, 6. Family history, 7. Review of systems, 8. Functional assessment or activities of daily living (ADLs).

23. B

When documenting complaints of pain, the nurse must be specific in her description of pain and must include details such as location, character, severity, timing, setting, aggravating and relieving factors, associated factors, and patient's perception of pain. In this case, 'stomach pain' is vague.

24. C

Setting provides information about how the pain started and what brought it on. The nurse may ask what the client was doing when the pain started.

25. C

Croup is the inflammation of the larynx, trachea and the bronchial tubes. The client produces a characteristic barking cough. It is categorized under childhood illnesses. The other options are a cluster under chronic illnesses.

26. C

Grav stands for Gravidity or the number of pregnancies the woman has had; term is the number of deliveries that reached 37 weeks or more, while preterm refers to the number of deliveries before the 37th week. Ab refers to the number of abortions or miscarriages, and living refers to number of children currently alive. The correct option is C.

27. D

The zoster vaccine is recommended to be given to people aged 60 and above. All options are expected vaccinations to be given during adulthood.

28. C

Health promotion practices are those that aim to maintain or start a healthy habit or lifestyle. In this case, asking about dental visits assesses health promotion practices.

29. D

Asking about routines prior to sex is insignificant unless the nurse has reasons to believe that the routine is pertinent to a case. All other options are appropriate questions.

30. B

The CAGE questionnaire is used to screen for excessive or uncontrolled alcohol intake. CAGE stands for Cut down, Annoyed, Guilt, Eye-opener. The nurse should ask instead if the client has ever been annoyed when criticized about his drinking.

31. B

To assess the client's perception of health, the nurse can ask about how the client views his/her current situation or what his/her health goals are. The nurse can also ask about his views of the future as well as his expectations of the staff and the facility.

32. D

Most common causes of childhood allergies are cow's milk, eggs, peanuts, soybean, wheat, tree nuts, and fish.

33. B

The HEEADSSS method of conducting an interview focuses on the assessment of the Home, Education and employment (not entertainment), Eating, peer-related Activities, Drugs, Sexuality, Suicide/depression, and Safety from injury and violence.

34. C

The HEEADSSS method has color-coded questions so that it will help identify the importance of the questions asked. Green colored ones are questions that are most important to ask.

35. B

The HEEADSSS method has color-coded questions so it will help identify the importance of the questions asked. Green colored ones are questions that are most important to ask. Texts in blue are additional important questions to ask if there is adequate time. Red ones dig deeper into a topic if it is called for.

36. D

For teenagers, the recommended number of hours of sleep at night is 9 hours.

37. C

Red questions in the HEEADSSS method are those that dig deeper into a topic if it is called for. Asking the client about his feeling of belongingness in the school or work is an example of a red question that delves into the topic of education or employment.

38. C

These questions assess coping and stress management. The nurse may also ask directly how the client copes with stress, or if the client has experienced any recent changes in mood lately.

39. B

When the nurse wants to review the cardiovascular system, she asks for known history or present conditions of palpitations, coldness of extremities, cyanosis and murmurs, dyspnea on exertion, high blood pressure or any limitation of activity.

40. A

This question is inappropriate because using the term 'husband' can cause confusion especially in a divorced woman. It is also making assumptions that the child's father is her current husband.

41. C

The OLD CART pneumonic stands for Onset, Location, Duration, Characteristic symptoms, Associated manifestations, Relieving/exacerbating factors, Treatments It is used to gather more focused and detailed data about a symptom or a complaint.

42. C

Relieving factors are the steps the patient has tried to experience relief from the symptom. Exacerbating factors are those that worsen a complaint.

43. A

The nursing process does not aim to establish a medical diagnosis. However, it contains a nursing diagnosis that specifies maladaptive health patterns or responses.

44. B

Consulting clinical literature has all of the above objectives but primarily, the reason for that is to make sound, evidenced-based decisions which will help develop an effective nursing care plan that in turn will ultimately benefit the client

45. C
Before finalizing your plan, it is important to discuss your assessment and plan with your patient and to seek out his or her opinions, concerns, and willingness to proceed with the interventions. During the planning phase, the patient should always take an active role.

46. D
The chief complaint is written in direct quotes. Taking Tylenol is part of Treatments. Mom and granny's heart attack is under family history.

47. A
Reliability is how a given test will yield similar results if done repeatedly over time.

48. B
Validity Indicates how closely a given observation agrees with "the true state of affairs," or the best possible measure of reality.

49. A
Identifies the proportion of people who test negative in a group of people known to be without a given disease or condition.

50. C
This intervention does not address the problem ineffective breathing pattern but of ineffective health maintenance

51. D
Identifying 4 out of 5 lifestyle changes and the strategies for those changes means that the nurse's health teaching has benefitted the client.

52. D
BMI is computed as weight of the client in kg divided by the square of the height in meters. The answer is 26

53. D
The nurse lists them in order of priority using the ABC's principle, Airway, Breathing and Circulation. Pain precedes knowledge deficit.

54. C
In the planning phase, the nurse involves the client in establishing goals, as well as develops strategies to address problems as specified in the nursing diagnoses.

55. B

The nursing process is ongoing as long as the client needs medical help. A lot of times, one problem is sufficiently addressed, while some concerns need to be reevaluated. In cases like these, some stages overlap each other for different problems addressed.

56. D

Anxiety is not an appropriate diagnosis because there is nothing in the assessment findings to support the diagnosis.

57. C

This cluster is best because it gives vital signs data and characteristics of pulse and heart rate

58. D

Greeting the client and using a formal title to address the client for the first time is most appropriate. Using "granny" and "dear" can depersonalize and demean unless rapport has been established and endearments are permitted by the client.

59. A

The client first gives consent before his medical information is released to anyone who does not provide direct care.

60. C

An expected outcome is measurable when a specific goal for the outcome yields accurate results, either expressed in percentage or ratio, or described as a completion of certain specific steps.

61. A

Self-reflection is looking into one's own way of thinking regarding certain situations. An example is determining one's biases before caring for others.

62. A

It is during the pre-interview phase that the nurse should review their clinical behavior and appearance. The nurse should appear for interview clean, neat, and wearing a conservative dress or a nurse uniform. A visible name tag can also help build trust in the patient. The nurse should show respect to the patient regardless of the circumstance as to why they were hospitalized, or their personal background.

63. B

To facilitate a successful interview, the nurse must learn to adjust the environment accordingly to provide for the patient's privacy and comfort. The ideal place for an interview is an empty room, and never within the hearing distance of others. Adjust the room temperature accordingly. Older patients appreciate warmer rooms. Ensure the patient's privacy when a private room is not available. The nurse can do this by closing the curtains, with the patient's permission.

64. C

While interviewing a patient, the nurse must take notes of important details using short phrases, but when the topic becomes sensitive or disturbing, the nurse must listen intently and put down their pens, while only mentally noting details. The nurse must directly face the patient and maintain eye contact during the entire interview process.

65. B

When meeting a patient for the first time, it is best to use a formal title to address the patient, like Mrs. Downey in this case. Unless the patient is a minor, the nurse must avoid addressing the patient by their first name unless permitted to do so by the patient or the family.

66. D

When greeting the patient, it is best to avoid words such as 'granny' or 'dear' because these can depersonalize and demean the patient.

67. B

When interviewing patients, the nurse must put into consideration the patients' cultural background and individual preferences. Using the right proxemics is important during interviews. The use of patient's intimate space is inappropriate. In most cases, the personal space is comfortable for the patient during interviews. The nurse must sit at eye level with the patient and move aside any obstructions in the way. The nurse may engage the patient in small talk to keep them at ease.

68. D

During the working phase of the interview, the nurse invites the patient's story to be able to extract more details about their chief complaint or presenting problem. The nurse can ask the patient to elaborate by using open-ended questions, such as "Tell me more about…"

69. A

When the patient fails to mention their perspective on their illness even after they have been given a chance to elaborate, the nurse may ask a follow-up question to explore this point of view. The nurse may ask how the illness has affected them, or how they have felt about their illness.

70. B

When the nurse needs to verify patient information using a series of questions, the nurse must remember to ask one question at a time because the patient may feel overwhelmed or confused and may give an inaccurate response.

71. B

The nurse must use the technique clarification when patients use ambiguous words or unclear associations. To seek clarification, the nurse may ask the patient what exactly they meant by those words with unclear meaning.

72. C
Validation is affirming or acknowledging the legitimacy of the patient's experience to make them feel at ease and to assure them that such emotions are understandable.

73. A
Telling an anxious patient that everything will be fine is giving false reassurance and is not therapeutic because it conveys that the nurse has not understood the extent of the patient's distress. Also, it prevents the patient from further verbalizing their feelings. The nurse may give therapeutic reassurance instead by providing information competently.

74. B, D
Empowered patients are more likely to follow health advice. The nurse can empower a patient by asking for their perspectives, conveying an interest in the patient and not just the problem, eliciting an emotional response, and revealing the limitation of the nurse's knowledge. The nurse must also encourage the patient to actively participate in their own care.

75. B
During hospitalizations or clinic visits, patients may feel anxious and vulnerable. To keep them at ease and in the know, the nurse must give them cues as to what would happen next so that they will know what to expect.

76. A, B, D
Silence during interviews can be disconcerting to novice nurses. The nurse must continue being attentive to the silent patient, encouraging them to elaborate more on the information they are sharing. The nurse must also refrain from asking a series of short-answer questions that can make a person silent as they collect their thoughts.

77. C
If a psychiatric or neurological disorder is suspected of a confusing patient, the nurse must not spend too much time asking for details of the patient's information, but rather shift to a mental status exam. The nurse must assess the patient's level of consciousness, orientation, memory, and their ability to comprehend.

78. C
Patients with impaired capacity are not the best person to provide information about their health. For patients whose capacity to comprehend and make decisions is impaired, the nurse must find a surrogate informant, who may be a family member or a healthcare proxy. The nurse must conduct the interview in the same manner as they would interview the patient.

79. A
When the nurse encounters a talkative person, the patient may provide a flow of information which is too much and too fast to comprehend and take note of. The nurse may use the technique

summarizing to validate the information and the concerns. All other techniques of therapeutic communication may be used as well but summarizing would be most useful.

80. D

Crying is usually a therapeutic response of a patient. The crying should be dealt with quiet acceptance. The nurse must respond in empathy and give the patient permission to cry. The patient must be offered a tissue and given time to recover. The nurse may acknowledge the feeling by telling the patient that it is good to express one's feelings. When the patient is in distress, the nurse must never leave them alone.

81. C

An advance directive is a document that states the patient's wishes and preferences for their care in the event that they become incapable of making a decision for themselves. The treatments in consideration are usually cardiopulmonary resuscitation, artificial feeding, hydration, and antibiotics. A Durable Power of Attorney is a legal document that designates a health care proxy who will make health care decisions for the patient when they become incapable of deciding for themselves. A DNR (Do Not Resuscitate) is a physician's order, with the permission of the patient, to withhold resuscitation attempts when the patient's heart stops.

82. C

When using interpreters, the nurse must avoid asking a relative or friend to act as interpreters. Doing so may violate the patient's privacy and may make the patient withhold pertinent information. The nurse must seek the services of qualified interpreters with knowledge of medical terms. In the presence of the interpreter, the nurse must interact with the patient and not the interpreter and must use simple language and short sentences. Assure the patient that all conversations will be interpreted for them.

83. C

When speaking with a patient with impaired hearing, the nurse must use a normal tone of voice and must speak clearly, making sure that they are facing the patient directly under a good light. The nurse must also remember to let the patient wear glasses if they have one. This makes lip reading easier. Background noise must either be reduced or eliminated.

84. C

A patient with severe cognitive disabilities, especially those with speech or language problems will benefit most from Augmentative and Alternative Communication (AAC) which utilizes all forms of communication except the oral form. Examples of AAC are picture and symbol communication boards or electronic devices.

85. B

Should there be an instance wherein a patient tells the nurse that they will provide information only if the nurse promises to keep the information confidential, the nurse must inform the patient that they could not make such a promise. The nurse must let the patient know that there are certain types of information that may need to be divulged to the appropriate people in the care team to protect the patient and others as well.

86. A

A comprehensive health assessment provides a full picture of the patient's health status as well as their needs for health promotion and maintenance, and risk reduction. A patient who is to be admitted to a long-term facility would need a comprehensive assessment so that they can be given the most appropriate care.

87. D

Patients who developed another problem while being cared for in a healthcare facility will need a focused or problem-oriented assessment because a prior comprehensive assessment has already been done. The nurse only gathers information to assess the patient's current concern.

88. B

A follow-up history is appropriate in assessing patients who are returning for re-evaluation. It is also needed when the nurse is following up on a concern identified by the nurse from an earlier shift. A follow-up history usually determines if a concern has been properly addressed or if a treatment plan has been successful.

89. D

A comprehensive assessment includes all components of the health history, as well as the complete physical examination. It is used to assess new patients, and it gives full information about a patient's health. It helps identify or rule out physical causes related to the health complaint of the patient.

90. A

Gathering emergency history is appropriate for urgent visits, such as that of the patient in the ER complaining of chest pain. Focused assessments address a particular symptom or body system.

91. A

Subjective data are those that the patient feels or what they tell the nurse. Objective data, on the other hand, are those that the nurse has observed or measured themselves.

92. B

Identifying data is a component of the adult health history whereby the nurse gathers data such as the patient's age, gender, occupation and marital status. Under this component, the nurse also identifies the source of the history and the source of referral.

93. C

The chief complaint is the primary reason or concern why the patient has sought care.

94. C

   When documenting a patient's chief complaint, the nurse must write a direct quote of the patient's words so that it is not subjected to the nurse's own opinion.

95. A, B, D

   When describing a symptom of the patient's present illness, the nurse should make sure that there are enough details that will enable them to make a nursing diagnosis. The seven attributes of a symptom include location, quality, quantity or severity, timing, the setting in which it happens, and the aggravating factors.

96. D

   When assessing the patient's present illness, the nurse must ask about a detailed description of the patient's reason for visit including any treatments or medications. When assessing the patient's intake of medications, the nurse must ask about the medications' name, dose, route, and frequency.

97. B, D

   When determining the patient's health maintenance efforts, the nurse should ask about the patient's immunization status, the screening tests they have undergone, the safety measures that they take, and the risk factors that they have for certain diseases.

98. C

   HEENT stands for Head, Eyes, Ears, Nose and sinuses, Throat and the pharynx. When the nurse is asking about the patient's use of hearing aids, they are reviewing the patient's HEENT.

99. A

   The hematologic system review assesses the patient's blood and their reaction to blood transfusion. Anemia is a disorder of the red blood cells.

100.   C

   A genogram provides a record that is visually informative of the disease patterns present in the family. It allows easy identification of diseases that are present within the family. It also provides a quick and accurate way of plotting the information provided by the patient.

101.   A

   The CAGE questionnaire is used to assess the patient's drinking or alcohol problem. CAGE stands for Cutting down, Annoyance if criticized, Guilty feelings and Eye-openers. This questions could also be used to assess illicit drug use.

102.   A

   Two or more affirmative answers to the CAGE questionnaire suggest alcohol abuse. If the patient answers yes to two or more questions, the nurse should further probe into the drinking problem by asking if there had been any blackouts, seizures or accidents that the patient experienced after drinking

103.   C

The Centers for Disease Control and Prevention recommends that older people aged 60 years old and above receive the shingles vaccine, whether they have had shingles in the past or not. The vaccine is not recommended for any other age group.

104.   B

Maternal use of DES or Diethylstilbestrol is linked to vaginal or cervical carcinoma. Asking female patients who were born before 1971 if they have knowledge of their mothers being exposed to DES assesses the patients' risk to these types of cancers.

105.   B

When gathering the patient's personal and social history, the nurse should ask about the patient's concept of self. To do this, the nurse asks them how a friend would likely describe them, or how they would handle a negative situation or emotion. Alternatively, the nurse asks about things that the patient would like to change in themselves.

106.   B

When the nurse is gathering data to assess the patient's role-relationships under the personal/social category of history-taking, the nurse asks the patient who they live with, who supports them, and if they feel safe in their relationships. The nurse also asks them to describe their relationships with others, as well as their jobs.

107.   C, D

Nurses must be careful when asking emotionally charged or sensitive questions, such as those that pertain to sexual health, domestic violence or abuse. To efficiently gather history on these topics, the nurse must resolve their own discomfort when probing into these matters to prevent skipping these parts of the history. The nurse must not be judgmental when learning about patient behaviors and must also explain the need for knowing certain information.

108.   A

When assessing the patient's sexual health, asking if they are sexually active can be ambiguous to the patient. Sometimes patients think that the nurse is asking them if they are the more active partner in a sexual act. The nurse should instead ask when was the last time the patient has had intimate physical contact with someone, and then explicitly ask them if that had involved sexual intercourse. Sometimes, it may be necessary to be precise with the definition of sexual intercourse. If the situation calls for it, the nurse must avoid using the term 'private parts' and define intercourse as 'when a man inserts his penis into a woman's vagina."

109.   A

Violence in the family can be a sensitive topic to explore during the interview. The nurse may start by asking normalizing questions such as "Is there any time in your relationship that you feel unsafe or afraid?". The nurse must ask these questions as if it is part of a routine interview.

110.   B, C

Nurses may suspect abuse if the injuries could not be appropriately explained by the patient, or if the patient has delayed getting treatment for trauma. The nurse must check the patient's records for repeated hospitalizations due to injuries and 'accidents'. Another sign of possible abuse is having a family member or anyone living with the patient who has an alcohol or drug problem. If the nurse notices that a patient's companion does not leave the patient's side and dominates the conversation, then the nurse must be alert for the possibility of abuse.

Behavior and Mental Status

Questions

1. A nurse is assessing several clients. Which of the following clients will need further and more thorough assessment of mental status?
    a. A tearful mother who is cuddling her baby with Down's syndrome
    b. A pre-school boy who believes his dead mother would soon wake up
    c. A husband who just lost his job eight months ago who looks unkempt and is always in solitude
    d. A woman who lost her husband to cancer 2 months ago and has since lived with her daughter

2. A woman who appears dazed is being seen in the emergency department because of a head trauma. The nurse asks, "Do you know where you are?" Which of the following parameters is the nurse assessing?
    a. Mood and affect
    b. Orientation
    c. Attention
    d. Memory

3. A novice nurse is trying to determine the difference between organic and psychiatric mental disorders. Which of the following is considered a psychiatric disorder?
    a. Delirium
    b. Alzheimer's disease
    c. Anxiety disorder
    d. Amphetamine abuse

4. The nurse is trying to assess the abstract reasoning of a client. Which of the following is an appropriate question to ask, or instruction to be given to the the client?
    a. "I will give you a simple test. You will see a series of figures. Which figure appropriately belongs on the spot of the question mark?"
    b. "What brought you here to the hospital?"
    c. "What are you thinking right now?"
    d. "What is the date today?"

5. The nurse is assessing the developmental competence of a 1-year-old child. Which of the following is an expected competence of child in using language to communicate?
    a. Differentiated crying
    b. Cooing
    c. One-word sentences
    d. Multi-word sentences

6. The nurse understands that as people age, hearing high frequency sounds is becoming more difficult. Which of the following is a manifestation of this change in hearing ability?
    a. The client has difficulty hearing the honking of car horns
    b. The client remains unmindful of the alarm ringing

c. The client cannot hear consonants well
d. The client disregards the barking of their neighbor's dog

7. The nurse is asking the client to recall four unrelated words she instructed the client to memorize 10 minutes ago. What is the nurse trying to assess?
   a. Thought content
   b. Thought process
   c. Remote memory
   d. New learning

8. The nurse asks the client, "Have you ever felt so sad that you thought of hurting yourself?" The client replies, "Yes." Which of the following follow-up question is NOT appropriate to ask?
   a. "How do you plan to hurt yourself?"
   b. "Do you have a gun at home?"
   c. "Would you like me to keep this just between us?"
   d. "How would you think other people will react if you were dead?"

9. The nurse is to utilize the Denver Developmental Screening Test to assess developmental competence. To which age group does this test apply?
   a. Elderly
   b. Adults
   c. Teenagers
   d. Infants and children

10. A novice nurse is trying to differentiate delirium from dementia. Which of the following concepts is INCORRECT?
    a. Delirium is acute while dementia is slow and progressive
    b. Delirium accompanies physical illness while dementia happens even in a state of physical health
    c. Alzheimer's is an example of delirium
    d. Delirium is usually resolved when underlying physical illness is treated.

11. The nurse is assessing for possible cognitive impairment in an elderly client. Which of the following actions in relation to the Mini-Cog test is INCORRECT?
    a. Ask the client to remember three unrelated words and ask the client to repeat each word after being mentioned
    b. Mention three related words
    c. Draw the face of a clock with the numbers
    d. Draw the hands of the clock so that time reads 12:45

12. A 70-year old Hispanic woman was admitted to the hospital a week ago due to dull upper right quadrant abdominal pain. She underwent cholecystectomy 2 days ago, and was in the ICU since

then. She scored 26 in the Mini-Mental state exam. She is found restless in bed but is quiet during visitation hours. She is uttering incomprehensible words that worsened at night. She got agitated when the nurse who has been caring for her for 6 nights in a row approached her to whom she says, "Who are you?" When asked, she remembers her name but not where she is, or the reason of her stay. She grabbed the nurse around 10pm telling the nurse, "Help me escape. My flower babies are gonna die if they won't see me today." Which of the following data describes appearance?

a. She is found restless in bed but is quiet during visitation hours
b. She got agitated when the nurse who has been caring for her for 6 nights in a row approached her to which she says, "Who are you?"
c. When asked, she remembers her name but not where she is or the reason of her stay.
d. She scored 26 in the Mini-Mental state exam

13. A 70-year old Hispanic woman was admitted to the hospital a week ago due to dull upper right quadrant abdominal pain. She underwent cholecystectomy 2 days ago, and was in the ICU since then. She scored 26 in the Mini-Mental state exam. She is found restless in bed but is quiet during visitation hours. She is uttering incomprehensible words that worsened at night. She got agitated when the nurse who has been caring for her for 6 nights in a row approached her to whom she says, "Who are you?" When asked, she remembers her name but not where she is or the reason of her stay. She grabbed the nurse around 10pm telling the nurse, "Help me escape. My flower babies are gonna die if they won't see me today." Which of the following data describes orientation?

a. She is found restless in bed but is quiet during visitation hours
b. She is uttering incomprehensible words that worsened at night
c. When asked, she remembers her name but not the place where she is or the reason of her stay.
d. She scored 26 in the Mini-Mental state exam

14. A 70-year old Hispanic woman was admitted to the hospital a week ago due to dull upper right quadrant abdominal pain. She underwent cholecystectomy 2 days ago and was in the ICU since then. She scored 26 in the Mini-Mental state exam. She is found restless in bed but is quiet during visitation hours. She is uttering incomprehensible words that worsened at night. She got agitated when the nurse who has been caring for her for 6 nights in a row approached her to which she says, "Who are you?" When asked, she remembers her name but not where she is or the reason of her stay. She grabbed the nurse around 10pm telling the nurse, "Help me escape. My flower babies are gonna die if they won't see me today." Which of the following is true of the client's mental status?

a. Dementia
b. Delirium
c. Depression
d. Paranoia

15. The nurse is assessing the level of consciousness of a client who has been confined to the ICU. He is observed to sleep most of the time. He awakens only to vigorous shake. He is also incoherent.

With these findings, what is the level of consciousness of the client?
a. Coma
b. Lethargy
c. Stupor
d. Obtundation

16. A client who has sustained blunt trauma to the head has decreasing level of consciousness. Yesterday, the client was observed to sleep most of the time. He awakened only to vigorous shake. He was also incoherent. Today he progressed to coma. Which of the following assessment findings alerted the nurse that the client is now in deep coma?
    a. Completely unconscious with no response to pain, and no motor response
    b. Completely unconscious with some reflex activity
    c. Completely unconscious with some reflex activity and purposeful movements
    d. Unconscious most of the time with some purposeful appropriate motor response

17. The nurse is assessing an elderly client. When the nurse asks the client how he'd been, the client responded with difficulty, uttering telegraphic words consisting mostly of nouns and verbs. What type of aphasia is the client most likely suffering from?
    a. Global aphasia
    b. Broca aphasia
    c. Wernicke aphasia
    d. Receptive aphasia

18. A client with laryngeal cancer is communicating with the nurse. He is observed to have difficulty speaking because his voice sounds hoarse. However, his articulation and language is normal. Which speech disorder is the client most likely suffering from?
    a. Dysphonia
    b. Dysarthria
    c. Aphasia
    d. Anhedonia

19. A psychiatric nurse is talking with a patient who had been running to and fro in the hallway. The client says, "I am the Queen of England today!" Which of the following correctly describes the client's affect?
    a. Elated
    b. Euphoric
    c. Flat
    d. Labile

20. A client arrives at the clinic appearing anxious and tired. She confides to the nurse that she used the stairs to come to the clinic because she has fears of being in an elevator. Which of the following anxiety disorders is the client most likely suffering from?

a. Obsessive-compulsive disorder
b. Social anxiety disorder
c. Agoraphobia
d. Generalized anxiety disorder

21. A 45-year old client comes is admitted to the hospital upon doctor's recommendation because of his complains of back pain that shoots down his leg. He states that the pain is more than 2 years now. Several tests and diagnostics procedures have been done to try to identify the cause but all results came back normal. The client has had 4 different jobs in 2 years. His mother was his only visitor in his 1-week stay at the hospital. Which of the following would prompt the nurse to start a mental health screening?
    a. History of a fall while playing soccer in college
    b. Family history of degenerative disc disease
    c. Present occupation as a manual laborer
    d. Indifference towards others and disinterest in hygiene

22. The nurse started interviewing the client who she notices is constantly looking around the room looking confused. As the client answers the nurse's questions, he pauses long enough as if trying to remember things. What should the nurse ask the client to assess orientation and memory?
    a. When was your last visit to the doctor? Do you know what date it is today?
    b. What do you think you'd do if you see a stranger looking inside your car?
    c. What kind of foods are fries, burger and pizza?
    d. Can you count backwards from 20?

23. A former beauty queen has been admitted because she has fainted due to severe hypoglycemia. As the nurse speaks with her, she noticed a blank expression to her face. What did the nurse assess when she observed the client's blank facial expression?
    a. Mood
    b. Affect
    c. Level of consciousness
    d. Attention

24. An 18-year old senior high school student was admitted after her parents observed her losing considerable weight and skipping meals. In her short 3-day stay, the nurse noticed that she just lies on the bed facing the wall and is barely responding to people talking to her. She seems to be sleeping most of the day. At one time, the nurse heard her sobbing. Which of the following best describes the client's actions?
    a. Depressed mood
    b. Blank affect
    c. Decreased level of consciousness
    d. Attention deficit

25. During a mental health screening on a hyperactive client, the nurse encourages the client to tell his story about a recent trauma. She asks the client what she is currently thinking and what she has to say about the traumatic experience. What is the nurse trying to assess?
    a. Judgment
    b. Memory
    c. Thought content
    d. Perception

26. The nurse is caring for a newly admitted client who couldn't remember who he is and where he is. The nurse aims to distinguish if the client has delirium or dementia. Which of the following is a correct statement regarding delirium and dementia?
    a. In delirium, there is an identifiable time of onset while in dementia, the onset may not be clear and typically reported to have happened in a span of months and ven years
    b. Dementia is reversible; delirium is progressive
    c. Delirium is due to as chronic disorder such as Alzheimer's; dementia is due to infection, effects of medication and myocardial infarction
    d. In delirium there is loss of memory of recent event while memory loss greatly varies in dementia

27. As an ICU nurse, it is your responsibility to frequently monitor clients' level of consciousness. One of the patients in the unit is a 60-year old woman who had been admitted due to stroke. You note that the client's eyes are closed. You call the client's name and the client opens her eyes and looks at you. When you ask how she is, she pauses and nods looking confused. The nurse understands that the best description of the client's level of consciousness is
    a. Lethargic
    b. Obtunded
    c. Stuporous
    d. Comatose

28. A patient in the outpatient department is looking unkempt, and is seen pacing the room while crying inconsolably. At times she sits down and covers her face with her hands. The client is exhibiting which kind of posture and motor behavior?
    a. Anxiety
    b. Agitated depression
    c. Depression
    d. Mania

29. When assessing grooming and personal hygiene of a client, the nurse notices that the client's shoes are not tied in the right foot. Her lipstick is smeared on the right side, as well as a smudge of dirt is observed on the client's same side. She recently sustained a head injury. These characteristics are typical of
    a. Schizophrenia

b. Mania
c. Obsessive compulsive behavior
d. Unilateral neglect

30. A hyperactive client is seen singing and dancing in the hallway. How would the nurse describe the affect of the patient?
    a. Flat
    b. Elated and euphoric
    c. Indifferent
    d. Apathetic

31. The nurse is aware of the different characteristics of speech. Which of the following accurately describes dysarthria?
    a. The patient has difficulty comprehending language. The patient hears or reads but do not understand the language, even his own speech.
    b. The patient completely understands language but cannot communicate back to respond either in writing or through speech
    c. The patient understands language perfectly and can write but is unable to produce speech either because of a muscle disorder in the area that produce speech, or of nerve damage that result to paralysis of muscles for speech
    d. The client both cannot discern language and cannot produce speech

32. The nurse is aware that it is essential to assess fluency. Which of the following accurately describes circumlocutions?
    a. "As I was rushing to get here, I forgot to take that (pause) thing that I use to put my belongings in"
    b. "I started digging with a bingbong"
    c. "walk…dog"
    d. The nurse asks the client to sign a document and the client rummages through her bag and replies, "wait I need to get a den"

33. The nurse is caring for a client with major depression. Which of the following is inappropriate to ask when assessing for suicide risk?
    a. Do you have any plans of harming yourself?
    b. How do you intend to kill yourself?
    c. When do you plan to carry out your plan?
    d. Have you talked to your lawyer about your will?

34. The nurse is trying to assess the thought processes of an alcoholic still in denial. During interview, the nurse notices the client pauses when trying to remember an event and then gives an answer that he seems unsure of. When verified with the wife, she denied that such event happened. The nurse understands that this is an example of

a. Flight of ideas
b. Incoherence
c. Confabulation
d. Paraphasia

35. A major depressive client on suicide precaution has been crying silently on her bed for the past week. At present, the nurse asks how she is and she replies, "I feel better now. The meds must be working. I'm gonna get a smoke a little later. You guys take it easy. Get yourself coffee or something." The nurse understands that this sudden change in affect means that
    a. The client is responding well to the medications
    b. The client is about to carry out her suicide plans
    c. The client is showing improvement in communication
    d. The client is looking into cigarette smoking as a coping mechanism

36. A nurse is interviewing a client with depression. She assesses the client for suicide risks. The nurse understands that the following are risk factors for suicide EXCEPT:
    a. Previous attempts
    b. Substance abuse
    c. Recent divorce
    d. With religious affiliation

37. A client tries to interact with client but with little success. She managed to have the client tell her that she couldn't find pleasure in anything anymore, whether it be food, recreation or even sex. The nurse understands that this accurately describes
    a. Apathy
    b. Anhedonia
    c. Aphasia
    d. Agoraphobia

38. A nurse is asking a client with dementia to tell her things that the nurse points at in the room. The nurse is assessing the client for which ability/parameter?
    a. Naming
    b. Constructional ability
    c. Coherence
    d. Memory

39. The nurse meets with a client and asks the latter to draw a clock with numbers and hands on a blank sheet of paper. Which ability is the nurse assessing?
    a. Naming
    b. Constructional ability
    c. Coherence
    d. Memory

40. The nurse conducting a mental health screening wants to assess abstract thinking abilities. Which of the following questions will help the nurse achieve this purpose?
    a. "What is the date today?"
    b. "Can you read this and do what it says?"
    c. "Can you tell me what apples and oranges have in common?"
    d. "Can you please count backwards in 3's starting from 30?"

41. A nurse is assessing a patient. After history taking and physical examination, the nurse decided that the patient needs to undergo a more thorough mental health screening. Which of the following parameters, if exhibited by the patient, will necessitate a mental health screening? Select all that apply.
    a. Chronic pain
    b. Personal history of acute pain
    c. Family history of fibromyalgia
    d. High symptom count
    e. Recent stress

42. A nurse assesses a patient in the clinic and suspects that the patient may have an anxiety disorder. Which high-yield screening question will indicate that the patient must undergo a psychiatric evaluation, diagnosis, and treatment for an anxiety disorder?
    a. "Over the past two weeks, have you ever felt down?
    b. "Over the past two weeks, have you ever felt little or no pleasure in doing things?"
    c. "Over the past two weeks, have you been unable to stop worrying?"
    d. "Have you ever felt guilty about drinking?"

43. A nurse is assessing a patient who was brought in by concerned neighbors after the patient was seen walking down the street without any footwear, and dressed in inappropriate clothes. As part of the assessment, the nurse asks the patient their name and the present date and time. Which parameter is the nurse currently assessing?
    a. Thought process
    b. Orientation
    c. Insight
    d. Judgment

44. A nurse wants to determine a patient's thought content as part of the mental status assessment. Which of the following details should the nurse ask the patient?
    a. What they presently think about
    b. Asking the patient to repeat a series of numbers
    c. Asking the patient what they would do should they find a lost wallet
    d. Asking the patient to elaborate on a story that they started telling the nurse

45. A nurse is assessing a patient's level of consciousness. The patient is immobile in bed with their eyes closed. The nurse tries to rouse the patient and asks for their name. The patient opens their eyes and looks at the nurse. The nurse asks for the patient's name again. This time, the patient responds after several seconds, and says, "Yeah, it's in my bag." Which of the following correctly describes the patient's level of consciousness?
    a. Drowsy
    b. Obtunded
    c. Stuporous
    d. Comatose

46. A nurse is attempting to rouse a stuporous patient. Which of the following is the likely reaction of the stuporous patient to the nurse's stimuli?
    a. No reaction
    b. Briefly opens their eyes after sternal rubbing
    c. Briefly awakens to make eye contact with the nurse, mumbles incomprehensible words
    d. Awakens, converses briefly with the nurse and falls back to sleep

47. A nurse is assessing several patients in the ward. With which of the following patient will the nurse need to perform a more detailed examination for possible mania?
    a. Overly energetic movements and story-telling
    b. Slumped slow movements
    c. Nail-biting, constantly looking around
    d. Looking away, no eye contact, no verbal response

48. A nurse is caring for a patient with obsessive-compulsive disorder. Which of the following will the nurse most probably observe in the patient's appearance and personal hygiene?
    a. Matted hair, untrimmed nails, with body odor
    b. Loud-colored Hawaiian top and very short underpants
    c. Neat, well-ironed formal attire during a clinic visit
    d. Neat and orderly clothing and makeup on one side of the body, and sloppy, dirty on the other side

49. Which of the following facial expression will the nurse most likely observe in a patient with paranoia?
    a. Hostile
    b. Elated
    c. Dull
    d. Flat

50. A nurse is taking a patient's history. The patient easily nods to mean they agree and shakes their head to disagree. When the patient is asked to elaborate, the nurse sees the patient struggling to make a verbal response. The verbal response is non-fluent and usually in just a noun-verb form

only. Which of the following most accurately describes the patient's symptoms?
a. Receptive aphasia
b. Expressive aphasia
c. Dyslexia
d. Global aphasia

51. A nurse is testing a patient for Aphasia. Which of the following will test for word comprehension?
a. Tell the patient to stand on one foot
b. Tell the patient to repeat a series of numbers
c. Ask the patient to read a quote from a book
d. Ask a person to write down their address

52. A nurse is assessing the mood of a patient with schizophrenia. Which of the following mood is associated with schizophrenia?
a. Deep melancholy
b. Joy
c. Euphoria
d. Detachment and indifference

53. A patient who has a chronic alcoholism is being interviewed by the nurse. The patient has been confined for three days now. The nurse asks the patient to recall their activities the day before. When asked about what he did before lunch, the patient paused for a while and tells the nurse that they and a friend went for a short walk. The nurse recalls that the patient was in his bed the day before reading a book in bed before lunch. Which of the following thought process did the patient exhibit?
a. Incoherence
b. Confabulation
c. Derailment
d. Circumstantiality

54. A nurse is interviewing a patient during history-taking. With every question, the patient talks for a long time with shifting topics that are loosely connected and seems to be satisfied with their answer. Which of the following correctly describes the patient's thought processes?
a. Blocking
b. Derailment
c. Incoherence
d. Circumstantiality

55. Which of the following patients exhibits echolalia?
a. A patient who repeats the words and phrases of the nurse
b. A patient who repeats words in a sentence
c. A patient who talks in short rhymes

d.   A patient who makes up new words and assigns them peculiar meanings

56. A patient with schizophrenia is found screaming in bed. The patient is pointing at their IV line and is shouting, "Snake! Snake!" Which of the following abnormalities in perception did the patient exhibit?
    a.   Persecution
    b.   Delusion
    c.   Hallucination
    d.   Illusion

57. A patient is seen slapping their arms and scratching different places on their extremities. When asked by the nurse what they are experiencing, the patient replies that bugs are biting them everywhere. Upon close examination, the nurse does not see any insects, nor are there any signs of insect bites on the patient's skin. Which of the following did the patient exhibit?
    a.   Gustatory hallucination
    b.   Tactile hallucination
    c.   Illusion
    d.   Delusion

58. A nurse wants to assess a patient's judgment. Which of the following questions will help check for judgment?
    a.   "What will you do if you if some stranger claims to own the bag that you are carrying?"
    b.   "How many children do you have?"
    c.   "What brings you to the clinic?"
    d.   "What do you think will happen if I open this box?"

59. A nurse asks the patient to repeat a series of four numbers and then lets them spell the word 'EIGHT' backward. Which of the following parameters is the nurse assessing in the patient?
    a.   Thought processes
    b.   Insight
    c.   Attention
    d.   Perception

60. A nurse wants to test a patient's attention using the digit span. Which of the following instructions should the nurse give the patient to follow?
    a.   Subtract 7 from 100, and keep subtracting
    b.   Repeat a series of two numbers until the series becomes five numbers in a row
    c.   Spell the word 'WOLRD' backward
    d.   Ask for the patient's mother's birthday

61. Which of the following sentences is considered a proverb that the nurse can use to test the patient's abstract thinking?

a. Do not scatter pebbles because they will be difficult to pick up one by one.
b. Turn off the lights when not in use.
c. Stop at a red light.
d. Don't cry over spilled milk.

62. A nurse is testing the abstract thinking of a patient using similarities. The nurse mentions the words "daisy" and "rose" and asks the patient how the two are alike. Which of the following patient responses refer to an abstract answer?
a. "Daisies are my favorite."
b. "The daisy is the rose's neighbor."
c. "Both have petals."
d. "Both are flowers."

63. A nurse assessing a patient gives the patient a pen and a sheet of paper and asks them to draw the face of a clock. Which of the following parameters is the nurse assessing?
a. Constructional ability
b. Attention
c. Abstract thinking
d. Perception

64. What is the current ratio of US adults who experience mental illness in a given year?
a. 1:10
b. 1:20
c. 1:5
d. 1:25

65. Which of the following is the 10th leading cause of death in the US, the 2nd leading cause of death among people who are aged 15-24?
a. Vehicular accident
b. Cardiovascular diseases
c. Diabetes
d. Suicide

ANSWERS

1. C
    Everyone at one time or the other feels sad, tearful, frustrated and disappointed. There may also be anorexia and insomnia due to these emotions. This is normal. A mental disorder already exists if the client's response to a painful or sad experience is more than what is normally manifested. There may be significant changes in behavior, emotion and cognition that persist for more than six months.

2. B
    Orientation refers to awareness of the environment in relation to self. The nurse can ask the client to identify a familiar person or place, or ask the client for the current date and time.

3. C
    Mental disorders are organic in nature if they are caused by a physical or medical disease. Examples of organic mental disorders are delirium, dementia, substance and alcohol intoxication and withdrawal. Psychiatric mental disorders are those without any organic causes. Some examples of psychiatric disorders are major depression, schizophrenia and anxiety disorder.

4. A
    Abstract reasoning tests assess how the client put deeper meaning to concrete or ideas. A simple test wherein the client determines the most appropriate figure for the missing part of the series is usually used to assess abstract reasoning. Asking the client what brought him to the hospital assesses thought processes. Asking what the client is currently thinking assesses thought content. The client may be asked the current date and time to test for orientation.

5. C
    Newborns' means of communication is crying. At 6 weeks, the baby coos. At one year, a child uses one-word sentences. A two-year-old uses several words to make a sentence. These are the developmental (language) competence expected at these ages.

6. C
    Age-related hearing loss is demonstrated by difficulty hearing high frequency sounds such as the pronunciation of consonants, making normal conversation a challenge to the elderly.

7. D
    The nurse may use the Four Unrelated Words Test to assess for new learning. The nurse asks the client to remember four unrelated words that the client should recall at 5- 10- and 30-minute intervals.

8. C
    Suicide thoughts should be divulged accordingly to the healthcare team so that suicide

precautions can be instituted immediately. The nurse cannot ensure confidentiality in this situation. She should inform the client that she would have to tell the healthcare team. All other questions in the options are appropriate to ask.

9. D

The Denver Developmental Screening Test is used to assess developmental competence of infants and children. It assesses gross motor, language, fine motor–adaptive and personal social skills. It will also help identify behavioral, language, cognitive, and psychosocial delays.

10. C

Alzheimer's disease is an example of dementia, a slow, progressive irreversible decrease in cognitive function. Delirium is a state of temporary confusional state or perceptual disturbance that usually accompanies acute physical illness.

11. B

The Mini-Cog test is done by asking the client to remember and repeat three unrelated words as the nurse says the words. The nurse also asks the client to draw the face of the clock with numbers, and then finally asks the client to draw hands that will indicate a specific time.

12. A

The client being found restless in bed but is quiet during visitation hours describes appearance.

13. C

Orientation refers to a patient's ability to correctly identify people, place, time or personal identity. During illness or confusion, the patient may exhibit impaired awareness and may fail to identify familiar people such as family and friends. They may also not remember where they are or why they were hospitalized.

14. B

The client is exhibiting signs and symptoms of delirium. Delirium is a state of temporary confusional state or perceptual disturbance that usually accompanies acute physical illness.

15. D

A client is obtunded when he sleeps most of the time, and when he is awakened only with a loud shout or a vigorous shake. The client may also ramble or be incoherent.

16. A

In deep coma, the client is completely unconscious. There is no response to pain and no motor response. In light coma, the client is also completely unconscious but there is some reflex activity without purposeful movement.

17. B

In Broca aphasia, the client understands language but responds with difficulty and with much effort. The client's speech consists of telegraphic words that are mostly just nouns and verbs.

18. A

A client with Dysphonia will have difficulty or discomfort in talking. The client will talk with abnormal pitch or volume. The cause of this disorder is usually a laryngeal disease, which in this case is cancer. Voice is hoarse or sounds whispered, but articulation and language are normal.

19. B

Euphoria is an excessively joyful or cheerful mood and is a sign of pathology. In comparison, elation reflects joy and optimism with possible overconfidence and increased in activity but is not pathologic. A flat affect is having the same facial expression regardless of topic, while a labile affect is having shifting expressions in a short span of time.

20. C

Agoraphobia is an irrational fear of being in a place where escape is difficult, such as the confined space of an elevator

21. D

Chronic pain is a common symptom of patients with anxiety, depression, or somatic disorders. In this case, the client is exhibiting signs and symptoms of depression

22. A

The nurse may need to assess memory and orientation by asking when his last hospital visit was, and asking the patient the present date, or his current location. (B) is assessing judgment. (C) assesses analysis and attention. (D) assesses for higher cognitive function.

23. B

Affect refers to an observable, usually episodic, feeling or tone expressed through voice, facial expression, and demeanor

24. A

Mood refers to a sustained emotion that describes a person's perception of the world, usually described as depressed, manic, and energetic. In this case, the client is exhibiting depressed mood.

25. C

When assessing thought content, the nurse tries to elicit what the client's thoughts are on a given time or on a particular situation

26. A

The onset of delirium is usually known and typically happens after a medical condition such as infections, heart attack, or after intake of certain medication. When the medical cause is identified and addressed, delirium usually subsides. The memory loss in patients with delirium varies greatly and may involve past and present events. On the other hand, the onset of dementia is a gradual process and may start as normal forgetfulness that progress into more confused and disoriented state. Patients also have difficulty remembering recent events.

27. B

Obtunded patients open their eyes and look at the nurse, but their response is slow and they look confused. Lethargic patients are drowsy but open their eyes and look at the nurse. They answer questions and might fall back to sleep in the middle of the conversation. Stuporous patients are unaware of what's around them and exhibit very little response even to painful stimuli. Comatose patients are unconscious and totally do not respond to any stimuli, even pain.

28. B

An agitated depressed client can be seen crying, pacing, wringing hands and covering face. A depressed client without agitation is usually slumped or lying in one place. An anxious patient appears tense and restless and may fidget with hands and legs. A manic patient shows energetic hyperactivity.

29. D

In certain conditions such as injury to the parietal cortex, or to the optic tract in homonymous hemianopsia, the client tends to neglect one side of his body.

30. B

Manic client's affect is usually that of euphoria and elation. It is often accompanied by goal-oriented energetic hyperactivity to the point of exhaustion.

31. C

Option (C) describes dysarthria. (A) describes Wernicke, sometimes also called receptive or fluent aphasia. (B) characterizes Broca or also called non-fluent or expressive aphasia. (D) refers to global aphasia.

32. A

Circumlocution is substituting phrases or sentences for a word that the client cannot think of, or using massive amounts of words to mean or describe something. (B) is an example of neologism, or invention of new words. (C) describes Broca's aphasia (D) describes paraphasia or the use of malformed words.

33. D

Asking a suicidal client to seek his lawyer's services to help arrange his will and testament is non-therapeutic. All other options are correct because asking about the details of his suicide plans will enable the nurse to intervene and prevent the attempt.

34. C

Confabulation is the fabrication of facts or events in response to questions in order to fill a memory gap. This is typical of Korsakoff syndrome in alcoholism.

35. B

Sudden change in affect in a depressive client to that of relief and euphoria can signal that the client has his suicide plans ready to be executed. The nurse enforces strict suicide precautions and institutes 24-hour monitoring.

36. D

Risk factors for suicide include prior suicide attempts; delusional or psychotic thinking, family history of suicide, mental disorders, or substance abuse; poor family and peer relationships, domestic violence, including physical or sexual abuse; access to firearms, ropes and controlled substances and recent trauma.

37. B

Anhedonia is loss of pleasure in daily activities.

38. A

Patients with dementia usually have difficulty naming common objects. Asking which things the nurse is pointing at assesses naming abilities.

39. B

The goal of constructional ability assessment is to let the client draw or copy complex objects into a blank sheet of paper.

40. C

Asking for similarities between or among things assesses for abstract thinking. The nurse can also ask the client to expound on a proverb.

41. A, D, E

As the nurse performs an assessment of a patient's condition, it may be necessary to conduct a more thorough mental health screening. Indicators that necessitate a more detailed investigation of a patient's mental status are the following: unexplained physical manifestation, high symptom count (several physical or somatic symptom), chronic pain, symptoms that persist for more than one and a half months, 'difficult encounter' with the patient, recent stress or trauma, extensive use of health services and drug or alcohol abuse.

42. C

If during the history-taking and patient examination, the nurse suspects that the patient may have anxiety, the nurse must ask high-yield screening questions, such as asking if the patient has been unable to stop worrying over the past two weeks. Alternatively, the nurse may also ask the patient if they ever felt nervous or anxious in the last two weeks or if they had any panic attack in the past month.

43. B

To assess for orientation, the nurse may ask the patient about their identity, the place, and the present date. This assessment is referred to as orientation to person, time, and place.

44. A

Thought content refers to what constitutes a person's thoughts, including delusions, obsessions and suicidal ideations. To obtain more information as to a patient's thought content, the nurse asks the patient what they are presently thinking about, or what they often think about.

45. B

Obtunded patients can be roused. They open their eyes and make eye contact with the nurse. Their response to the nurse's questions is slow and maybe inappropriate. They appear somewhat confused.

46. B

Stuporous patients are unresponsive and immobile most of the time, and they awaken or respond only briefly when vigorous physical stimulation is applied.

47. A

When the nurse assessing a patient observes overly energetic, agitated movements and loud, fast and excited speech, the nurse must further examine the patient for mania.

48. C

Patients with obsessive-compulsive disorder will exhibit excessive fastidiousness, especially if their compulsion is maintaining orderliness and cleanliness. Patients with depression will have an unkempt appearance. Patients who have mania will be in loud-colored and inappropriate clothes, and women will be wearing excessive make-up. Patients with unilateral neglect will have one side of their body looking neat, while sloppy on the other side.

49. A

Patients with paranoia will exhibit anger, hostility, suspiciousness or evasiveness and their facial expressions will show these emotions. Patients with mania look elated. A flat affect is characteristic of schizophrenia. Finally, patients with dementia will most likely have a dull affect.

50. B

A patient with expressive aphasia will exhibit non-fluent effortful speech with intact comprehension. On the other hand, a patient with receptive aphasia will have impaired language comprehension but with fluent speech. Global aphasia has both receptive and expressive aphasia manifestations. Dyslexia is difficulty with reading comprehension, spelling, and writing.

51. A

   To test for word comprehension, the nurse gives a simple command and asks the patient to follow that command. For example, the nurse may ask the patient to raise their hands, stand on one foot or point to their nose.

52. D

   Patients with schizophrenia will have a flat affect and a detached and indifferent mood. Those with depression will be melancholic. On the other hand, patients with mania will exhibit euphoria.

53. B

   Confabulation is the fabrication of facts or events to fill in memory gaps. It is evident in patients with schizophrenia, dementia, and aphasia.

54. B

   Derailment or loosening of associations is also referred to as tangential speech. It is characterized by speech with shifting, loosely connected or unrelated topics. The patient may talk with a lack of focus and without going back to the original topic of conversation. Patients with schizophrenia exhibit derailment.

55. A

   A patient who exhibits echolalia will repeat the words and phrases of others. Perseveration is the repetition of words or ideas in their speech. Patients who speak based on rhymes rather than meaning exhibit clang association.

56. D

   An illusion is a misinterpretation of a real external stimulus, which in this case, is the IV line, mistaken for a snake.

57. B

   Hallucinations are false or unreal experiences that feel real for the patient. Hallucinations may be tactile (felt on the skin superficially), gustatory (taste), olfactory (smell), auditory (hearing), visual, or somatic (pain). It occurs in people with schizophrenia, delirium, dementia, PTSD, and alcoholism.

58. A

   To assess for judgment, the nurse determines a patient's response or decision regarding an important situation. The nurse may use family matters or those that pertain to jobs, finances or interpersonal relationships.

59. C

   Tests of attention check the patient's ability to focus and pay attention to a simple task such as spelling a word backward.

60. B

   To perform the digit span test, the nurse asks the patient to repeat a series of two numbers until the series grows to a 5-digit series. The nurse should avoid choosing consecutive numbers, numbers with a pattern, or numbers that are familiar to the patient.

61. D

   Asking a patient to explain or interpret a proverb is a test of abstract thinking. A proverb will have an abstract meaning. A patient with poor abstract thinking will understand that "don't cry over spilled milk" means not to shed tears if the milk is accidentally spilled. In people with good abstract thinking, the proverb will be interpreted as moving on after a past mistake.

62. D

   Categorizing similar things or ideas is an abstract skill. In this situation, the patient recognizes that the words "Daisy" and "Rose" pertain to the category of flowers. On the other hand, saying that both have petals is a concrete answer.

63. A

   Constructional ability is a reflection of higher cognitive function. To test for constructional ability, the nurse instructs the patient to copy figures of increasing complexity in a clean blank sheet of paper. Alternatively, the nurse tells the patient to draw the face of the clock. Patients with poor constructional ability will draw distorted images.

64. C

   Twenty percent of adults or 1:5 adults in the US experience mental illness in a given year. One in every 25 experience a serious mental illness that interfered with their normal life in a given year. (source)

65. D

   Suicide is the 10th leading cause of death in the US and the 2nd leading cause of death among people who are aged 15-24. The rate of suicide is highest in people who are aged 45-54 years old.

Preparation for Physical Examination, Assessment Techniques, and Safety

Questions
1. Which type of patient data will the nurse obtain through physical examination?
   a. Laboratory results
   b. Family history
   c. Objective data
   d. Subjective data

2. Which of the following is best for the nurse to do to avoid making their patient anxious when an examination of a body part is taking a long time?
   a. Make notes and continue with the examination.
   b. Appear calm and continue with the examination.
   c. Tell the patient, "I would like to take extra time examining your abdomen, but it doesn't mean there is anything wrong."
   d. Tell the patient, "I could not feel the borders of your liver. Please give me more time to examine it."

3. A nurse is palpating the patient's abdomen and feels a mass that is the size of a fist. The patient asks, "What are your findings?" Which of the following response is best for the nurse to say?
   a. "I feel a hard mass the size of the fist. Let's hope it's not cancer."
   b. "I feel something hard in your abdomen. The physician will re-examine you, and he will order more tests to know what it is."
   c. "I feel a tumor in the lower part of your abdomen. I'm sure there's nothing to worry about."
   d. "It may be an ovarian tumor. You will undergo more tests to verify my suspicion."

4. Which of the following reflects the proper way of doing a physical examination?
   a. Start in the area that is preferred by the patient
   b. If a part of the examination is missed, avoid going back to the patient to re-examine them
   c. Appear calm and organized even if feeling inexperienced
   d. Tell the patient what possible disorder they may have based on the physical examination findings

5. How should the nurse adjust the bed after they are done with the physical examination?
   a. Raise the bed to its highest position
   b. Lower the bed
   c. Lower the side rails
   d. Elevate the head and foot of the bed

6. Which type of lighting is most appropriate to use when assessing the jugular venous pulse?
   a. Perpendicular lighting
   b. Tangential lighting
   c. UV light
   d. Diffused lighting

7. Which of the following actions shows that the nurse is respectful of the patient's privacy?
    a. Lowering the bed to its lowest position
    b. Dimming the light for examination
    c. Closing the doors and curtains
    d. Politely asking that the volume of the television be turned down

8. During a physical examination of a patient, a nurse uses their middle finger to quickly tap against the distal third of the middle finger of their other hand that is touching the patient's chest. Which of the following techniques of examination is the nurse using?
    a. Inspection
    b. Palpation
    c. Percussion
    d. Auscultation

9. The nurse wants to assess the genitals of a female patient. Which of the following position should the nurse help the patient assume?
    a. Sitting
    b. Supine
    c. Left side-lying
    d. Lithotomy

10. Which of the following technique is best to use when performing a physical examination on a patient?
    a. dirty-to-clean
    b. Head-to-toe
    c. Proximal-to-distal
    d. Lower body first then the upper body

11. When is the best time to start the general survey part of the physical examination?
    a. When the patient is sitting up
    b. Toward the end of the examination
    c. Upon meeting and greeting the patient
    d. When the patient is completely undressed

12. The nurse is to perform an ophthalmoscopic examination on a patient, as part of the HEENT assessment. Which of the following is a correct preparation for an ophthalmoscopic examination?
    a. Darken the room
    b. Turn on bright lights
    c. Ask the patient to blink several times
    d. Obtain cotton balls

13. Which position should the nurse help the patient assume during the examination of their abdomen?
    a. Partly turned to their left side
    b. Semi-fowler's
    c. Lithotomy
    d. Supine

14. Which of the following equipment is installed and mounted on a wall, and measures height?
    a. A Snellen chart
    b. A sphygmomanometer
    c. A goniometer
    d. A stadiometer

15. In which of the following situations should the nurse use personal protective equipment (PPE)? Select all that apply.
    a. Assisting a patient with diarrhea to use a bedpan
    b. Obtaining a urine specimen from the patient
    c. Dressing a patient's surgical wound
    d. Helping a patient to transfer to a wheelchair
    e. Turning the patient to their side

16. In which situation is hand hygiene necessary? Select all that apply.
    a. Before touching a patient
    b. After glove removal
    c. Before removing protective gown
    d. At the end of patient care before leaving the room
    e. Before and after wound cleaning

17. All the patient's body fluids are considered infectious EXCEPT:
    a. Semen
    b. Amniotic fluid
    c. Sweat
    d. Urine

18. Where should the nurse stand to be able to perform a physical examination most effectively?
    a. At the foot of the bed
    b. Near the head of the bed
    c. By the patient's right side
    d. By the patient's left side

19. A nurse auscultates over an arterial vessel and hears a turbulence. What is the right documentation entry for the nurse's findings?

    a. Bruit
    b. Thrill
    c. Pulse
    d. Murmur

20. When performing a physical examination on a patient, the nurse should follow the order: inspection, palpation, percussion, auscultation, except in the examination of the patient's:
    a. Chest
    b. Head
    c. Abdomen
    d. Back

21. Which of the following set of tasks should the nurse do before leaving the patient who they have just examined? Select all that apply.
    a. Raise the bed to its highest position
    b. Place the patient's belongings within reach
    c. Place the call bell/light within reach
    d. Dispose of any waste properly
    e. Perform handwashing

22. How should the nurse adjust the bed before leaving a patient at the end of physical examination
    a. Raise the side rails and lower the bed to its lowest position
    b. Raise the side rails and raise the bed to its highest position
    c. Raise the head of the bed
    d. Lower the head of the bed

23. What is the best way of ensuring the patient's privacy when the nurse is transitioning their examination from the chest to the abdomen?
    a. Cover the chest and expose the abdomen
    b. Expose the patient's abdomen down to their knees
    c. Expose the patient's chest down to their hips
    d. Expose both the chest and the abdomen and cover both legs

24. Which of the following is an example of a blood-borne disease?
    a. Diphtheria
    b. Heart attack
    c. Stroke
    d. HIV

25. In which of the following situations should the nurse perform handwashing?
    a. In between counting the pulse and taking the temperature
    b. In between examining the head and the chest

c. In between auscultation of the chest and abdomen
d. Before beginning the physical examination

26. A student nurse is mastering the skill of inspection as part of the physical examination of a client. Which of the following is INCORRECT about the concept of inspection?
    a. It is a general survey of the client from the whole body to specific areas
    b. It is imperative to inspect both sides of the body
    c. Each side should be perfectly symmetrical
    d. Inspection requires adequate lighting and appropriate instruments

27. The nurse wants to assess a client's temperature without a thermometer at hand. Which of the following is a correct technique?
    a. Use the fingertips placed on the neck
    b. Use the back of the hand and feel the neck
    c. Use the palm and lightly grip the upper arm
    d. Grasp the wrist with the thumb and forefinger

28. The nurse is aware that when palpating a body part, intermittent pressure is better than continuous pressure. In which situation should the nurse use both hands to palpate a client using intermittent pressure?
    a. Feeling for varicose veins
    b. Checking for warmth on a swollen extremity
    c. Checking for tenderness on the lower right quadrant of the abdomen
    d. Doing the Leopold's maneuver to check the position of the baby in a pregnant woman

29. The novice nurse assesses the abdomen of the client by using percussion. Which of the following parameters will percussion NOT accurately assess when examining the client?
    a. Organ size
    b. Organ density
    c. Organ location
    d. Pain

30. The nurse wants to assess the client's lung for pneumothorax by percussing the chest. Which of the following techniques is incorrect?
    a. Hyperextend the finger pad of the middle finger (pleximeter) of the non-dominant hand and place it firmly against the skin
    b. Rest the wrist of your non-dominant hand gently on the client's body
    c. Snap your wrist to strike the pleximeter with the fingertip of the middle finger of the dominant hand
    d. Hit just behind the nail bed or the distal interphalengeal joint when striking the pleximeter

31. The nurse wants to assess the client's back using percussion. Which of the following techniques

reflects that further teaching is necessary?
a. When striking the pleximeter, use moderate and quick striking force
b. Percuss twice in every location
c. Use a stronger percussion stroke for thin underweight clients
d. Use the same striking force as you move to another location

32. A novice nurse is to perform percussion of the client's abdomen. She reviews her concept on the technique, and determines the components of the sound waves that the technique is producing. Which of the following reflects correct knowledge of percussion?
a. Amplitude is the number of vibrations per second
b. Pitch is the loudness or softness of a sound
c. Quality is the timbre or the distinctiveness of sounds
d. Duration is the time in between two percussion strokes

33. A nurse is assessing a client with emphysema. Which of the following percussion sounds of the chest will most likely be noted by the nurse?
a. Resonant
b. Hyperresonant
c. Tympany
d. Dull

34. The nurse is percussing the abdomen of the client. As she moves to the right upper quadrant just below ribcage, she notes a dull sound. Which of the following is a correct interpretation of the percussion sound?
a. It is expected. The dull sound is because of the liver.
b. It is expected. The dull sound is produced by the spleen.
c. The area should produce tympany.
d. The area should produce resonance.

35. The nurse is about to perform a physical examination on a client. She reviews the proper techniques of percussion. Which of the following is a correct concept regarding percussion?
a. Denser structures will produce louder, deeper and longer sounds
b. An air filled structure will produce softer, higher and shorter sounds
c. Thicker body walls will produce softer sounds
d. The percussion sound will depend largely on the thickness of the body wall

36. The nurse is doing a physical examination of a client. The nurse wants to assess the bowel sounds. Which of the following is the correct technique of auscultation?
a. Use the diaphragm of the stethoscope and press deep over the abdomen
b. Use the bell of the stethoscope and press deep over the abdomen
c. Use the diaphragm of the stethoscope and place firmly over the abdomen
d. Use the bell of the stethoscope and place firmly over the abdomen

37. The nurse is preparing to auscultate the chest of the client. Which of the following actions of the nurse would need a correction of her auscultation techniques?
    a. Asking the client to turn off his radio
    b. Rubbing the diaphragm with the palm of the hand to warm it prior to use
    c. Wetting the hairy part of the chest to be used for auscultation
    d. Place stethoscope over the gown to avoid unnecessary exposure

38. The nurse is preparing for a physical examination of a client. Which of the following reflects IMPROPER preparation of the setting or area of examination?
    a. The nurse turns off the television
    b. The nurse spreads the curtains of the partition properly
    c. Push one side of the bed against the wall to secure the client
    d. Use tangential lighting when assessing body contours

39. The nurse is to assess the client's abdomen. Which of the following equipment is UNNECESSARY?
    a. Stethoscope
    b. Tape measure
    c. Skin marking pen
    d. Tuning fork

40. The nurse is using the ophthalmoscope to assess the client's eyes. Which of the following techniques is correct when adjusting the focus?
    a. Rotate the lens selector dial
    b. Bring your eyes nearer the viewing aperture
    c. Angle the ophthalmoscope farther from the client's face
    d. Position the scope well below the brow

41. The nurse wants to assess the client's range of motion. Which of the following equipment should she prepare?
    a. Doppler sonometer
    b. Goniometer
    c. Monofilament
    d. Bladder scanner

42. The nurse who is assessing the client's blood pressure cannot hear Korotkoff sounds well because of ambient noise. Which equipment should the nurse have on hand to facilitate the examination?
    a. Doppler sonometer
    b. Diopter
    c. Monofilament
    d. Bladder scanner

43. The nurse with a cough is to examine a patient. Which of the following actions by the nurse is incorrect?
    a. She covers her nose and mouth with a surgical mask
    b. She washes her hands before client contact
    c. She washes her hands after client contact
    d. She keeps a distance of 2.5 feet when examining the client

44. As the nurse begins the physical examination, she ensures that she is doing the right techniques. In which of the following actions would the nurse need further teaching?
    a. Using an icebreaker when she senses that the client is tense
    b. Making the client completely undress and then change into a hospital gown
    c. Writing down the examination sequence
    d. Summarizing findings at the end of the examination

45. A nurse is to assess a pre-school and proceeds to prepare the child for physical examination. Which of the following is necessary for the nurse to perform?
    a. Asking the child which equipment she prefers the nurse to use
    b. Allowing the child to play with equipment
    c. Asking the child to completely undress and change into a gown
    d. Being quick in the examination so as not to bore the child

ANSWERS.

1. C
    As the nurse performs a physical examination of a patient, they obtain objective data. Objective data are those that are observed by the nurse.

2. C
    To avoid causing undue alarm in the patient when an examination of a body part is taking a long time, the nurse must reassure the patient that although the assessment is taking time, it does not mean that anything is wrong. Saying nothing can cause apprehension in the patient. Telling the patient what the nurse could not do may also cause the patient to think that something is wrong.

3. B
    When the patient asks about the result of an examination, the nurse must give an objective answer, but not their suspicion of a medical condition. It is the physician's role to make a diagnosis. The nurse may, however, tell the patient that more tests would be performed to make the diagnosis definite.

4. C
    When doing a physical examination, the nurse must appear calm and organized even if they feel that they lack experience doing the physical examination. The nurse may tell the patient that the examination is taking more time but that it does not mean that there is something wrong. Should the nurse forget a part of the examination, they can return to re-examine the patient again. The nurse must avoid interpreting their findings.

5. B
    After the nurse is finished with the physical examination, they should lower the bed so that the patient can get off the bed safely if they are left on their own.

6. B
    Tangential lighting is most appropriate to use when assessing body structures because it shows contours, elevations, and depressions of body structures, such as the distention of the jugular veins and the pulsations of the apical pulse.

7. C
    Showing respect to the patient by being sensitive to the patient's privacy needs is a very important responsibility of the nurse. Before beginning the physical examination, the nurse must close the door, draw the curtains, and drape the patient appropriately.

8. C

   To perform percussion during a physical examination, the nurse uses a plexor finger, usually the middle finger to rapidly strike or tap the distal third of the middle finger of their other hand that is touching the patient. The striking motion produces a sound which the nurse uses to make an assessment of the underlying tissues.

9. D

   To perform a pelvic examination on a female patient, the nurse helps the patient assume a lithotomy position. To put a patient in a lithotomy position, the nurse should help the patient lie on their back, with the hips flexed, abducted and externally rotated, and the knees flexed.

10. B

    When performing a physical examination on a patient, the nurse must be organized and proceed with the assessment of the patient from head to toe.

11. C

    The general survey begins at the beginning of patient contact and should continue throughout history taking and physical examination.

12. A

    To perform an ophthalmoscopic examination, the nurse should darken the room because it helps in pupillary dilation and makes the fundi of the eyes visible.

13. D

    When performing an examination of the patient's abdomen, the patient must be flat in bed. The nurse may need to lower the head and foot of the bed to put the patient in a supine position during an abdominal examination.

14. D

    A stadiometer measures height. It is installed and mounted on the wall at the correct height to be able to make accurate measurements. A Snellen chart is used to assess vision. A sphygmomanometer is used to measure blood pressure. A goniometer measures the angles of a joint's range of motion.

15. A, B, C

    In any situation where there is a possibility of being in contact with the patient's body fluids, the nurse must strictly observe standard precautions and use personal protective equipment (PPE). PPEs include gloves, gowns, and protection for the mouth, nose, and eyes. They should be used accordingly when anticipating contact with the patient's blood, body fluids, secretions and excretions, including non-intact skin and mucous membranes.

16. A, B, D, E

The Centers for Disease Control and Prevention recommends hand hygiene in the following key situations:

- Before touching a patient
- At the end of patient care before leaving the room
- After contact with the patient's body fluids
- Before doing an aseptic procedure
- When performing a care procedure from a contaminated area to a clean area of the patient's body
- After removing gloves and personal protective equipment

17. C

Sweat is not a carrier of blood (or body fluid) borne pathogens. On the other hand, the following fluids are considered infectious: blood, semen, vaginal secretions, and cerebrospinal, synovial, pleural, peritoneal, pericardial, and amniotic fluids.

18. C

There are several advantages of doing a physical examination by the patient's right side. It makes the assessment of jugular pressure more reliable. It also makes the palpation of the apical pulse as well as the kidneys easier.

19. A

A bruit is a sound of turbulent blood flow heard over an artery with the use of a stethoscope.

20. C

During the examination of a patient's abdomen, the nurse performs auscultation after inspection so that palpation would not alter bowel motility and give inaccurate findings.

21. B, C, D, E

Before leaving a patient who has just been examined, the nurse must promote safety in the patient. The nurse must place personal belongings and the call bell/light within the patient's reach. They should also dispose of waste properly and then wash their hands.

22. A

To ensure the safety of the patient and prevent falls after performing a physical examination, the nurse must raise the side rails of the bed and lower the bed to its lowest position. Raising the side rails prevents them from rolling over the bed and falling while lowering the bed also helps to prevent falls when getting off the bed.

23. A

When doing an examination, the nurse must ensure the patient's privacy by covering the finished part and exposing only the part that is to be examined next.

24. D

Blood-borne diseases are those that are transmitted through blood. Examples of blood-borne diseases are Human Immunodeficiency Virus (HIV) infection and Hepatitis B.

25. D

Nurses should perform handwashing before touching a patient. Handwashing is also recommended before transitioning from a dirty area to a clean area, after removing the gloves that were in contact with the patient's body fluid, and before doing any aseptic technique, among others.

26. C

One side of the body is nearly symmetrical to the other side but not perfectly symmetrical.

27. B

When assessing temperature, the nurse may use the back of the hand to feel for hotness or coldness because the skin there is thinner and more sensitive to temperature.

28. D

In Leopold's maneuver, the nurse uses both hands to palpate various places in the abdomen to determine fetal position.

29. D

Percussion will help map out organ size, location and density but it will not accurately assess pain. Palpation is more appropriate to use in this situation.

30. B

The wrist of your non-dominant hand should be lifted up and not touch the client's body.

31. C

The thickness of the client's chest wall affects percussion sounds. Use a stronger percussion stroke for obese clients.

32. C

Amplitude or intensity is the loudness or softness of a sound. Pitch or frequency is the number of vibrations per second. Quality is the timbre or the distinctiveness of sounds, and duration is the length of time the sound is heard.

33. B

A client with emphysema has overdistended lungs filled with air. Doing percussion of the client's chest will produce hyperresonant sounds.

34. A

The liver is located at the right upper quadrant of the abdomen. Percussing this area just below the ribcage will produce a dull sound because the liver is a massive organ.

35. C

Thicker body walls will produce softer sounds, hence the need a stronger striking force in obese clients. An air-filled structure will produce louder, deeper and longer sounds. Denser structures will produce softer, higher and shorter sounds. The percussion sound will depend not only on the thickness of the body wall, and the correct techniques but more on the characteristics of the underlying structures.

36. C

The diaphragm of the stethoscope is best to use in assessing high-pitched sounds such as breath, bowel, and normal heart sounds. The bell on the other hand is best to use to hear soft, low-pitched sounds such as heart murmurs. The nurse should place the stethoscope firmly against the client's skin because pressing deeper may distort bowel sounds.

37. D

When auscultating, the nurse must ensure that room is quiet to reduce background noise. Rubbing the diaphragm to warm it before use will prevent shivering in a client. Hair on the chest will produce crackling sound. Wetting the area for auscultation will prevent crackling. Listening over clothing will produce artifacts or unwanted and distorted sounds.

38. C

When preparing for examination, the nurse should ensure that both sides of the client are accessible. All other options reflect correct preparation.

39. D

When assessing the abdomen, the nurse will need a stethoscope and a tape measure. To mark a specific location for a procedure or reference, the nurse uses a skin-marking pen. A tuning fork is used to assess hearing acuity.

40. A

Rotating the lens selector dial will adjust the focus of the ophthalmoscope.

41. B

A goniometer measures range of motion.

42. A

The nurse would need a Doppler sonometer, which would amplify pulse and blood pressure measurements.

43. D

   When a nurse has cough, it is necessary for her to use a surgical mask to cover her nose and mouth to avoid transmitting microorganisms to her patients. It is also proper for her to do handwashing before and after examination. The nurse should keep a comfortable distance between the client and herself while doing the examination. Standing 2.5 feet away will make the client out of reach so that examination cannot be accomplished properly.

44. B

   The correct technique is to ask the client to undress leaving underpants on and change into a gown because this will make him feel more comfortable and not exposed. Inform him that he will have to remove the underpants when it is time to examine the genitals.

45. B

   Allowing the child to play with the equipment will reduce anxiety in the child. The nurse should not allow the child to choose which equipment to use, but may offer choices for the same equipment (e.g. choosing the color of the earpiece of the stethoscope rather than asking to choose between stethoscope and an otoscope). Although a pre-school is willing to undress, ask the child to leave underpants on. It is important not to rush to prevent undue anxiety in the child.

General Survey, Vital signs, and Pain

Questions

1. The nurse is assessing the child playing across the playroom. The nurse observes that the child is squatting on the floor, with the upper body slightly leaning forward while being braced by the extended arms. Which of the following correctly describes the child's position?
    a.   Fetal position
    b.   Tripod position
    c.   High-fowler's position
    d.   Semi-fowler's position

2. The nurse is observing a client as he walks. Which of the following details indicate a need for further assessment?
    a.   The feet are approximately the same width as the shoulders
    b.   The client steps forward with a slight forward swing of the opposite arm
    c.   The client maintains balance when walking
    d.   As the client steps forward, there is slight shuffling gait

3. The nurse performing an examination of the client makes several observations. Which of the following observations warrants additional evaluation?
    a.   Walk is smooth and even
    b.   Body length from the top of the head to the pubic line is equal to the length of the pubic line to the soles of the feet
    c.   The client smiles when talking to the nurse and looks out the window with hands clasped tightly when the nurse is not looking
    d.   Wears a coat over wool clothes that winter day

4. The nurse measured the height and weight of a client and proceeded to compute the client's body mass index or BMI. Her computations revealed a BMI of 36. What is the correct interpretation of her findings?
    a.   Underweight
    b.   Normal
    c.   Overweight
    d.   Obesity class II

5. The nurse is assessing the weight of the client. She notes a decrease of weight from her baseline 3 months ago. Which of the following will not be considered a factor in the unexplained weight loss?
    a.   Heart failure
    b.   Recent infection
    c.   Chronic illness
    d.   Recent weight loss regimen

6. The nurse took the clients weight and height. The client weight is 150 lbs and the height is 170cm.

What is the client's BMI?
a. 23.6
b. 32.6
c. 28.2
d. 40.1

7. The nurse is assessing the abdomen of a male adult client. She noted that the waist circumference is 41 inches. The nurse prepares a health teaching on the health risks of obesity. Which of the following is NOT a risk factor?
a. Cardiovascular disease
b. Thyroid disease
c. Dyslipidemia
d. Type 2 diabetes

8. A client who experienced physical trauma has increased temperature unresponsive to antipyretics in the absence of an acute infection. Which body part most likely was traumatized that resulted to this finding?
a. Abdomen
b. Lower back
c. Chest
d. Head

9. The nurse wants to measure the temperature of a confused client. She wants to use an invasive method to obtain measurements closest to the core temperature. Which of the following available method is the most appropriate to use?
a. Oral
b. Rectal
c. Tympanic membrane thermometer
d. Glass thermometer

10. The nurse is assessing the pulse of the client. Which of the following is a factor that can acutely affect pulse rate?
a. Weight
b. Height
c. Activity
d. Hormonal change

11. A nurse is receiving endorsements from the nurse of the ending shift. The client's record reads, pulse: 88 bpm, +3. What is the correct interpretation of +3?
a. Full, bounding
b. Normal
c. Weak

d.   Absent

12. The nurse assessing the client obtained BP measurements: 120/80. What is the client's pulse pressure?
    a.   120
    b.   80
    c.   40
    d.   200

13. The nurse is reviewing her concepts of factors that can increase blood pressure. Which factors can lead to an increase in BP?
    a.   Decreased cardiac output
    b.   Decreased peripheral vascular resistance
    c.   Decreased arterial wall elasticity
    d.   Decreased viscosity

14. The nurse wants to assess the blood pressure of a thin and frail elderly. Which of the following is correct to consider?
    a.   Use a thigh cuff
    b.   Use a pediatric cuff
    c.   The length of the cuff should be 90% of arm circumference
    d.   Use a normal adult cuff

15. A nurse from the adult medical ward has been temporarily assigned to the pediatric ward. The nurse is careful to note the difference of vital signs measurement techniques. Which of the following reflects a correct technique in obtaining vital signs of a pediatric client?
    a.   Take the radial pulse for a full minute for infants and pre-schoolers
    b.   Use an oral glass thermometer on a distressed 1-year old
    c.   Take the apical pulse of a 7-month old baby in one full minute
    d.   Count for the respiratory rate in the pre-schooler who is crying

16. A nurse is caring for a 70-year old female client admitted due to pneumonia. The client's temperature indicates that she is hypothermic. What is the correct interpretation of her findings?
    a.   The nurse needs to obtain a new measurement using a different method and instrument
    b.   Understand that in the elderly, a client's reaction to acute infection may differ from that of an adult.
    c.   The elderly sweat more than adults
    d.   The elderly is misdiagnosed

17. The nurse has finished assessing a19-year old female client and obtained the following findings. Which of the following requires further evaluation?
    a.   BP= 110/70

    b.   RR= 16

    c.   Temp= 36.6 oC

    d.   SaO2 = 95%

18. Several nurses are taking the blood pressure of their clients. Which of the following correctly explains the results of a faulty blood pressure measurement?
    a. Positioning the arm above the heart results to a falsely high reading
    b. Pushing the stethoscope over the brachial artery results to falsely low diastolic pressure
    c. Inflating cuff not high enough results to falsely high systolic pressure
    d. Halting in the middle of deflation to restart inflation results to falsely low diastolic pressure

19. A nurse is assessing the general appearance of a male client, who is thin and tall. He also has elongated arms. Upon further assessment, the nurse notes that the arm span is greater than the height and there is sternal deformity. With the assessment findings, which condition should the nurse suspect?
    a. Cushing syndrome
    b. Marfan Syndrome
    c. Anorexia nervosa
    d. Acromegaly

20. While on the examination table, the nurse notes that the client's face is round and that she is specifically obese on the trunk and upper back. However, her extremities are markedly thin. There is also some prominent moustache-looking facial hair. Which condition is the client most likely suffering from?
    a. Cushing syndrome
    b. Achondroplastic dwarfism
    c. Anorexia nervosa
    d. Acromegaly

21. Pain is the fifth vital sign, and understanding how pain is generated, felt and relieved is very important in the care of patients. In the review of the concepts of pain, which of the following correctly describes the pathway of pain?
    a. In the initial phase called transduction, the injured tissue releases neurotransmitters, which sends the pain signal through the afferent nerve fibers to the spinal cord
    b. In the second phase or transmission, the pain message from the afferent nerve fibers reaches the brain in the absence of opioids in the spinal tract
    c. In the third phase, perception, the person becomes aware of the pain; this is because the cerebellar structures account for emotional response to pain
    d. In the fourth phase, moderation, the body is equipped with its own analgesia to halt the pain

22. The nurse is reviewing her concepts of the types of pain. Which of the following is a cause of neuropathic pain?

a. Fracture
b. Chemical burn
c. Sciatica
d. Toothache

23. A client is complaining of pain in the upper quadrant of the abdomen after eating fried or fatty food. After further examination and diagnostic procedures, the client was diagnosed with cholelithiasis. Which type of pain is the client experiencing?
    a. Somatic
    b. Deep somatic
    c. Visceral
    d. Cutaneous pain

24. The client with atherosclerosis is complaining of chest pain. There is also pain radiating to his jaw and left arm. What type of pain was felt at the jaw and upper arm?
    a. Somatic pain
    b. Deep somatic pain
    c. Visceral pain
    d. Referred pain

25. A client with cancer reports a moderate pain sensation at least an hour before her scheduled dose of narcotic. What type of pain is the client experiencing?
    a. Referred pain
    b. Malignant pain
    c. Nonmalignant pain
    d. Breakthrough pain

26. A middle-aged female client has been recently diagnosed with fibromyalgia after coming to the clinic complaining of pain and easy fatigability for the past 8 months. Which type of pain is the client suffering from?
    a. Acute pain
    b. Chronic malignant
    c. Chronic nonmalignant
    d. Breakthrough pain

27. The nurse is preparing a teaching material for nursing students. She wants to discuss pain felt by the fetus to infancy. Which of the following concepts is important to include in her teachings?
    a. Fetuses feel pain by the 14th day from being conceived when the fetal heart starts to beat
    b. Pre-term infants are more sensitive to painful stimuli than full term infants
    c. Repetitive pain caused by repetitive procedures can make a person less sensitive to pain later in life
    d. Infants do not remember pain

28. A nurse in a hospice center is caring for several clients in pain. Which of the following concept in elderly pain perception is INCORRECT?
    a. Pain is part of the aging process
    b. The elderly is less sensitive to painful stimuli
    c. People with dementia experience pain
    d. Older people tend to underreport pain experience

29. A nurse is considering gender as a factor affecting pain sensation. Which of the following reflect an accurate finding regarding gender differences in pain perception?
    a. During puberty, more females than males experience migraine
    b. Men are stoic in manifesting pain; women are more expressive
    c. Men are more likely to suffer from fibromyalgia
    d. After puberty, more males experience migraines than females

30. While conducting health history, the nurse wants to know the alleviating and aggravating factors of the client's pain. Which of the following is the most appropriate question to ask the client to elicit this information?
    a. "How much pain do you have now?"
    b. "How would you describe your pain?"
    c. "Are you having any pain right now?"
    d. "What makes your pain better or worse?"

31. The nurse is using the PQRST method of pain assessment. Which question will help identify timing?
    a. "Can you rate your pain from 0-10, with 10 as the most severe?"
    b. "Where do you feel the pain?"
    c. "When did the pain start?"
    d. "Can you describe your pain?"

32. A nurse wants to assess the client's pain in relation to effects on mood, mobility and sleep for the past day. Which pain assessment tool is most appropriate to use?
    a. The Initial Pain Assessment
    b. The Brief Pain Inventory
    c. The short form Mc-Gill Pain questionnaire
    d. The faces pain scale

33. An elderly client is complaining of pain that fluctuates in intensity in a day. Which pain scale is the most appropriate to use to assess for the client's pain?
    a. Numeric scale
    b. Descriptor scale
    c. Faces scale

d.   The Brief Pain Inventory

34. A nurse is assessing pain in a pre-school child using the Revised Faces Pain Scale (FPS-R). Which of the following reflects correct technique in using the scale?
    a.   "These faces show different people having pain."
    b.   Point to the first face on the left and say, "this face shows very much pain"
    c.   Ask the child to point the face that shows how much it hurts at that current time
    d.   Provide a score from 0-6 with 0 corresponding to the first face on the left

35. A client arrived in the ER complaining of throbbing pain at the lower back felt since the night before. The physician has ordered several diagnostic tests and prescribed pain medications PRN. Which of the following is the best nursing action if the client still complains of pain while waiting for laboratory results?
    a.   Administer pain medications
    b.   Defer pain medications until after test results are back
    c.   Provide comfort measures while waiting for laboratory results
    d.   Position accordingly to reduce pain

36. A client of Chinese descent appears stoic to pain. However, upon further assessments, the nurse finds that he is manifesting poorly controlled pain. Which of the following reflect poor control of pain? Select all that apply.
    a.   Tachycardia
    b.   Decreased cardiac output
    c.   Hypoventilation
    d.   Diarrhea
    e.   Urinary frequency

37. The daughter of an elderly client is worried that the chronic pain her mother is experiencing may lead to negative consequences. Which of the following is a long-term effect of chronic pain?
    a.   Decreased appetite
    b.   Unrestful sleep
    c.   Diminished quality of life
    d.   Increase in blood pressure

38. The nurse assesses a client and uses objective data to assess the client's pain. Which of the following assessment findings are consistent with chronic pain behaviors? Select all that apply.
    a.   Guarding
    b.   Rubbing
    c.   Moaning
    d.   Diminished activity
    e.   Sighing

39. A 2-month old infant has just undergone surgery and is now in the recovery room. The nurse wants to assess the neonate's pain using the CRIES pain scoring. The baby has high-pitched cry and her vital signs are increased to 25% from pre-operative values. The baby also requires 20% O2 for increasing SaO2 . He is grunting and grimacing and is constantly awake. What is the neonate's CRIES score?
    a. 6
    b. 7
    c. 8
    d. 9

40. The nurse is having difficulty assessing pain in a client with dementia. Which of the following tool is most appropriate to use?
    a. CRIES
    b. PAINAD
    c. FLACC
    d. The Brief Pain Inventory

41. A female client seeks medical attention for a lump she feels on her lower abdomen. As soon as the nurse greets the client, she says, "It sure was a long walk from the parking lot to here!" When the nurse takes her vital signs, the BP was 140/90, RR: 22, PR: 96 bpm. What is the most appropriate nursing action?
    a. Report findings to the doctor immediately
    b. Administer antihypertensive STAT
    c. Retake vital signs after 15 minutes
    d. Document findings and report findings to the doctor

42. A woman walks into the emergency department with a worried look and is seen biting her fingernails. She is constantly on the lookout for something or someone and cannot maintain eye contact. From these findings, the client is showing evidence of which problem?
    a. Pain
    b. Anxiety
    c. Depression
    d. Attention deficit

43. A nurse is assessing the vital signs of a patient seen in the outpatient department. Which item in the room calls the attention of the nurse and probably necessitates retaking measurements after 30 minutes?
    a. A wet umbrella by the side of the client
    b. An empty can of energy drink in the client's belongings
    c. An empty package of lunch from a fast food chain
    d. A paperback book being read by the client

44. When the nurse assesses a client's BP, she is sure to correct which of the following situations?
    a. The arm where measurement is to be taken is at heart level
    b. Client is sitting comfortably with his legs crossed
    c. The room is comfortably cool
    d. The patient has waited for the nurse for 15 minutes

45. Who of the following nurses needs to reevaluate her BP taking skills?
    a. A nurse taking the measurement 30 minutes after her client takes his anti-hypertensives
    b. A nurse waiting to take measurements of his client who excused himself to smoke
    c. A nurse taking the BP on the right arm of a patient with a right fistula
    d. A nurse using a thigh cuff on a morbidly obese client

46. The nurse is assessing the BP of a 72-year old client with hypertension. She noticed that as she auscultates the pulse during measurement, the pulse seemed to skip some beats between systolic and diastolic pressure. What is the most probable cause for this?
    a. It is a common finding in elderly clients especially those with hypertension and it is called an auscultatory gap.
    b. The client has an arrhythmia called atrial fibrillation
    c. The BP cuff was wrapped too tight around the client's arm
    d. The nurse failed to hear all Korotkoff sounds due to inexperience

47. The nurse is careful when assessing the blood pressure of the client. Which of the following can cause a false low blood pressure?
    a. Cuff too large or too wide
    b. Arm is below heart level
    c. Deflating the cuff too quickly
    d. The cuff is too loose or is uneven

48. A coherent, responsive client comes to the clinic looking comfortable and with no signs of distress. Upon assessment, the nurse notes that the client's BP is 160/100. Retaking after 15 minutes yielded the same results. The physician orders antihypertensives and 40 minutes after administration, the nurse finds the client with cold and clammy skin. BP reading is 110/70. How would the nurse interpret her findings?
    a. It is an expected outcome because the client has taken medication to decrease her BP
    b. 110/70 is within normal range and should document her findings promptly
    c. Her BP dropped drastically and the physician needs to be informed immediately
    d. Her BP after medication is within normal and the nurse should continue assessing the client for probable causes of her cold, clammy skin.

49. The nurse is taking the vital signs of a 24 year old frail underweight patient with tonic-clonic seizures. Which of the following nursing actions needs further improvement?
    a. The nurse obtains BP measurements using a pediatric cuff

b. The nurse takes the client's temperature using an oral thermometer
c. Nurse counts number of respiration while the patient is watching TV
d. The nurse simultaneously assesses the pulse rate of both arms

50. The morning shift's nurse documentation says that the client has a pulse deficit of 10 beats. The nurse understands that the pulse deficit is
    a. The difference between the client's actual pulse and 60
    b. The difference between the client's actual pulse and 100
    c. The difference of the apical rate and the pulse rate when taken at the same time for a full minute
    d. The difference of the apical rate and the pulse rate when taken after the other on a given time.

51. The nurse plans to take the rectal temperature of several clients. To which of the following patients is the procedure contraindicated?
    a. A 5-year old with bacterial pneumonia
    b. A client with heart failure on full bed rest
    c. A 23-year-old camper with Lyme's disease
    d. A newborn with imperforate anus

52. A nurse is doing a sponge bath on a febrile client when suddenly the client started to shiver. What is the best nursing response?
    a. Finish the sponge bath to quickly lower body temperature.
    b. Discontinue the bath and dress the client warmly.
    c. Make the water for the bath 1 degree colder
    d. Make the water for the bath 1 degree warmer

53. A client is reporting severe pain of the shoulders. A series of tests was made to determine the cause. All results came out normal. After psychiatric evaluation, the client did not have symptoms of depression, anxiety, somatization or conversion. What is the most probable nature of his pain?
    a. Somatic
    b. Neuropathic
    c. Idiopathic
    d. Psychogenic

54. A 35-year old client has just undergone a cesarean operation to deliver her baby. She reports pain in the surgical site 24 hours after the surgery. What type of pain is the client most likely experiencing?
    a. Somatic
    b. Neuropathic
    c. Idiopathic
    d. Psychogenic

55. A client was admitted at the emergency department due to a head injury sustained from a vehicular accident. Upon assessment, the nurse noticed irregularity in the patient's breathing pattern. The client's breathing exhibits long pauses, increased and decreased rate, deep or shallow breathing with no identifiable pattern. The nurse understands that this type of breathing is called
    a. Ataxic respiration or Biot's
    b. Kussmaul's respiration
    c. Cheyne-Stoke's respiration
    d. Hyperventilation

56. A client sees a nurse due to complaints of dizziness and tingling sensation around the mouth. She says she experiences this especially after singing in their church choir for a long period, or sometimes if she is exhibiting extreme emotion such as anger. Which type of respiration is most likely responsible for the client's symptoms?
    a. Ataxic or Biot's breathing
    b. Kussmaul's respiration
    c. Cheyne-Stoke's respiration
    d. Hyperventilation

57. A client comes seeking help in the outpatient department regarding the pain on her lower back. According to her, the pain became increasingly more difficult to treat. At first she was relieved by analgesics. And then they didn't work anymore. A doctor prescribed vicodin. After some time, she couldn't feel any relief with vicodin. The reason for her visit is to get prescription for a stronger pain reliever. Which of the following pertains to the client's experience?
    a. Dependence
    b. Addiction
    c. Inappropriateness
    d. Tolerance

58. During documentation of assessment findings, the charge nurse calls the attention of the nurse regarding which of the following entries?
    a. Client appears to be in no acute distress, and is well-nourished
    b. He has intercostal muscle retraction when breathing
    c. Client weighs 130 lbs and is 5'7" tall, BMI 20.4, VS: RR: 20, PR: 88, BP: 110/80, right arm sitting, temp, 36.7 °C tympanic
    d. Four extremities in full range of motion

59. A 16 year old student reports pain as 8 in a scale of 1-10. The nurse observes the client lying on the bed comfortably while watching television. Vital signs are normal. The client has pain meds PRN. What is the best nursing action?
    a. Hold the pain meds because the client may get addicted to the medication
    b. Administer pain meds as ordered
    c. Reassess pain level after 30 minutes

    d. Cut the pain medication's dose in half

60. The nurse is to take the apical pulse of the client with no known heart abnormalities. The nurse places the diaphragm of her stethoscope over
    a. 2nd intercostal space, right midclavicular line
    b. The hollow part of the crease between forearm and lower arm
    c. Below the patient's left nipple
    d. 5th intercostal space, left midclavicular line

61. A patient who was rushed to the emergency department has just been diagnosed with cerebrovascular accident or stroke. As the nurse performs an urgent assessment, which of the following would most likely be included in the general survey findings?
    a. Fidgeting
    b. Agitated
    c. Facial asymmetry
    d. Scissoring gait

62. A patient is seen in the ER because of trauma to the head. The nurse assesses the patient's level of consciousness by determining their orientation to different parameters. Which of the following questions assesses for orientation?
    a. "Can you describe your pain?"
    b. "Can you remember what you did before the accident?"
    c. "Do you feel anxious?"
    d. "Do you know where you are and the date today?"

63. A nurse is caring for several patients in the ward. Which of the following patients would most likely show agitation and restlessness?
    a. The patient with depression
    b. The patient with an anxiety attack
    c. The patient in pain
    d. The patient with paralysis of the lower extremities

64. A nurse is assessing a patient with chronic obstructive pulmonary disease or COPD. Which of the following posture is commonly assumed by patients with COPD to ease their breathing efforts?
    a. Flat on bed
    b. Sitting and slightly leaning forward with the arms braced
    c. Lying on their right side
    d. Semi-fowler's

65. A patient with diabetes was admitted due to increased blood sugar levels. Which of the following would the nurse most likely note of the patient's breath during the physical examination?
    a. Acetone smell

b. Alcohol scent
c. Halitosis
d. Ammonia-like smell

66. On a summer day, a patient comes to the clinic wearing several layers of clothes. Which of the following can the patient's wearing of excess clothing suggest?
    a. Spastic movements of cerebral palsy
    b. Paralysis of stroke
    c. High blood sugar of diabetes
    d. Cold intolerance of hypothyroidism

67. The patient is seen sitting in a tripod position. The nurse is observing the patient for paleness, sweating, and shortness of breath. Which of the following is the nurse assessing for?
    a. Cardiac or respiratory distress
    b. Pain
    c. Anxiety
    d. Hyperglycemia

68. Which of the following is the best way to count the patient's respiratory rate?
    a. Directly look at the patient's abdomen and count the rate of breathing
    b. Tell the patient that you will be counting how many times they breathe in a minute and then count the rate
    c. Directly look at the patient's chest and count the rate of breathing
    d. After counting the radial pulse, count the respiration while still holding the patient's wrist

69. A nurse is to measure a patient's blood pressure. Which of the following should the nurse ensure before taking blood pressure measurements?
    a. The radial pulse should be palpable before beginning to take measurements
    b. A cuff with a width that is about 40% of the arm circumference of the patient is available
    c. The length of the inflatable bladder should be at least 100% of the circumference of the patient's upper arm
    d. If the patient is seated, the arm of the patient should be at waist level

70. Which of the following patients would need to wait before their blood pressure measurement is taken?
    a. A patient who is seen in the emergency department with a head trauma
    b. A patient who just finished an energy drink
    c. A patient with a fistula on the right arm
    d. A patient with an active IV line on the left arm

71. Which of the following is a correct technique of determining the right pressure for cuff inflation during blood pressure measurements?

a. To determine how much pressure is needed to inflate the cuff, estimate the systolic pressure by percussion first
b. Feel for the radial artery and inflate the cuff until the radial pulse disappears
c. Note where the brachial pulse disappears and add 30 mm Hg
d. Deflate the cuff promptly and completely and wait for at least 15 minutes

72. The nurse takes blood pressure measurements twice on both arms and notes a difference of 15 mm Hg. Which of the following should the nurse do?
a. Take the BP again in 30 seconds
b. Take the BP again after 30 minutes
c. Inform the physician of the findings
d. Document the results and administer an anti-hypertensive

73. Which of the following errors of BP measurement leads to falsely high readings?
a. Cuff that is too wide
b. Repeating assessments too quickly
c. Pressing the stethoscope too hard on the pulse
d. Arm below heart level

74. A nurse is taking the radial pulse of an adult patient and finds it irregular. Which of the following is best for the nurse to do next?
a. Retake the pulse on the other hand
b. Place the stethoscope on the left midclavicular line 5th intercostal space and count the apical pulse for a full minute
c. Count the carotid pulse instead
d. Place the stethoscope on the right midclavicular line 3rd intercostal space and count the apical pulse

75. The nurse is taking the vital signs of a patient with a seizure disorder. Which of the following situations indicate that the nurse needs further teaching?
a. The nurse takes the radial pulse for one full minute
b. The nurse takes the BP measurement on the arm without an IV line
c. The nurse counts the breath while pretending to still count the pulse
d. The nurse obtains an oral thermometer to get the temperature

76. Which of the following way of using a rectal thermometer is INCORRECT?
a. Place the disposable cover over the probe and lubricate it
b. Ask the patient to lie on their side with the hip flexed
c. Insert the thermometer 3-4 inches into the anal canal
d. Wait 10 seconds before obtaining a reading

77. A patient has a fever. Which of the following symptoms when noticed by the nurse suggest a

falling body temperature?
a.   Feeling cold
b.   Sweating
c.   Goosebumps
d.   Shivering

78. Which of the following describes chronic pain?
a.   It is a pain that is not associated with cancer or any medical condition and is persisting for 3-6 months
b.   It is a severe pain
c.   It arises quickly and is short lived
d.   It is a signal that the body or a body part is injured, diseased or inflamed

79. The nurse is assessing a patient who is complaining abdominal pain. The nurse would like to know the location of the pain. Which question is the most appropriate to ask the patient to know the location of the pain?
a.   "When did you feel the pain begin?"
b.   "Does the pain come and go?"
c.   "Where do you feel the pain?"
d.   "Can you point where exactly you feel the pain?"

80. A nurse is assessing the pain of a patient who had undergone abdominal surgery. The nurse asks the patient to describe their pain, with 0 as having no pain, and 10 as the worst pain imaginable. Which pain scale did the nurse utilize to assess the severity of the patient's pain?
a.   Visual analog scale
b.   Combination pain scale
c.   Numeric pain rating scale
d.   Verbal pain rating scale

81. A nurse is assessing a patient who presented with right upper quadrant pain that radiates to the right shoulders. The patient describes the pain as gnawing, felt after eating. The patient reports that they feel nauseous. Which of the following is the associated manifestation of the patient's pain?
a.   Gnawing
b.   Felt after eating
c.   Radiation to the shoulders
d.   Feels nauseous with the pain

82. A patient diagnosed with multiple sclerosis reports burning sensation in their scalp. The patient denied putting anything on their scalp or experiencing any head trauma. Which of the following types of pain is the patient most likely manifesting?
a.   Somatic pain

b. Neuropathic pain
c. Psychogenic pain
d. Idiopathic pain

83. The nurse is assessing the effectiveness of pain management in the patient using the 4 A's of monitoring patient outcomes. Which of the following pair of patient outcomes and manifestations are correct?
a. Analgesia – Acetaminophen 500mg q4h relieves the pain
b. Activities of daily living – nausea
c. Adverse effects – cannot tolerate standing
d. Aberrant drug-related behaviors – morphine 2.5-10 mg SC q6h effective in relieving pain

84. A nurse is performing a physical examination on a female patient. The patient is well rested. The nurse obtained the patient's blood pressure and got a reading of 140/90 mm Hg. The patient tells the nurse that she took her blood pressure measurements at home and the last reading was 118/80. The equipment used by the patient was in good condition, and the patient's ability to take BP measurements has been verified. Which of the following is the likely explanation of the patient's hypertension?
a. Ineffective anti-hypertensive medication
b. White coat hypertension
c. High-cholesterol meal prior to clinic visit
d. Strenuous exercise the day before

85. A nurse is taking the blood pressure readings of an obese patient. There is no available BP cuff that is appropriate for their size. Which of the following should the nurse do next?
a. Defer the blood pressure measurements
b. Obtain a thigh cuff
c. Inform the physician
d. Inform the head nurse

ANSWERS

1. B

   The client is assuming a tripod position when he leans forward while the upper body is propped or supported by the arms.

2. D

   Shuffling gait indicates a pathologic condition such as Parkinson's disease. The client needs further evaluation. All options describe normal gait.

3. C

   Even though the client is smiling at the nurse, her gestures suggest anxiety. This should be explored further by the nurse. All options describe normal behavior.

4. D

   The following are the correct interpretation of BMI:
   Underweight < 18.5 kg/m2
   Normal weight 18.5 to 24.9 kg/m2
   Overweight 25 to 29.9 kg/m2
   Obesity (class 1) 30 to 34.9 kg/m2
   Obesity (class 2) 35 to 39.9 kg/m2
   Extreme obesity (class 3) ≥ 40

5. A

   Heart failure will most likely result to weight gain, not weight loss because of fluid retention secondary to the altered pumping mechanism of the heart.

6. A

   Step 1. Convert into proper unit of measurements: 150lbs/2.2 = 68.18 kg; 170cm/100= 1.7m
   Step 2. Use the formula weight in kg/ height in meters squared
   Step 3: compute: 68.18kg/1.7m2 = 68.18/2.89 =23.59

7. B

   Obesity does not cause thyroid disease. Decreased thyroid function causes weight gain.

8. D

   Damage to the hypothalamus, which is located in the brain, will result to altered thermoregulation. The client most likely suffered brain/head trauma.

9. C

   The most accurate, appropriate and the least invasive method to use for measuring temperature in a confused client is the temporal artery thermometer. However, in its absence, the next option is the tympanic membrane thermometer.

10. C

Activity acutely affects pulse rates. An increase in activity will result in a faster pulse rate. Hormonal changes can also affect pulse but not acutely. For example, girls in puberty will have increased rate than boys of the same age.

11. A

The correct interpretation of a +3 pulse is full and bounding.
3+—Full, bounding
2+—Normal
1+—Weak, thread
0—Absent

12. C

Pulse pressure is obtained by subtracting the diastolic pressure from the systolic pressure. 120-80=40 mmHg.

13. C

With decreased arterial wall elasticity (stiff and rigid vessels) blood pressure increases. A decrease in cardiac output, peripheral vascular resistance and blood viscosity increases blood pressure.

14. B

To obtain accurate readings, the nurse should ensure the bladder width and length of the cuff is 40% and 80% of the client's arm circumference respectively. If the client is thin and frail, it may be necessary to use a pediatric cuff, and likewise in an obese client, a thigh cuff may be more appropriate to use on the arm.

15. C

For very young pediatric clients (0-2 years old), take the apical pulse one full minute in consideration of normal irregularities in rhythm. The best method for acquiring temperature readings in a distressed infant is with a temporal artery thermometer or a tympanic membrane thermometer. A glass thermometer may break inside the mouth of a distressed infant. Resting respiratory rate is the most accurate to obtain.

16. B

In the care of the elderly, it is important to understand that the client's reaction to acute infection may differ from that of an adult. (e.g. temperature regulation may be altered and they sweat less than adults).

17. D

Normal oxygen saturation is 97-99%. However, SaO2 > 95% is considered normal if the client also has normal hemoglobin. An SaO2 of 95% means that the client needs to be evaluated further. All other findings are normal.

18. B

Pushing the stethoscope over the brachial artery results to falsely low diastolic pressure. All other options describe the opposite of correct concepts.

19. B

Marfan Syndrome is a genetic disorder wherein the client appears thin and tall with abnormally long limbs and fingers. There is also sternal deformity called pectus excavatum.

20. A

A person with Cushing syndrome would have central obesity manifested by fat deposits around the trunk and the upper back. There is also the characteristic moon-facie (round face), thin limbs and hirsutism (facial hair).

21. A

In the initial phase, transduction, the injured tissue releases neurotransmitters and sends the pain signal through the afferent nerve fibers to the spinal cord. In the second phase or transmission, the pain message from the spinal cord reaches the brain in the absence of opioids in the spinal tract. In the third phase, perception, the person becomes aware of the pain; this is because the cortical structures account for emotional response to pain. In the fourth phase, modulation, the body produces its own analgesia to halt the pain.

22. C

Sciatica is a neuropathic pain, which is pain caused by a disease or damage to the somatosensory nervous system. Other diseases that cause neuropathic pain are AIDS, diabetes mellitus, shingles, amputation and chemotherapy. All other options are examples of nociceptive pain.

23. C

The pain that the client is experiencing visceral, caused by impaction of the bile duct by gallstones. Visceral pain is produced by damaged or diseased organs.

24. D

Referred pain is pain that originated from another area with the same source of innervation.

25. D

Breakthough pain is moderate to intense pain felt before a scheduled dose of analgesia, or end-of-dose medication failure.

26. C

Having pain for longer than 6 months categorizes the client's pain under the chronic type. Since the cause is non-cancer by nature, it is subcategorized as nonmalignant.

27. B

Pre-term infants are more sensitive to painful stimuli than full term infants because nuerotransmitters that inhibit pain sensation are still inadequate. Fetuses feel emotional pain by the 30th week of gestation. Repetitive pain caused by repetitive procedures can make a person hypersensitive to pain later in life. The saying that "Infants do not remember pain" is a myth.

28. A

Pain is not a part of the aging process. It is usually the result of a disease or pathology. The elderly is less sensitive to painful stimuli. Older people tend to underreport pain experience. People with dementia experience pain, too.

29. B

Men are stoic in manifesting pain while women are more expressive. Women are more likely to suffer from fibromyalgia. During puberty, there is equal prevalence of migraines in boys and girls. However, after puberty, more females experience migraines than males.

30. D

Asking the client for any behavioral, pharmacologic and non-drug related interventions that make the pain worse or go away will identify alleviating and aggravating factors of pain.

31. C

Asking the client when the pain started, its duration and frequency will identify the timing of the pain.

32. B

The Brief Pain Inventory assesses the client's pain in relation to effects on mood, mobility and sleep for the last 24 hours. It is scaled 1-10.

33. B

Some elderly clients, especially those with fluctuating intensity of pain are having difficulty describing their pain using a numeric pain scale. The best tool to use in this situation is the descriptor scale that puts description of the intensity of pain with or without corresponding numbers.

34. C

At the beginning of the assessment, the nurse tells the child that the faces show how much something can hurt. Point to the face at the extreme left and tell the child that the face shows no pain, to increasing pain as you point farther to the right. Indicate that the face on the right shows very much pain. Ask the child to point to the face that shows how much he is hurting at that moment. From the left, assign 0, 2, 4, 6, 8 and 10 respectively to each of the faces. Provide a score.

35. A

In clients with acute pain, it is essential to administer pain medications to provide symptomatic relief. Comfort measures and proper positioning should also be carried out but medicating the client takes priority.

36. A, C, D

Physiologic manifestations of poorly controlled pain include tachycardia, increased cardiac output, hypoventilation, ileus, and urinary retention, among others.

37. C

Long-term effects of chronic pain are those that result from constant or repetitive sensations of pain experienced over a period of at least 6 months. Examples of these effects are diminished quality of life, depression, isolation and impaired mobility, among others.

38. B, D, E

When experiencing chronic pain would usually just rub the painful part or sigh. The client may also have reduced activities and appetite. Grimacing, moaning, guarding and verbalization of pain are some behaviors related to acute pain experience.

39. D

All parameters in the CRIES neonatal post-operative pain measurement score are assigned the score of 2 except for the client's % O2 for increasing SaO2, which garners a score of 1. Since there are 5 parameters, four have scores of 2 and only one has a score of 1. The score is 9.

40. B

The nurse best assesses pain of the client with dementia with the PAINAD scale. The PAINAD scale assesses five parameters namely breathing, vocalization, facial expression, body language, and consolability. Each parameter has 3 levels of intensity with scores 0-2. Total score obtained can be any number form 0-10. For scores 4 and above, pain medication is indicated.

41. C

After physical exertion, vital signs are expected to elevate because of increased metabolism. Retaking vital signs after the client has rested will yield more accurate results.

42. B

When assessing the client's general appearance, watch for signs of anxiety such as worried look, fidgety movements, cold and moist palms, inexpressive or flat affect, poor eye contact, and slow psychomotor movements.

43. B

In any situation wherein blood pressure may elevate without pathologic causes (e.g. physical exertion, recent cigarette smoking, use of caffeinated beverages), the BP needs to be measured again after the effects of such wanes.

44. B

All options are correct except that which the client has his legs crossed. Crossing the legs can falsely increase BP.

45. C

BP measurements cannot be taken on the arm with an AV fistula, previous brachial artery cutdowns, lymphedema, burns or that arm which has just been irradiated

46. A

An auscultatory gap is a silent interval that may be present between the systolic and the diastolic pressures and is usually caused by arterial stiffness, atherosclerotic disease, and wide pulse pressure.

47. A

BP cuffs that are too large or wide can give false low BP readings. B, C, and D all cause false high readings

48. C

A sudden fall in blood pressure can be harmful. A drop of just 20 mm Hg (in this case— a decrease of 40 mmHg in systolic and 30mmHg diastolic) can cause dizziness, fainting, and cold sweats due to decreased blood supply to the brain.

49. B

For clients with episodes of tonic-clonic seizures, the use of oral thermometers is dangerous. When the client experiences seizures, the jaw is clenched and the risk of breaking the thermometer while still in the client's mouth is high.

50. C

The pulse deficit is the difference between the rates of the heart and a peripheral pulse when taken simultaneously in a minute.

51. D

Using a rectal thermometer on a newborn with imperforate anus will harm the client and is therefore contraindicated.

52. B

When a febrile patient starts to chill and shiver during a sponge bath, the procedure should be discontinued immediately and the patient dressed warmly. Shivering further increases the body temperature and is therefore avoided.

53. C

Pain is idiopathic in nature when there is no identifiable cause. Somatic pain is brought about by tissue damage. Neuropathic pain is brought about by damage to the nerves or the central nervous system. Psychogenic pain is caused by psychiatric conditions, culture and norms, and even personality.

54. A

Somatic pain is brought about by tissue damage. Neuropathic pain is brought about by damage to the nerves or the central nervous system. Psychogenic pain is caused by psychiatric conditions, culture and norms, and even personality. Pain is idiopathic in nature when there is no identifiable cause.

55. A

Ataxic breathing is characterized by unpredictable irregularity in rate, rhythm quality. It can be a combination of apnea, bradypnea, hyperpnea, deep, shallow or labored breathing.

56. D

In hyperventilation, deep rapid breathing causes carbon dioxide to be expelled more rapidly than the body can produce. This in turn causes vasoconstriction that decreases blood supply to the brain. The client then experiences lightheadedness, tingling sensations and even loss of consciousness.

57. D

Tolerance is a type of adaptation to a medication wherein the drug's supposed effect decreases over time.

58. A

Using words like 'no distress', 'in distress', 'well-nourished' and 'developed' can be vague and should be avoided. Provide more specific description like "Client weighs 130 lbs and is 5'7" BMI 20.4, normal" for 'well-nourished', for example.

59. B

Pain is a subjective data and nurse should rely on verbal feedback from client. In this case, the nurse administers the medication as ordered.

60. D

The 5th intercostal space left midclavicular line is the location where the apical pulse is best heard. Using the client's left nipple as a landmark for the location is not reliable.

61. C

Facial asymmetry is a common finding in patients who had cerebrocardiovascular accident, Bell's palsy or other injuries of the cranial nerves.

62. D

To check for the patient's orientation as part of the assessment for level of consciousness, the nurse may ask the patient to say their name, where they are, and the present date.

63. B

Patients with anxiety attacks would exhibit agitation and restlessness. Patients with pain, paralysis or depression usually avoid movements.

64. B

Patients with COPD or chronic obstructive pulmonary disease have difficulty breathing because of overinflated lungs. The patient with COPD would usually sit and lean slightly forward with their arms braced to be able to breathe more efficiently.

65. A

A patient who is experiencing diabetic ketoacidosis or very high blood sugar levels will have a fruity scent or acetone-smelling breath. An alcoholic patient will have an alcohol-smelling breath. Halitosis is the noticeably unpleasant breath odor. An ammonia-like breath will be evident in patients who have uremia.

66. D

Patients who are wearing excess clothes that are too warm for the weather may be experiencing cold intolerance, such as those with hypothyroidism. Excess clothing may also be an attempt to hide a patient's frail body in anorexia, or needle marks in drug abusers.

67. A

Shortness of breath, chest tightness, pallor, diaphoresis, and sitting in a tripod position are signs of cardiac or respiratory distress.

68. D

When counting the patient's respiratory rate, the nurse must be inconspicuous because informing the patient that their breathing will be counted, or showing the patient that their breathing is being observed may change the pattern and rate of their breathing. The best strategy to use is to count the patient's breathing while still holding the patient's wrist after counting their radial pulse.

69. B

Before taking blood pressure measurements, the nurse must ensure that the width of the cuff of the inflatable bladder is about 40% of the patient's upper arm circumference, and its length about

80% of the patient's upper arm circumference. The nurse must also ensure that the brachial pulse is viable and that the arm is positioned comfortably where the brachial artery is at heart level.

70. B
Blood pressure measurements cannot be obtained within 30 minutes of drinking caffeinated beverages. Examples of caffeinated beverages are coffee and energy drinks. The nurse should also not obtain BP measurements in the arm with fistulas or IV lines, but they can do so in their other arm.

71. C
To determine how much pressure is needed to inflate the cuff during BP measurements, the nurse must estimate the systolic pressure by palpating for the brachial artery first. The cuff is inflated until the brachial pulse disappears and this pressure is noted. The nurse then adds 30 mm Hg to this pressure. The cuff is deflated promptly and completely before re-inflating the cuff after at least 15 seconds.

72. C
If the nurse notes more than 10 mm Hg difference in pressure between the left and right arms, the nurse must retake the BP. If the pressure difference is confirmed, then the readings must be duly documented, and the physician informed accordingly. A pressure difference of more than 10 mm Hg suggests subclavian steal syndrome, aortic dissection, and supravalvular aortic stenosis.

73. D
When the BP measurement is taken in an arm below heart level, the nurse obtains a false high reading. On the other hand, using a cuff that is too wide, repeating assessments too quickly or pressing the stethoscope too hard on the brachial pulse will result in false low readings.

74. B
If the nurse palpates for the radial pulse and finds it irregular, the apical pulse must be counted instead. The nurse must place the diaphragm of the stethoscope on the left midclavicular line, 5th intercostal space, which is also the point of maximal impulse where the apical pulse is heard best in an adult patient. The apical pulse is counted one full minute.

75. D
Oral temperatures are contraindicated in patients with seizure disorders, and in those who are unconscious or unable to close their mouths. The possibility of sudden jaw movements can break the glass thermometer and cause injury to the patient.

76. C

When obtaining a rectal temperature, the nurse should place a disposable cover over the probe and lubricate it. The patient is positioned on their side with their hips flexed. The lubricated probe is inserted 3-5 cm or about 1.5 inches into the anal canal to the direction of the umbilicus. The nurse has to wait for at least 10 seconds before obtaining a reading.

77. B

Sweating and feeling hot accompany a falling body temperature. Feeling cold, shivering, and goosebumps, on the other hand, suggest a rising body temperature.

78. A

Chronic pain is defined in several ways. Chronic pain can be a pain unassociated with cancer or any other medical condition that persists for 3-6 months. It is also defined as pain lasting for one month longer than a course of an illness, or recurring pain that is felt at monthly intervals. Acute pain, on the other hand, is associated with a physical cause and is a signal that a body part is injured, diseased or inflamed. It arises quickly but it short-lived.

79. D

When assessing about the location of pain, the nurse must ask the patient to point exactly where it hurts because the patient's use of lay terms may not be accurate to localize the site of origin of the pain.

80. C

The numeric pain rating scale describes pain in numerical terms with 0 as the absence of pain, and 10 as the worst pain.

81. D

The associated manifestations of pain refer to other symptoms accompanying the pain.

82. B

Neuropathic pain is the result of injury to nerves either of the central or peripheral nervous system. In multiple sclerosis, the myelin sheaths of the central nervous system nerves are damaged, causing neuropathic pains, such as the burning sensation felt in the scalp.

83. A

The nurse may use the 4A's of monitoring patient outcomes when managing pain. Analgesia refers to the effectiveness of pain relieving measures. Activities of daily living refers to how the pain and relieving measures affected the patient's daily activities. Adverse effects refer to the undesirable and harmful effects of the pain medication administered to the patient. Aberrant drug-related behaviors pertain to aberrant behaviors brought about by the abuse of prescribed pain medications.

84. B

White coat hypertension refers to hypertension in people who have lower or normal blood pressure at home or in more relaxed settings. It is related to anxiety, and it is more common in female patients.

85. B

When there is no available cuff size for an obese patient, the nurse may use obtain a thigh cuff.

Substance Abuse and Domestic and Family Violence Assessments

Questions
1. A nurse is asking a client who had been in a recent vehicular accident what type of alcohol he had taken, and how much of it he had the night of the accident. The client says he took hard liquor, about half a pint of it. About how many standard drinks did the client take?
    a. 1
    b. 2
    c. 4
    d. 6

2. Which of the following is a systemic negative effect of alcohol?
    a. It stimulates the parasympathetic nervous system
    b. It increases blood pressure and afterload
    c. It decreases estrogen that in turn lead to breast cancer development
    d. It can deter the development of cirrhosis

3. A nurse is providing counseling to a group of teenagers. Four out of ten of the members confessed to using illicit drug. The nurse knows that the most common abused drug is
    a. weed
    b. speed
    c. The big H
    d. LSD

4. A client confides to the nurse that she fakes pain and exaggerates intensity just to get a prescription of oxycodone. Which of the following is a factor that leads to abuse of prescription medications?
    a. Affordability of the medications
    b. Lax laws that regulate dispensing
    c. Increased marketing of medications for off-label uses
    d. Inadequate prescribing

5. A 54-year old male employee tells the occupational health nurse that he consumes about seven standard drinks in one party night. What is the correct categorization of the client's drinking pattern?
    a. Moderate drinking
    b. At-risk drinking
    c. Hazardous drinking
    d. Harmful drinking

6. A nurse is trying to determine the pattern of alcohol drinking in a male client. Which of the following is NOT included in the diagnostic criteria of problematic alcohol use?
    a. Strong craving or desire to drink alcohol
    b. A great amount of time is spent obtaining, using and recovering from alcohol
    c. Important activities in the home, community and work are disregarded or missed because of

alcohol use

    d. Alcohol is taken in a very large amount in a single event in a year

7. A client is being interviewed by the nurse prior to being admitted for hepatitis. According to the client, he is taking whiskey about double of what he used to take last year. He confesses to have missed several important occasions because he had been "really busy". He admits to sometimes driving after taking a few drinks. For the past few months, he has taken a liking to bourbon and whiskey mix that he takes in the morning to "fuel (him) up". With the assessment findings mentioned, what is the severity of the client's problematic drinking pattern?

    a. Mild

    b. Moderate

    c. Severe

    d. Cannot be determined

8. An alcoholic client who has undergone rehabilitation has not had any of the criteria met for problematic alcohol drinking pattern for more than a year now. He confides though that the urge to drink is still there but that he manages to control himself through the strategies he learned in the center. What type of remission is the client in?

    a. Early remission

    b. Late remission

    c. Sustained remission

    d. Exacerbation

9. A nurse is conducting health teachings to a group of pregnant women on alcohol intake during pregnancy. Which of the following should NOT be included in her teaching plan?

    a. 18% of women drink on the first trimester without knowing that they are pregnant

    b. Only one standard drink per day is allowed because an intake more than that pose significant harm to the baby

    c. Alcohol toxicity results in physical, learning, and behavioral problems in a fetus

    d. A safe dose for the pregnant woman is already toxic to the baby

10. Although alcoholism in the elderly is less likely than other adult groups, the risk of being negatively affected by alcohol is increased. Which of the following is NOT a factor for this risk for alcoholism in the elderly?

    a. More tissue in the body in which the alcohol is concentrated

    b. Decreased kidney and liver function

    c. Increased intake of therapeutic drugs that may react with alcohol

    d. Fewer situations for alcoholism to be detected; they no longer work or drive

11. The AUDIT is a questionnaire that helps identify drinking and alcohol abuse and dependence disorders. It specifically assesses current alcohol use and works with all applicable age, gender and culture. The AUDIT questionnaire covers three parameters. Which of the following does not

belong to the group?
a. Alcohol consumption
b. Drinking behavior or dependence
c. Age related response
d. Negative effects of alcohol

12. The nurse is assessing a client for alcohol use disorders using the standard clinical diagnostic criteria. To determine whether there is a problematic pattern of alcohol use causing clinically significant impairment or distress, the nurse asks if alcohol is the cause of several results. Which of the following results does NOT belong?
a. Risk for bodily harm
b. Relationship trouble
c. Risk for financial ruin
d. Run-ins

13. A nurse wants to assess a pregnant woman for possible alcohol use. Which questionnaire is specific to women in identifying at-risk drinking?
a. CAGE
b. AUDIT
c. TWEAK
d. 4R's

14. Prescription drug abuse is increased among teen and young adult groups. Which of the following concept is NOT true of prescription drug abuse?
a. The person takes a medication that is prescribed for someone else
b. The person takes more than what is prescribed
c. The person takes the medication for longer than prescribed
d. The person takes over-the-counter medications more than five times a day

15. The National Institute on Drug Abuse (NIDA) has found out that teenagers abuse drugs to keep them awake studying. Which drug according to NIDA is abused this way?
a. marijuana
b. ADHD drugs
c. Heroin
d. Alcohol

16. A nurse is caring for a drunk driver who had been in a vehicular mishap. The police officer who brought him to the clinic said that he failed the breath analyzer test. Which of the following is true of the breath analysis?
a. It detects any amount of alcohol at the end of expiration after a deep inhalation
b. It is the same as blood alcohol concentration (BAC)
c. It is the basis for legal interpretation of drinking.

    d.   Normal values indicating no alcohol are 0.00.

17. A client admitted due to chronic alcoholism has his blood drawn for analysis. Which biomarker Is most commonly used in assessing alcohol drinking?
    a.   Bilirubin
    b.   Serum protein gamma glutamyl transferase (GGT)
    c.   Creatinine
    d.   Mean corpuscular volume (MCV)

18. The nurse is using the Short Michigan Alcoholism Screening Test—Geriatric Version (SMAST-G) in assessing an elderly client for possible alcohol abuse. Which of the following scores indicates that the client is at risk for having a problematic alcohol abuse pattern?
    a.   1
    b.   2
    c.   4
    d.   6

19. The nurse is using the Short Michigan Alcoholism Screening Test—Geriatric Version (SMAST-G) in assessing an elderly client for possible alcohol abuse. Which of the following question is NOT included in this test?
    a.   Has a relative, friend, doctor, or other health care worker been concerned about your drinking or suggested that you cut down?
    b.   Have you ever increased your drinking after experiencing a loss in your life?
    c.   Has a doctor or nurse ever said they were worried or concerned about your drinking?
    d.   Have you ever made rules to manage your drinking?

20. A nurse is assessing a client in the ICU using the AUDIT-C questionnaire and gathered a score of 2 from the client. What is the interpretation of this score?
    a.   High risk
    b.   Moderate risk
    c.   Low risk
    d.   No risk

21. A female client confides to the nurse that her partner drags her and then forces her to have sexual relations with him against her will. Which of the following is the partner committing?
    a.   Paraphilia
    b.   Sexual violence
    c.   Coercive tactics
    d.   Threats of sexual violence

22. The social workers brought in a 6-year-old child who appears unkempt and pale. She is indifferent to the nurse's questions. Her weight and height are below expected range of girls her age. Her

mother, a known alcoholic, cares for her at home. She is not attending school. Which of the following accurately describes the situation?

a. Physical abuse
b. Child neglect
c. Sexual abuse
d. Domestic abuse

23. A child confides to the school nurse that she sees his neighbor strip naked by his window every time he sees her playing alone in their backyard. The nurse informs the child's parents and the authorities of which case?

a. Child abuse
b. Coercive tactic
c. Sexual abuse - sodomy
d. Sexual abuse – indecent exposure

24. A nurse reports a colleague whom she has heard telling an elderly bedridden client, "…serves you right, you old hag!" The nurse's colleague has committed which type of elderly abuse?

a. Physical abuse
b. Psychological abuse
c. Abusive contact
d. Risk for emotional abuse

25. The nurse admits a male teenager who had been a victim of domestic violence. He was hit with a block of wood to the head, and is bleeding in the site of impact. What type of injury did the client sustain?

a. Laceration
b. Incision
c. Ligature compression
d. Blunt-force trauma

26. A client sustained a wound after being batted by a metal pipe to the arm. What type of injury did the client sustain?

a. Cut
b. Ligature
c. Laceration
d. Strangulation

27. The abuse of adolescence results to negative impacts. Which of the following is considered short-term negative consequence of teen relationship violence?

a. Decreased self-esteem
b. Poor academic performance
c. Disordered eating behaviors

d. Unintended pregnancies

28. The school nurse is assessing a first grader. Included in her assessment findings are height and weight below normal range for age, unkempt appearance, wounds on several body parts in various stages of healing. Upon conversation with her teacher, the nurse noted that she is not performing well, and is behind in all subjects. Which of the assessment findings will necessitate the nurse and the supervisor to call the authorities?
    a. Height and weight below normal range for age
    b. Unkempt appearance
    c. Wounds on several body parts in various stages of healing
    d. Poor academic performance

29. A psychiatric nurse has volunteered to do health teachings to several young clients with violent behaviors. Which of the following should the nurse assess importantly?
    a. History of childhood physical abuse
    b. Financial status of parents
    c. Community resources
    d. Support groups available

30. A nurse wants to assess if the client have ever been in an abusive dating relationship. Which of the following questions is most appropriate to ask?
    a. Have you ever used contraception when you date?
    b. Is there any unsafe place you have been to?
    c. Have you ever felt unsafe in a relationship?
    d. Have you been subjected to a forceful sexual act?

31. A 22-year old was rushed to the ER because of a gaping wound to the face made by a sharp blade. What type of injury did the client obtain?
    a. Laceration
    b. Incision
    c. Abrasion
    d. Contusion

32. A male teenage client has been rescued by police. He was found confined to a room of his uncle's house. His uncle had physically abused him for years. As the nurse examines the client in the clinic, she notes 2 small circular ecchymotic looking marks about 2 inches apart on the abdomen. As she examines the back, she notes 2 more pairs of similar marks. What type of injury did the client most likely sustain based on the marks?
    a. Penetrating injury
    b. Blunt-force trauma
    c. Patterned injury
    d. Hematoma

33. A nurse preparing for her duty reads the client's record. The client is a victim of abuse. The document read, "several ecchymotic marks on the right upper arm." Which of the following correctly describes ecchymosis?
    a.   A superficial round blotch that is non-elevated, bluish or purplish in color.
    b.   An accumulation of blood in an organ, space or tissue caused by damaged or ruptured blood vessels
    c.   Caused by active bleeding from a ruptured vessel whether within the body or outside the body
    d.   Pinpoint round non-elevated purplish-red skin-deep hemorrhage that turns bluish and then yellowish as it heals

34. A client was assessed for violence and abuse to which he tested negative. However, as the nurse examines the client, she notes ecchymosis on different parts of the body. Which factor most likely contributed to the client's condition?
    a.   Use of warfarin
    b.   Use of steroids
    c.   Prolonged immobility
    d.   Self-inflicted injuries

35. A nurse is assessing several clients with signs of bruising. Which of the following indicates a possible abuse that necessitates the nurse to inform the authorities?
    a.   Ecchymosis on the upper thigh of a 7-month old infant who tested negative for dengue and Rocky Mountain spotted fever
    b.   Petechiae on both the client's arm after 2 days of having elevated temperature
    c.   Hematoma on the perineal area of a mother with a 3-day old child.
    d.   A bruise on the arm of a school-aged child who said he sustained the injury after he fell from a chair

36. A nurse is documenting assessment findings of a client who suffered injuries from physical abuse. Which of the following is an incorrect technique of documentation?
    a.   The nurse writes in direct quotes (verbatim) as the client says
    b.   Taking photographs of the injuries of an unconscious client without consent
    c.   Taking photographs of the injuries of a conscious client after asking for consent
    d.   The nurse estimates the age of the bruises by color

37. The nurse assessing the client for domestic violence wants to determine societal factors. Which of the following factors is considered a societal stressor?
    a.   Legal status
    b.   Lack of access to health care
    c.   Poverty
    d.   Gender roles

38. A nurse is examining a pre-school child. Bruising in which area should alert the nurse to possible abuse?
    a. Arm
    b. Leg
    c. Neck
    d. Buttocks

39. Maltreatment in the US comes in many forms. Which of the following is the most prevalent?
    a. Neglect
    b. Physical abuse
    c. Sexual abuse
    d. Parental substance abuse

40. A nurse examines a client who is a victim of physical abuse. The nurse notes cord-like bruising around the neck. Which forensic term is most appropriate to use in the documentation of this assessment finding?
    a. Strangulation
    b. Manual compression of the neck
    c. Ligature marks
    d. Ecchymosis

ANSWERS

1. D

   A pint of hard liquor is equivalent to around 11 standard drinks. Half a pint means that the client consumed 5-6 standard drinks.

2. B

   Alcohol stimulates the sympathetic nervous system. It increases blood pressure, which in turn causes increased afterload. It also increases the risk of breast cancer because it increases estrogen. Alcohol abuse can cause cirrhosis.

3. A

   The 'weed' or marijuana is the most commonly abused drug. Speed is a street name for amphetamine. The Big H is heroin. LSD is a hallucinogen.

4. C

   Factors that contribute to abuse of prescription medications include prescribing for someone who really does not need it, increased marketing of medications for off-label uses, and the increase in prescription as a response to inadequate treatment of pain in the past.

5. B

   At-risk drinking pattern is having more than 14 standard drinks in a week, or more than 4 drinks per occasion for men, and + 7 in a week and at least three standard drinks per occasion for women.

6. D

   There are 11 diagnostic criteria for problematic alcohol use pattern. One of the criteria is that alcohol should be used in larger amounts than standard, more frequently for longer periods. All options except D are included in the criteria.

7. B

   There are three levels of severity of problematic alcohol use. The client's drinking problem is mild if 2-3 of the 11 criteria are met. The level is moderate if 4-5 symptoms are present. The problem is severe if klsix or more symptoms are evident. In this scenario, the client exhibited five symptoms, which makes the severity of the problem moderate.

8. C

   A person is in sustained remission if he had previously met criteria for problematic alcohol drinking pattern but has since not manifesting those criteria for at least 12 months (except for the criteria on craving). Craving or urge may still be present.

9. B

   No amount of alcohol is safe during pregnancy. All other options reflect correct information.

10. A

There is less tissue and muscle mass in the elderly for faster metabolism of alcohol. Blood concentrations increase faster and for longer. There is also decreased kidney and liver function. The elderly also tend to have prescribed medications that react with alcohol. There are also less situations that will necessitate testing for alcoholism.

11. C

The AUDIT questionnaire covers three parameters, namely: alcohol consumption, drinking behavior or dependence and negative effects of alcohol.

12. C

Alcohol abuse results to risk for bodily harm, relationship trouble, role failures and run-ins. financial ruins is more of a result of gambling problems.

13. C

The TWEAK questionnaire is specific to women in identifying at-risk drinking. TWEAK assesses tolerance, worry, eye-opener, amnesia and cut down.

14. D

Prescription drug abuse happens when a person takes a medication that is prescribed for someone else, takes more than what is prescribed, or for longer than prescribed. Over the counter medications do not need a prescription.

15. B

Drugs for Attention Deficit Hyperactivity Disorder are usually abused by 1 out of 8 teens because they use the drug to keep them awake for studying. This is according to The National Institute on Drug Abuse (NIDA).

16. A

The breath alcohol analysis detects any amount of alcohol at the end of expiration after a deep inhalation. It complements the results of blood alcohol concentration (BAC) that is the basis for legal interpretation of drinking. Normal values of BAC indicating no alcohol are 0.00.

17. B

The biomarker that is most commonly used in assessing alcohol drinking is the serum protein gamma glutamyl transferase (GGT). Sudden elevation of this biomarker after obtaining normal levels indicates that the client relapsed and is drinking again.

18. A

The Short Michigan Alcoholism Screening Test—Geriatric Version (SMAST-G) is used in assessing an elderly client for possible alcohol abuse. Getting a score of 2 or more indicates a current alcoholism problem. Scoring 1 may indicate a potential problem or risk.

19. A

The question in option A is included in the AUDIT questionnaire and not in SMAST-G.

20. C

A score of < 2 in the AUDIT-C questionnaire means that the client has a low risk response to alcoholism.

21. B

Sexual violence is committed when a person uses physical means to force another to engage in a sexual act against her will or if a sexual act is forced on another who has no capacity to consent because of illness, disability or alcohol or substance use.

22. B

Neglect is failing to provide for the child's basic needs such as food, shelter, clothing, education, security, love and belongingness. It is also failure to attend to medical needs.

23. D

Indecent exposure is a form of sexual abuse wherein the abuser intentionally shows his/her sexual organs to public or a person.

24. B

A psychological or emotional abuse happens when an elderly is traumatized after being exposed to threats, forced submission or controlling behavior. It includes humiliation, embarrassment, social isolation and damage to client's property.

25. D

Blunt-force injury is a non-penetrating trauma that is caused by impact or physical attack, which in this case caused by the block of wood.

26. C

When the skin breaks because of the impact of a blunt trauma, the injury is called laceration. The wound edges of a laceration are jagged and irregular.

27. D

The abuse of adolescence results to short-term and long-term negative impacts. Some short-term consequences are: early and unintended pregnancy, alcohol and substance abuse, depression and thoughts of suicide, smoking, and other risky behaviors. Long-term effects are decreased self-esteem, poor performance in school and disordered eating behaviors among others.

28. C

Wounds or fractures (seen in x-rays) in various stages of healing suggest physical abuse. Any suspicion of physical abuse should be reported to the authorities.

29. A

A history of childhood physical abuse is important to assess because childhood physical abuse is found to be the most consistent predictor of youth violence.

30. C

Asking the client if she has felt unsafe in a relationship will helps identify dating violence.

31. B

An incision is a linear cut or wound made by a sharp object such as a blade.

32. C

Patterned injuries leave distinct and patterned marks on the skin. In this situation, the patterned injuries are caused by a stun or tazer gun.

33. A

An ecchymosis is a superficial round blotch that is non-elevated, bluish or purplish in color. A hematoma is an accumulation of blood in an organ, space or tissue caused by damaged or ruptured blood vessels. Hemorrhage is caused by active bleeding from a ruptured vessel whether within the body or outside the body. Petechiae are pinpoint round non-elevated purplish-red skin-deep hemorrhage that turns bluish and then yellowish as it heals.

34. A

Use of blood thinners such as warfarin and heparin can cause ecchymosis formation. Other medications such as valproic acid, prednisone, and clopidogrel have the same effect. Prolonged use of bilberry, garlic, ginger, and ginkgo can also lead to bleeding tendencies as manifested by ecchymosis.

35. A

Infants who have not yet attempted to walk will not have bruises unless they are with medical conditions that result to bleeding problems. Suspect abuse in this case, and duly inform the authorities.

36. D

Estimating the age of the bruises through color is not recommended because published evidence does not support dating injuries by color alone. Taking photographs of the injuries of an unconscious client is allowed.

37. C

Societal stressors such as poverty contribute to problems in relationships that result to domestic violence.

38. C

Bruising on the neck, torso, ears of a pre-school child are likely intentional.

39. A

   According to the Child Protective Services, neglect is the most prevalent type of maltreatment, followed by physical abuse, and sexual abuse.

40. C

   Ligature marks are caused by compression of the neck by cord-like objects, such as rope or an electrical cord.

Nutrition and Hydration

Questions

1. A nurse is conducting a health teaching about the possible effects of obesity from childhood to adulthood. Which of the following is NOT a possible result of childhood obesity that persisted until adulthood?
    a. Type 2 diabetes
    b. Hyperthyroidism
    c. Hypertension
    d. Dyslipidemia

2. The nurse assesses several young children. On one assessment, she documents that a 4-year old child is obese. Which of the following BMI (body mass index) correctly reflects her documentation?
    a. BMI > the 85th percentile based on age- and gender-specific BMI charts
    b. BMI > 95th percentile based on age- and gender-specific BMI charts
    c. BMI of 25 or greater
    d. BMI of 30 or greater

3. The nurse is preparing for an evidence-based health teaching for some students. Which of the following concepts on nutritional assessment is NOT evidence-based?
    a. There is no significant increase in obesity rates in the recent years after previous rates of steady increases
    b. Being overweight or obese in childhood will result to also being overweight or obese during adulthood
    c. If previously obese children become non-obese as adults, the risks of developing cardiovascular diseases still persists
    d. There is no risk of being obese as an adult if one is not obese as a child.

4. A nurse is assessing the nutritional status of babies from birth to the first year of life. Which of the following concept is INCORRECT regarding nutrition and growth in the first year of life?
    a. Newborns grow fastest during the first four months of life.
    b. There is normal weight loss up to 8% of body weight in the first few days of life
    c. Infants are expected to have doubled their birth weight by the first year of life
    d. By their first birthday, infants have increased their length by 50%

5. A novice nurse is assigned by the head nurse to teach a group of young mothers on the advantages of breastfeeding. Which of the following should be included in her teachings? Select all that apply.
    a. It prevents overfeeding
    b. It reduces risks of allergy and food intolerance
    c. It has low amounts of iron
    d. It contains antibodies
    e. It does not contain Vitamins C and E

6. A nurse is counseling a mother who just delivered a healthy baby. The nurse emphasizes that

the baby should not be fed skimmed or low-fat milk on the first 2 years of life for which of the following reasons?
a. They do not contain proteins
b. They lack essential fatty acids for proper brain development
c. They are difficult to digest
d. They cause allergies

7. Adolescents are at risk for nutritional deficiencies. The nurse is aware of the reasons why this is so. Which of the following reflects correct concept of the reasons for poor nutritional intake in the adolescent? Select all that apply
a. Preference for sweet foods and beverages
b. Skipping meals
c. Preference for processed and fast food
d. Preference for large meals over small meals
e. Small intake of fruits and vegetables

8. The nurse is learning about nutritional problems in adolescence. Which of the following contributes to obesity that is not related to food intake?
a. Inactivity related to watching television and internet use
b. Peer pressure
c. Use of recreational drugs and alcohol
d. Preference for fast foods

9. A nurse is preparing her nursing care plans and she is including ways on how to prevent sarcopenic obesity in the elderly. Which of the following measures will prevent sarcopenic obesity in the elderly?
a. Limit fast food intake
b. Encourage resistance exercises
c. Do not allow sweetened beverages
d. Increase weight bearing exercises

10. A client who is a known Catholic informs the nurse that they are celebrating Holy week. Which food should not be included on his meal tray on Friday?
a. Beef and vegetable dish
b. Corn and crab soup
c. Pork stew
d. Cheese pizza

11. A nurse is doing her morning rounds. She observes her client who is a Seventh Day Adventist is about to be served her breakfast. Which of the following on the client's tray will she request to be replaced?
a. Omelette

   b. Watermelon
   c. Coffee
   d. Bread

12. A nurse wants to perform a nutritional assessment that focuses on which foods the client eats and how many times those foods are eaten in a day, week or month. Which assessment tool is best for the nurse to use?
   a. 24-hour recall
   b. Food frequency questionnaire
   c. Food diaries
   d. ChooseMyPlate

13. A nurse asks the client to make a food diary. Which of the following shows that the client understood the nurse's instructions?
   a. The client lists different foods and indicates how frequent she eats the food
   b. The client lists the food she ate after eating for three consecutive days
   c. The client writes down all the food she ate from yesterday
   d. The client lists the food she plans to eat in the next 3 days

14. A client has lost 2 lbs in the last three days. Which of the following findings is associated with rapid unintentional weight loss?
   a. Exercise
   b. Fasting
   c. Water therapy
   d. Diarrhea

15. A nurse is observing several mothers feeding their infants. Who of the following should receive further instructions?
   a. Mother who cuts a hotdog into half-inch sizes
   b. Mother who mashes a pumpkin in a bowl
   c. Mother who purees a mango
   d. Mother who nips some bread and feeds her child using bare hands

16. A nurse is preparing a nutritional assessment for several pregnant mothers. She wants to emphasize prevention of delivering low birth weight babies. Which of the following factors should NOT be included in her teachings?
   a. Hyperglycemia during pregnancy
   b. Alcoholism
   c. Multiparity
   d. Pregnancy in adolescence

17. A nurse is reviewing the health database of several clients to retrieve information on unintentional

weight loss. Which of the following data reflects significant weight loss?
a.   Current weight: 120 lbs; weight 6 months ago: 136 lbs
b.   Current weight: 130 lbs; weight 3 months ago: 126 lbs
c.   Current weight: 130 lbs; weight 3 months ago: 136 lbs
d.   Current weight: 120 lbs; weight 1 months ago: 116 lbs

18. The nurse is making nutritional assessments of elderly clients in a facility. Which of the following are expected age-related changes regarding nutrition?
a.   Height decreases in women and not in men beginning age 40
b.   Arm span is more accurate to measure than height in people aged 60 above who are bedridden or confined to a wheelchair
c.   TSF measurements are accurate in the elder elderly population
d.   Waist-to-hip ratio and not BMI is the best indicator of obesity in this age-group

19. The nurse is assessing a client's tongue for signs of nutritional deficiencies. Which pair of tongue characteristic and manifestation is accurate?
a.   Papillary atrophy – iron
b.   Pale – riboflavin
c.   Purplish colored tongue - niacin
d.   Beefy red tongue – Vitamin B complex deficiency

20. The nurse is conducting a physical examination. As she checks the client's eyes, she notes a foamy dry-looking spot on the cornea. The nurse expects that the physician will order which supplementation?
a.   Vitamin B complex
b.   Vitamin A
c.   Vitamin C
d.   Vitamin D

21. Which of the following nutrients will hasten healing?
a.   Potassium
b.   Protein
c.   Fats
d.   Vitamin D

22. Which of the following can cause weight gain?
a.   Malignancy
b.   Anorexia
c.   Hyperthyroidism
d.   Fluid accumulation

23. Which of the following is NOT a factor for malnutrition?

    a.   Lack of teeth
    b.   Adolescence
    c.   Alcoholism
    d.   Drug abuse

24. Which of the following parameters in the nutrition screening checklist will garner a score of 4 points if the patient answers yes to that item in the checklist?
    a.   I eat fewer than two meals a day
    b.   I don't have enough money to buy the food that I need
    c.   I eat alone most of the time
    d.   I take 3 or more prescribed or over-the-counter drugs each day

25. What is the recommended daily fruit intake?
    a.   6-11 servings
    b.   2-4 servings
    c.   3-5 servings
    d.   <2 servings

26. The nurse is assessing the skin of the patient's upper chest and notices bruise-like discoloration. The physician confirms that those discolorations are ecchymosis and they are caused by poor nutrition. The nurse knows that the physician refers to which nutrient as extremely lacking in the patient's diet?
    a.   Protein
    b.   Iron
    c.   Vitamin K
    d.   Vitamin B complex

27. The nurse is examining the patient's upper extremities and notices that the patient's nails are brittle and spoon-shaped. The patient also looks pale. The nurse is to provide teaching regarding proper nutrition. Which of the following nutrients will the nurse encourage the patient to take more to help correct the anemia and the spoon-shaped nails?
    a.   Vitamin K
    b.   Vitamin B
    c.   Protein
    d.   Iron

28. A patient is being assessed by the nurse in the clinic. The patient is severely underweight with evident muscle wasting. Which of the following nutrients would the nurse encourage the patient to consume more?
    a.   Protein
    b.   Carbohydrates
    c.   Fats

d.   All of the above

29. Which of the following is a sign of fluid volume deficit?
    a.   Jugular vein distention
    b.   Increased BP and pulse
    c.   Decreased skin turgor
    d.   Increased venous filling

30. The nurse is assessing a patient who presents with difficulty breathing in the emergency department. Upon further examination, the nurse notices jugular vein distention. Auscultation of the patient's chest reveals fine crackles. The nurse should prepare to care for a person with:
    a.   Fluid volume deficit
    b.   Fluid volume excess
    c.   Anemia
    d.   Paresthesia

31. A male elderly patient tells the nurse that in the last few days, he could not put on his shoes because they suddenly felt so tight when worn. The nurse assesses the patient further and notices that the patient has edema of the lower extremities. Which of the following is best for the nurse to do?
    a.   Encourage decreased intake of protein
    b.   Promote exercise
    c.   Inform the physician of your findings
    d.   Provide teaching on the importance of proper dieting

32. The nurse is getting the patient's nutrition history. Which of the following questions would provide information about the patient's food pattern?
    a.   "Are you on a special diet?"
    b.   "Who prepares food?"
    c.   "Is there enough money for food?"
    d.   "Do you have any problems with chewing?"

33. Which of the following is NOT included in the proper way of measuring height?
    a.   Have the patient remove their wallets, keys and anything heavy in their pockets
    b.   Use a stadiometer that is installed and mounted on the wall
    c.   Ask the patient to stand erect away from the wall
    d.   Take the patient's height

34. Which of the following will determines if a balance beam scale is properly calibrated?
    a.   The big counterweight can be slid to the side
    b.   The small counterweight can be slid to the side
    c.   The counterweights are at zero, and the pointer is in the middle

d. The counterweights are in the middle, and the pointer is also in the middle

35. A nurse is assessing the patient's upper body and notices that the patient has an enlarged neck. Upon palpation, the nurse finds that the thyroids are enlarged. Which of the following conditions does the enlarged thyroid suggest?
    a. Lack of potassium
    b. Lack of sodium
    c. Lack of iodine
    d. Lack of iron

36. The nurse is assessing a patient's vital signs. Which of the following will the nurse note on a patient who is dehydrated?
    a. Bounding pulse
    b. hypothermia
    c. Tachycardia
    d. Decreased respiratory rate

37. A patient is being examined by the nurse. The patient, a known chronic alcoholic, is complaining of difficulty breathing and fatigue. The nurse notices that the patient's abdomen is distended. Upon palpation of the abdomen, the nurse feels a fluctuant sensation. Which of the following is a correct documentation entry for the patient's enlarged abdomen?
    a. Distended abdomen due to overeating
    b. Enlarged abdomen due to constipation
    c. Distended abdomen due to lack of iron
    d. (+) ascites

38. A patient who came in for his annual checkup has their weight and height taken. The patient is 172 cm tall and weighs 70 kg. Calculate the patient's Body Mass Index (BMI).
    a. 29.3
    b. 14.9
    c. 27.3
    d. 23.7

39. A patient's Body Mass Index (BMI) is 28.2. Which of the following appropriately describes the patient's weight status?
    a. Underweight
    b. Normal
    c. Overweight
    d. Extreme obesity

40. Which of the following patients need to limit their sodium intake to 1,500 mg a day?
    a. A 54-year old patient with hypertension

b. A 5-year-old patient with upper respiratory tract infection
c. A 17-year old patient with mild diarrhea
d. A 35-year old post-partum mother

41. A patient with anorexia nervosa has a BMI of 15.5. Which of the following signs and symptoms would most likely manifest in this patient?
a. Hypertension
b. Amenorrhea
c. hyperkalemia
d. Oily skin

42. A patient was recently diagnosed with bulimia nervosa of the nonpurging type. Which of the following manifestation is UNLIKELY to be observed in the patient?
a. Binge eating
b. Exercise
c. Fasting
d. Induced vomiting

43. A patient undergoing a weight reduction program is doing the recommended exercises. He tells the nurse, "I am giving my best shot, but I realized it's harder than I previously thought." Which stage of the Change Model is the patient in?
a. Precontemplation
b. Contemplation
c. Preparation
d. Action

44. A patient with bone pain has been determined to have a calcium deficiency. Which of the following foods would the nurse recommend to increase the patient's calcium levels?
a. Bacon
b. Carrots
c. Kiwi
d. Kale

45. A patient is on a potassium-restricted diet. Which of the following food items on the patient's meal tray would need to be replaced?
a. Raisin
b. Lettuce
c. Apple
d. Eggplant

ANSWERS

1. B
   Childhood obesity that persists until adulthood increases the risk for Type 2 diabetes, hypertension, dyslipidemia, and carotid artery atherosclerosis. It does not result to hyperthyroidism.

2. B
   A BMI > 95th percentile based on age- and gender-specific BMI charts is considered obesity in children. BMI > the 85th percentile based on age- and gender-specific BMI charts is considered overweight. For adults, a BMI of > 30 is considered obesity and a BMI of 25-29 is considered overweight.

3. B
   Scientific evidence shows that there is leveling of obesity rates in the most recent years as compared to previous years where there are significant increases in rates. There is also a correlation between childhood and adult obesity but childhood obesity does not absolutely result to adulthood obesity. If previously obese children become non-obese as adults, the risk for cardiovascular diseases and type 2 diabetes is the same for those who were never obese.

4. C
   Birth weight doubles by the fourth month of life and triples by the end of the first year. All other options reflect correct concepts.

5. A, B, D
   Breastfeeding has numerous advantages. It prevents overfeeding, reduces risks of allergy and food intolerance and has antibodies. Compared to cow's milk, it contains iron and vitamins C and E.

6. B
   Babies up to 2 years of age should not be fed skimmed or low-fat milk because the babies need essential fatty acids for proper brain development.

7. A, B, C, E
   Reasons for poor nutritional intake in the adolescent includes preference for sweet foods and beverages, processed and fast food, skipping meals and reference for small intake of fruits and vegetables, among others. Due to increased metabolism during adolescence, there should be three main meals and at least 2 snacks in a day.

8. A
   Genetics and inactivity are some factors that are not related to food intake and are contributory to obesity.

9. B
   Sarcopenic obesity is the result of a decrease in muscle mass that is accompanied by an increase

in body fat. Resistance training is recommended to strengthen muscles and reduce body fat.

10. C

Catholics are forbidden to eat pork on Good Friday, the Friday of their Holy Week.

11. C

Seventh Day Adventists do not drink alcoholic beverages and caffeinated drinks.

12. B

A food frequency questionnaire is a nutritional assessment that focuses on which foods the client eats, and how many times those foods are eaten in a day, week or month.

13. A

A food diary is a list of all foods eaten in at least three consecutive days, ideally Thursdays to Saturdays. The client writes all foods consumed right after eating to ensure accuracy.

14. D

Diarrhea and acute infections can cause rapid unintentional weight loss. Exercise, fasting and water therapy are intentional and therefore incorrect.

15. A

When feeding young children, avoid serving foods that are choking hazards. Examples of these foods are hotdog bits, hard candies, popcorn, grapes, small berries, and nuts.

16. A

Factors that can lead to delivering low birth weight babies are multiparity, pregnancy in adolescence, alcohol and drug use during pregnancy, persistent vomiting and anemia among others. Maternal hyperglycemia can cause large-for-gestational-age babies.

17. A

Unintentional weight loss is significant when the client loses >5% of body weight in 1 month, >7.5% of body weight in 3 months, or >10% of body weight in a 6-month period.

18. B

Arm span is more accurate to measure than height in people aged 60 above who are bedridden or confined to a wheelchair. Height decreases in both men and women beginning the age of 30. TSF measurements are not accurate indicators in the elder elderly population because of sagging skin and decreased muscle mass; therefore, BMI and waist to hip ratio are indicators that are more reliable.

19. D

Beefy red tongue indicates vitamin B complex deficiency. A pale tongue indicates iron deficiency.

Magenta or purplish tongue means there is riboflavin deficiency. Atrophied papilla indicate multi-nutritional deficiencies.

20. B

A foamy dry-looking spot on the cornea is called a Bitot's spot. It is caused by Vitamin A deficiency. The patient with Bitot's spot will be given Vitamin A supplementation.

21. B

For proper recovery from wounds or injury, the body needs all nutrients it can get. But to hasten the healing process, the body particularly needs more protein because proteins are the building blocks for tissue repair.

22. D

Fluids have weight. If fluids are retained in the body, the patient gains weight. Malignancy, anorexia, and hyperthyroidism cause weight loss.

23. B

There are many factors that can lead to malnutrition. Some of these factors are the lack of financial resources, old age, lack of teeth, ill-fitting dentures, alcoholism and drug addiction. Adolescence is not a known factor of malnutrition.

24. B

Among the items in the nutrition screening checklist, the parameter, I don't have enough money to buy the food that I need, scores 4 points, indicating that finances play a significant role in meeting the patient's nutritional needs.

25. B

The recommended daily intake of fruits is 2-4 servings a day. For proper nutrition, 6-11 servings of grains and cereals, 3-5 servings of vegetables and 2-3 servings of both meat and dairy are recommended to be included in a person's daily diet.

26. C

Vitamin K is necessary for proper blood clotting. When the body is Vitamin K deficient, there is increased bleeding tendency as manifested by petechia or ecchymosis.

27. D

Iron is a nutrient needed in blood production. Without sufficient iron, the patient will look pale and feel tired most of the time. The patient with iron-deficiency anemia will also have spoon-shaped brittle nails.

28. D

Evident muscle wasting in the patient can be caused by a deficiency of protein, carbohydrates, and fats. The nurse must encourage the intake of foods rich in these nutrients.

29. C

Skin turgor is used to determine the if the patient is dehydrated. The nurse pinches the skin for a few seconds and releases it. When the skin rebounds quickly, the patient is said to have good skin turgor. If on the other hand, the skin is released and slowly recoils back, then the patient has poor skin turgor. Decreased skin turgor is a manifestation of fluid volume deficit.

30. B

Signs of fluid excess in a patient are sudden weight gain, edema, increased BP, bounding pulse, jugular vein distention, rales or crackles, and dyspnea, among others.

31. C

Signs of rapid weight gain in just a few days suggest water retention due to possible cardiac or peripheral vascular disease. It is not related to poor nutritional intake. The cause of edema of the lower extremities needs further assessment.

32. A

During nutrition history-taking, the nurse may ask how many meals and snacks are eaten in a day, inside and outside of the home to determine the patient's food pattern. The nurse may also ask about any special diet or supplements to know more about their food patterns.

33. A

During height measurements, the nurse must ask the patient to remove their shoes and hat, and undo any hairstyle that adds height. The nurse then asks the patient to stand erect, facing away from the stadiometer. Ideally, the stadiometer should be mounted on the wall. Finally, the nurse measures the patient's height.

34. C

A balanced beam scale is calibrated when the counterweights are at zero, and the pointer is at the mid-level or center position.

35. C

An enlarged thyroid suggests possible iodine deficiency or thyroid malfunction or malignancy.

36. C

Dehydrated patients would have tachycardia, a weak pulse, a decreased blood pressure and an elevated temperature.

37. D

Ascites is fluid that has accumulated in the abdomen. It causes abdominal distention. Ascites is a manifestation of several diseases, such as advanced liver, kidney or heart disease. In this case, the patient's alcoholism caused their liver disease. Ascites is a sign of liver failure.

38. D

The formula for calculating Body Mass Index (BMI) is weight in kg divided by the square of height in meters.

BMI= _Weight(kg)_ = __70kg__ = __70kg__ = 23.7
         Height2 (m2)   1.722   2.9584

39. C

People with a BMI of <18.5 are considered underweight. The normal BMI is 18.5 – 24.9. People with a BMI of 25.0 to 29.9 are considered overweight. A BMI of more than 30 is considered obesity.

40. A

The recommended daily allowance of sodium is 2300mg a day. However, people with hypertension, diabetes or kidney disease or those aged 51 years old and above should limit their salt intake to 1,500mg per day.

41. B

Patients with anorexia nervosa would not have enough nutrients, body mass and fat to perform normal body processes. Some of the biologic complications of anorexia nervosa are amenorrhea, hypoglycemia, hypotension, hypokalemia and dry skin, among others.

42. D

Patients with bulimia nervosa of the nonpurging type will engage in binge eating and then compensate with behaviors that reduce weight such as fasting and exercise. They do not induce vomiting, unlike those with the purging type.

43. D

In the action stage of the Change Model, the patient is seen actively performing activities or doing a behavior toward the desired change. The patient may give verbal cues that tell the nurse what they are doing and the challenges they are facing as they act on the change.

44. D

Milk, dairy products and dark leafy vegetables such as collards, mustard greens, and kale are rich in calcium. On the other hand, low to zero calcium content foods are bacon, carrots, and kiwi, among others.

45. A

Raisins are rich in potassium. Patients who are on a potassium-restricted diet should avoid bananas, raisins, apricots and baked beans, among others.

The Integumentary System

Questions

1. The nurse is assessing an elderly client and notices dark red to purplish discoloration on the client's forearm. When assessed further by the nurse, the client states that he occasionally bumps into the door frame. There is no indication of physical abuse. The nurse documents her finding as:
    a. Chloasma
    b. Striae gravidarum
    c. Senile purpura
    d. Vernix caseosa

2. A nurse is caring for a client with melanoma. The nurse knows that certain cultural/racial groups are more prone to developing melanoma than others are. Which cultural/racial group has the highest incidence of melanoma?
    a. Hispanics
    b. Asians
    c. African-Americans
    d. Whites

3. A concerned client comes to the clinic after the scar from her arm laceration has elevated in a matter of weeks that grew beyond the boundaries of the flat scar. The nurse provides correct information by saying that the client's scar has undergone which process?
    a. Skin tag formation
    b. Depigmentation
    c. Melasma development
    d. Keloid formation

4. An elderly client is complaining of painful skin in one area of the chest. Upon careful examination, the nurse notes vesicular lesions on the chest. Which of the following conditions should the nurse suspect?
    a. Eczema
    b. Acne
    c. Herpes zoster
    d. Xerosis

5. Pigmented lesions are a cause of concern especially if changes are noted in a short span of time. The Pneumonic ABCDE is used to guide assessment of pigmented lesion and identify possible melanomas. Which of the following reflects INCORRECT concept on the assessment of pigmented lesions?
    a. Asymmetry or half of the lesion does not look like its other half
    b. Color variation or lesions that have multiple shades of brown, blue, black and red
    c. Discoloration or the appearance of either lighter or darker area around the lesion
    d. Evolution or the rapid changing of the lesion in terms of color, shape, or condition

6. A nurse is assessing pallor in a black client, the nurse would expect the skin of the client to look or appear:
    a. Pale
    b. Yellowish brown
    c. Reddish
    d. Ashen

7. The nurse is assessing a client for nutritional deficiency, especially long standing iron deficiency. Which of the following finding would be consistent with chronic iron-deficiency anemia?
    a. Clubbed nails
    b. Spoon-shaped nails
    c. Diaphoresis
    d. Yellowish tone of the skin

8. A nurse assessing a client with heart failure has edema of the lower extremities. Upon palpation, the nurse leaves a dent on the skin that is about 6mm deep. It takes about 15 seconds for the indentation to rebound. What is the grade of the client's edema?
    a. 1+
    b. 2+
    c. 3+
    d. 4+

9. The nurse is assessing for cyanosis on several clients. Which of the following findings would NOT be a reliable indication of hypoxemia?
    a. Bluish discoloration around the mouth of a neonate
    b. Bluish discoloration of the lips of a Mediterranean client
    c. Yellowish hue to the extremities of a client who sustained trauma to the extremity ten days ago
    d. Bluish hands and feet of a newborn

10. The nurse is examining a client, and notes yellowish discoloration of the skin, sclera and mucous membranes. Which of the following findings will be consistent with hyperbilirubinemia?
    a. Tea-colored urine
    b. Pinkish urine
    c. Fatty stool
    d. Dry mucous membrane

11. A nurse is assessing a newborn. As she turns the baby to the side, she notices that the dependent side is flushed red, while the upper side is pale. Which of the following correctly describe this phenomenon?
    a. Harlequin color change
    b. Erythema toxicum

c. Acrocyanosis
d. Cutis marmorata

12. An elderly client has red brownish raised and rough looking skin lesions on the face and forearms, with silvery plaques on the top. According to the client, a few years back, they were just flat reddish brown skin discoloration. The nurse asks for possible risk factors for this condition. Which of the following is the most appropriate response of the nurse?
    a. "Do you eat shellfish"
    b. "Do you spend a lot of time outdoors?"
    c. "What supplementations are you taking?"
    d. "Do you take steroids?"

13. The nurse notes that the client's skin is yellowish-orange hue especially noticeable in the forehead, palms and soles. Upon further assessment of the sclerae, conjunctiva and oral mucosa, there are no yellowish discolorations. Which of the following findings will be consistent with the client's condition and should NOT cause an alarm to the nurse?
    a. Tea-colored urine
    b. Grey colored stool
    c. Dull pain in the right upper quadrant of the abdomen
    d. Massive intake of carrot and mango shake

14. A client, who is complaining of extreme fatigue and dizziness when standing, also noted bronzing or tanning of the skin, especially the scars, areas around the nipples, inner thighs, buttock and axillae. Which of the following conditions does the nurse consider?
    a. Uremia
    b. Addison's disease
    c. Hyperbilirubinemia
    d. Vitiligo

15. A mother brings her child to the clinic because of lesions on the face that started a week ago looking like an 'insect bite' that become fluid filled. In matter of days, it has spread. The lesions have erythematous base and honey-colored crusts. The nurse knows that the manifestations are consistent with which condition?
    a. Impetigo
    b. Vitiligo
    c. Eczema
    d. Atopic dermatitis

16. A nurse is caring for a client with rubeola or measles. Which of the following skin characteristics indicates rubeola?
    a. Red-purplish maculopapular rash that starts after a few days of fever appearing first on the face and then gradually spreading all over the body

b. Pink, finer papular rash appearing from the face and spreading all over the body
c. Vesicular lesions appearing first on the trunk that later erupts, crusts and scabs over
d. Erythematous lesions that forms vesicles with irregular borders; may weep, crust over and itch intensely

17. A client comes to the clinic complaining about some lesions on her upper lip. Upon further questioning, the client denies any fever before appearance of the lesion, although she noted some tingling and pulling sensation in the area where the lesion appeared. The lesions started as a tight vesicle that scabbed over. Which condition is the client most likely suffering from?
    a. Herpes zoster
    b. Labial herpes simplex
    c. Tinea Versicolor
    d. Erythema migrans

18. A nurse is assessing the client's skin when she notices a bull's eye or target rash. Which of the following is an appropriate response by the nurse to assess for possible causes of the rash?
    a. "Have you been exposed to a person recently who have had similar rash?"
    b. "Have you been to the woods lately?"
    c. "What antibiotics did you take the past week?"
    d. "Does the rash itch at night?"

19. A teenager has developed tinea pedis. Which of the following reflects a correct concept of tinea pedis or athlete's foot?
    a. There is severe itch of the heels of the feet
    b. The lesions are small and fluid-filled found more in between toes
    c. The feet are always dry
    d. Cooler climate encourage the condition

20. A nurse looks at the pressure ulcer of the client on the buttocks. She notes that the skin is intact with localized erythema that does not blanch when pressed. What stage is the pressure ulcer at?
    a. Stage 1
    b. Stage 2
    c. Stage 3
    d. Stage 4

21. The nurse reviews the anatomy of the skin and knows that the following are functions of the skin EXCEPT:
    a. It allows excretion of products of metabolism such as uric acid and carbon dioxide.
    b. Helps in regulating body temperature
    c. Serves as a protective barrier against pathogens and injuries
    d. Provides sensory perception (touch, pain, pressure, temperature)

22. The nurse is assessing jaundice on a dark-skinned baby. The nurse is sure to check which part of the baby to observe for the yellowish discoloration?
    a. The sclera
    b. The palms
    c. The gums and inner lips
    d. The clavicle

23. Which of the following when observed in a newborn necessitates informing the physician immediately?
    a. Peripheral cyanosis
    b. Central cyanosis
    c. Jaundice after 5 days
    d. Dark round spots on the lower back and buttocks

24. The nurse is seen pinching the forearm of the client and observing the skin spring back. Which assessment parameter is the nurse checking?
    a. Mobility and turgor
    b. Presence of Edema
    c. Observing for blanching of the skin
    d. Checking for petechiae

25. A client with right-sided heart failure is admitted to your unit. You notice that there is edema of the lower extremities. When you press the swelling on the extremities, there is a 4mm indentation. How would you describe the edema of the client?
    a. Dependent edema, non pitting
    b. Anasarca, pitting +2
    c. Periorbital edema, pitting +2
    d. Dependent edema, +2

26. A nurse is assessing a client complaining of painful blister-like lesions on his chest. The vesicles are painful to touch and confined to just the upper right side of his chest. Upon history taking, the client has had chicken pox when he was a child. Based on his history and the description of his skin lesions, what disorder would the nurse primarily suspect the client has?
    a. Reinfection with chicken pox
    b. Herpes zoster
    c. Psoriasis
    d. Atopic dermatitis

27. A community nurse is tending to a 75-year old bedridden patient. He is incontinent and is wearing adult diapers. His wife, a frail 77-year old woman states that she is having difficulty changing his diapers due to his sheer size. The patient gets changed only when the daughter helps out after office hours. The nurse notes on inspection of the buttocks that the skin is soaked with urine, but

the skin is still intact. Which of the following is the client at highest risk of developing?
a.   Skin infection
b.   Urinary tract infection
c.   Incontinence
d.   Skin maceration

28.   A patient with full blown AIDS is severely emaciated. The nurse aims to assess his risk for developing pressure ulcer. Which assessment tool is most appropriate to use?
a.   The CAGE questionnaire
b.   Faces scale
c.   The Braden scale
d.   The Glasgow coma scale

29.   A housewife from a depressed area of the city summons a community health nurse to check on her husband who is confined to bed because of advanced Alzheimer's disease. She states that her husband seems to sleep most of the days and nights. He is wearing an adult diaper that is changed just once a day. She is concerned that her husband is developing a wound on his sacral area. Upon assessment, the nurse notes that the wound has extended into the muscles. Which of the following assessment findings is accurate?
a.   A high Braden scale score
b.   Stage 2 pressure ulcer
c.   Stage 3 pressure ulcer
d.   Stage 4 pressure ulcer

30.   Upon inspection of the hair of a school-aged child, the nurse sees very tiny oval-shaped silvery bits attached to the hair shafts. The child is constantly scratching her head and is unkempt. Which of the following is the most accurate assessment finding?
a.   The child has dandruff
b.   The child is suffering from psoriasis
c.   The child's hair is extremely dirty
d.   The child has pediculosis capitis

31.   A patient is diagnosed with long-standing iron-deficiency anemia. In addition to pallor of the skin and easy fatigability, which of the following characteristics of the nails do you expect to see?
a.   Clubbing of the nails
b.   Spoon-shaped nails
c.   Pitted nails
d.   Thick, dry, layered nails

32.   A 60-year old farmer is seeking consultation for a mole that has gone bigger in the past month. Client states it has become lighter in color and seems to spread. As the nurse assesses the client, the nurse understands that among skin lesions, which has the highest chance of being malignant

and lethal?
a. Actinic keratosis
b. Basal cell carcinoma
c. Melanoma
d. Telangiectasias

33. A 9-year old boy is accompanied by his mother to the clinic because of skin lesions that seem to itch severely especially at night. Upon close examination, the nurse notes tiny brown burrows, papules and pustules aligned in a linear fashion. She noted them on the hands, wrists and across the abdomen. Which of the following is the most likely cause of the boy's lesions and itch?
a. Tinea corporis
b. Pediculosis corporis
c. Scabies
d. Small pox

34. Freckles are an example of what skin lesion?
a. Papule
b. Vesicle
c. Macule
d. Nodule

35. A nurse is assessing a client with systemic lupus erythematosus. The nurse notices a reddish rash on the both cheeks that crosses the bridge of the nose. What rash is the nurse referring to?
a. Urticarial rash
b. Butterfly rash
c. Slapped cheeks
d. Periorbital purpura

36. A patient recently diagnosed with psoriasis is seen by the clinic nurse. The nurse notes scaly reddish, silvery patches on the client's elbows and knees. Which statement by the patient necessitates further nursing intervention?
a. "I am careful not to scratch these scales."
b. "They are quite unsightly. I usually wear long sleeves and pants."
c. "I am sure to garden first thing in the morning, when the sunshine is light, wearing only cotton clothes."
d. "I now know how to apply the ointment my friend gave me."

37. The nurse is unsure of a lesion she found on her client's leg. She consults a nursing literature and decides if her client has a spider angioma or a spider nevi. Which of the following is an accurate distinction between the two?
a. Spider angioma: There is positive pulsation on the center of the lesion; spider nevi: no pulsation
b. Spider angioma: often seen in the lower extremities; spider nevi: usually found in the face and

upper trunk

c. Spider angioma: accompanies varicose veins; spider nevi: accompanies pregnancy, liver disorders

d. Spider angioma: bluish in color; spider nevi: reddish in color

38. A client recently traveled to a tropical country. He stated that he didn't enjoy much of his stay because he'd been bugged by mosquitoes. After a few days, he developed fever, joint pains, stomach pains and is passing black stools. He was tested positive for dengue hemorrhagic fever. Which of the following lesion would the nurse expect to see on the client's body?
    a. Ecchymosis
    b. Spider angiomas
    c. Spider nevi
    d. Petechiae.

39. A client had recently been involved in a car accident. He is recuperating in the hospital. The nurse notes a purplish discoloration of the skin with some tinge of yellow and green. The client states the area is still painful. Which skin lesion is the client most likely exhibiting?
    a. Petechiae
    b. Purpura
    c. Ecchymosis
    d. Urticaria

40. A patient with HIV has advanced to the AIDS stage. Upon examination of the oral mucosa, the nurse notes white patches on the oral mucosa and the tongue. Which of the following is the most likely cause of the patches?
    a. Oral candidiasis/moniliasis
    b. Koplik's spot
    c. Herpes simplex
    d. Vitiligo

41. The nurse is performing a physical examination on a patient and is assessing the patient's sensation of touch, pain, temperature, and pressure on their skin. The nurse's findings are aligned with which function of the skin?
    a. It provides non-verbal cues
    b. It allows sensory perception
    c. It gives identity
    d. It allows repair of wounds

42. A patient is being examined by the nurse. The nurse notices that the patient's skin is bluish. Which of the following should the nurse do to determine if the bluish discoloration is central or peripheral in nature?
    a. Check oxygen levels in the patient's arterial blood

 b. Check if the hands and feet are bluish

 c. Check if the environment is warm

 d. Check if the skin is warm

43. The nurse wants to determine if the patient has jaundice. Which of the following sources of light is best to use to assess for jaundice?

 a. Light coming from a penlight

 b. Natural light

 c. Yellowish artificial light

 d. Tangential lighting

44. The nurse is assessing an African-American male for jaundice. Which of the following is the best way of assessing for jaundice in this patient?

 a. Check the color of the sclera

 b. Check the color of the hard palate

 c. Check the color of the arms

 d. Check the color of the legs

45. Which of the following conditions can cause the skin to feel cool to touch?

 a. Hypothyroidism

 b. Hyperthyroidism

 c. Cellulitis

 d. Allergic reaction

46. A nurse is assessing the lower extremities of the patient with chronic heart failure. Both legs are swollen. The nurse exerts pressure on one leg with the tip of their finger and finds that they could make a depression 6mm deep. Which of the following is the correct documentation of the nurse's findings?

 a. Non-pitting edema

 b. 1+ pitting edema

 c. 2+ pitting edema

 d. 3+ pitting edema

47. Which of the following predispose a patient to pressure sore development? Select all that apply.

 a. Increased metabolism

 b. Impaired mobility

 c. Shearing forces

 d. Moisture

 e. Dry skin

48. A nurse used the Braden Scale to assess a patient's risk for pressure sore development using parameters such as sensory perception, moisture, activity, mobility, nutrition, and friction and

sheer. The patient scored 11. Which of the following is the correct interpretation of the patient's pressure sore risk assessment?

a. The patient has no risk
b. There is a mild risk
c. There is a moderate risk
d. There is a high risk

49. The patient who is being seen by the nurse in the clinic has a pearly white lesion on the face that looks translucent. The patient tells the nurse that they have noticed it several months before and has not changed much in those times. Which of the following would the nurse likely suspect of the patient's skin condition?

a. Basal cell carcinoma
b. Squamous cell carcinoma
c. Melanoma
d. Dermatitis

50. Which of the following is NOT a risk factor for the development of melanoma?

a. Heavy sun exposure
b. Severe allergies, especially in childhood
c. Atypical moles
d. Immunosuppression

51. A nurse is assessing a patient's mole using the ABCDE-EFG method. The mole has changed rapidly in the last three months, and is now 7mm in diameter, with irregular borders. It is discolored with gradations of blue and black. Which of the following is a correct documentation entry for the nurse's findings?

a. A- 7mm
b. B- irregular borders
c. C- changing rapidly
d. E- gradations of blue and black

52. A nurse is assessing the patient's face for erythema. In which of the following situations would the nurse most likely observe the presence of erythema?

a. Fifth disease
b. Decreased venous return
c. Dehydration
d. Carotenemia

53. A male Caucasian patient comes to the clinic for a wellness check-up. As the nurse performs a general survey and inspects the patient's skin, the nurse notices a yellowish hue of the palms and the skin. Which of the following will suggest to the nurse that the patient has carotenemia and NOT jaundice?

a. The patient's lips are pale
b. The patient's soles are pale
c. The patient's sclerae are yellow
d. The patient's sclerae are white

54. The nurse is assessing the skin on a patient's back. She noticed two light brown patches on the skin about 1 cm in diameter, not raised but with irregular borders. Which of the following refers to the patient's skin condition?
a. Acanthosis nigricans
b. Tinea versicolor
c. Café-Au-Lait spots
d. Vitiligo

55. A patient is being seen by the nurse in the clinic. The nurse's assessment of her skin suggests vitiligo. Which of the following descriptions of skin conditions is consistent with vitiligo?
a. Desquamated painful skin
b. Scaly skin with white plaques
c. Depigmented skin that appears extensive making it very apparent on the patient's face and arms
d. Presence of hypopigmented, slightly scaly macules found on the neck and upper arms

56. A nurse is caring for a patient with atopic eczema. In which of the following locations would the nurse most likely note the patient's skin lesions?
a. Extensor surfaces
b. Flexor surfaces
c. Anterior and posterior chest
d. Face

57. A patient comes to the emergency department with a fever. The patient complains of malaise. As the nurse examines the patient's skin, she notices a target-shaped reddish discoloration in the patient's inner upper arm. The patient further claims that they had a camping trip two days before. Which of the following conditions does the target-shaped skin lesion suggest?
a. Mycosis fungoides
b. Herpes simplex
c. Tinea versicolor
d. Lyme disease

58. Which of the following lesions will have an annular or arciform shape?
a. Tinea faciale
b. Small-vessel vasculitis
c. Herpes zoster
d. Tinea corporis

59. A university male student comes to the clinic for his annual checkup. The student complains of severe itching of his toes, especially the area in between the digits. Upon inspection, the nurse notes linear cracks in the skin; some have signs of minimal bleeding. The student claims that he uses the gym shower. Which type of depressed skin lesion best describes the patient's skin condition?
    a. Erosion
    b. Excoriations
    c. Fissure
    d. Ulcer

60. A novice nurse is assessing the skin of the patient's thighs and is now unsure which vascular lesion the patient has. Which of the following will correctly guide the nurse's assessments?
    a. Spider angioma – pressure on the center does not cause it to blanch
    b. Spider vein – bluish, diffuse pressure blanches the veins
    c. Cherry angioma – fiery red, solitary, with variable shape
    d. Spider vein – ruby red, round and flat

61. A patient is on their third day of recovery from a blunt trauma incident caused by a baseball bat to the arm. The lesion of the patient's arms appear bluish and purplish and is relatively large, covering most of the outer upper arms. When pressed, the patient feels pain, but the area does not blanch with pressure, and no pulsations are noted. Which type of lesions does the patient most likely have?
    a. Petechiae
    b. Purpura
    c. Ecchymosis
    d. Spider vein

62. A patient has been recently diagnosed with a peripheral vascular disease. Which of the following manifestations are consistent with this condition?
    a. Striae, purpura or ecchymoses, moon facie
    b. Strawberry tongue, cherry red lips, desquamation of the palms and soles
    c. Dystrophic brittle toenails, hairless shins, pallor of the extremities
    d. Jaundice, spider angiomas, terry nails, pruritus

63. A 5-year-old patient presents to the pediatric clinic with fever and generalized vesicular lesions. The mother of the patient described the lesions as similar to dewdrops on a leaf and the first vesicles that appeared were on the abdomen. The patient is seen scratching the lesions. Which of the following lesions does the patient most likely have?
    a. Varicella
    b. Rubeola
    c. Rubella

d. Coxsackie A

64. A nurse is visiting an older patient in their home. Upon assessment, the nurse finds pressure ulcers on the patient's buttocks and bony prominences of the lower extremities. There is full-thickness skin loss with tissue destruction and necrosis. The patient's muscles are exposed. Which of the following is the correct staging of the patient's pressure ulcer?
a. Stage I
b. Stage II
c. Stage III
d. Stage IV

65. A nurse is assessing the digits of a patient with a diagnosis of congenital heart disease. The nurse notes that the patient's fingernails are curved downward and does not form a relatively straight line with the nail fold. Upon palpation, the nurse finds the nailbeds spongy. Which of the following nail conditions does the patient most likely have?
a. Paronychia
b. Clubbing of the fingers
c. Onycholysis
d. Terry nails

ANSWERS

1. C

    Senile purpura are bruise-looking dark red to purplish discoloration on the client's forearm caused by minor trauma. This happens because of the fragility of the superficial blood vessels.

2. D

    The whites have 10 times higher incidence of melanoma than African Americans and about 5 times higher than Hispanics.

3. D

    Keloid formation is the elevation and thickening of a scar that grows beyond the boundary of the flat scar.

4. C

    Herpes zoster or shingles is caused by the reactivation of dormant varicella virus in a nerve branch. It is manifested by skin pain and vesicular lesions along the area of innervation by the affected nerves.

5. C

    ABCDE in pigmented lesion assessment stands for Assymetry (half of the lesion does not look like its other half, Border irregularity (poorly defined or irregular margin), Color variation (have multiple shades of brown, blue, black and red, Diameter greater than 6mm and Elevation or evolution (rapid changing of the lesion in terms of color, shape, or condition)

6. D

    Assessing pallor in a black client can be challenging at first. The nurse should look for the skin tone where a reddish hue is reduced. In this case, the client would appear gray or ashen.

7. B

    Spoon-shaped nails, pallor, easy fatigability, increased heart rate and dizziness are some of the manifestations of chronic iron deficiency anemia.

8. D

    Grading of edema are as follows

    1+ Mild pitting; slight indentation; no perceptible swelling of the leg

    2+ Moderate pitting; indentation subsides rapidly

    3+ Deep pitting; indentation remains for a short time; leg looks swollen

    4+ Very deep pitting; indentation lasts a long time; leg is very swollen

9. B

    Mediterranean people have a natural bluish hue to the lips and therefore assessing for cyanosis by looking at the lips is not reliable. Circumoral cyanosis in a neonate is a sure sign of hypoxemia.

Yellowish skin on a previously traumatized skin indicates resolution of an ecchymosis. Bluish hands and feet in a newborn is called acrocyanosis and is normal.

10. A

People with hyperbilirubinemia will have yellowish discoloration of the skin, sclera and mucous membranes. Because conjugation of bilirubin is impaired and bile pigments remain in the blood, the skin appears yellowish, the stool become clay or grey colored, and urine will be dark or tea-colored.

11. A

Harlequin color change occurs when a newborn is turned to the side, and the dependent side becomes flushed red, while the upper side becomes pale.

12. B

The client's manifestations are consistent with actinic keratosis and they are caused by sun exposure. Asking if the client spends a lot of time outdoors assesses this risk factor.

13. D

The client's manifestations are consistent with carotenemia, or the increased amounts of carotenoids in the blood due to the consumption of carotene rich foods such as carrots, mango and papaya.

14. B

Addison's disease is a disease of the adrenal gland wherein there is inadequate production of cortisol and aldosterone. The client feels weak and dizzy and will have hypertension, hyponatremia, hyperkalemia and hypercalcemia. There is also marked bronzing of the skin especially the scars, areas around the nipples, inner thighs, buttock and axillae.

15. A

Impetigo is a highly infectious bacterial infection of the skin that starts as a fluid-filled vesicle that erupts to form an erythematous base with honey-colored crusts when the lesions dry.

16. A

Rubeola or measles is characterized by red-purplish maculopapular rash that starts after a few days of fever appearing first on the face and then gradually spreading all over the body. Option B describes German measles or Rubella, option C describes varicella zoster or chicken pox and option D describes atopic dermatitis.

17. B

The lesions of labial herpes simplex or cold sores are found on the lips. There is tingling and pulling sensation in the area where the lesion appears. The lesion starts as a tight vesicle that scabs over.

18. B

A bull's eye or target rash is characteristic of Lyme's disease, caused by a ricketssia transmitted by deer ticks. Asking if the client has been to the woods or if he has gone camping will help provide clues to the client's condition.

19. B

Tinea pedis or athlete's foot is a fungal infection that manifests as lesions that are small and fluid-filled in between toes. There is intense itch. Warm environment, moist, covered feet encourage the growth of fungi that cause tinea pedis.

20. A

Stage 1 pressure ulcer: the skin is intact with localized erythema that does not blanch when pressed
Stage 2: there is erosion of the dermis or epidermis, area painful and erythematous
Stage 3: The ulceration extends to the subcutaneous tissue, appears whitish, creamy
Stage 4: The ulceration extends to the muscles and bones; may have tunneling, foul odor

21. A

The skin does not excrete carbon dioxide. It excretes water, electrolytes, sugar and uric acid

22. C

Assessing jaundice in dark-skinned babies is a challenge because their color makes it difficult to see the yellowish tint. It is best to check the gums and inner lips for jaundice. If still in doubt, bilirubin test should be performed

23. B

Central cyanosis is a bluish tint to the skin of the entire body especially observable in the tongue and mucosa. It signifies decreased oxygenation and is a serious condition that needs immediate medical attention. A, C, and D are normal occurrences. (A) is due to decreased capillary flow, (B) is called physiologic jaundice and (D) is also known as Mongolian spots.

24. A

Lifting the skin of the client and watching how fast it springs back is assessing for mobility and turgor. Normally, the pinched skin promptly goes back into place. Poor turgor signifies dehydration.

25. D

Dependent edema is fluid accumulation in the interstitial spaces of the lower part of the body (the legs, ankles and sacrum). Pitting edema can be translocated when pressed and will leave an indentation mark. If the depression made is 2mm, the scale is +1; 4mm: +2, 6mm: +3, 8mm: +4. Anasarca is generalized edema.

26. B

The lesions of herpes zoster appear as serous fluid filled vesicles that are confined within a demarcated area of the body and are painful to touch. They can be mistaken for chickenpox because the lesions of both look the same. In chickenpox however, the lesion spreads all over the body and are not painful.

27. D

Skin maceration is the softening and breaking down of the skin due to prolonged exposure to moisture or due to soaking.

28. C

The Braden scale is a tool used to assess risk factors for developing pressure sores. It provides a score for every level of the following parameters: sensory perception, moisture, activity, mobility, nutrition, friction and shear. The lower the Braden score, the higher the risk.

29. D

The client has stage 4 pressure ulcers when the extent of damage involves muscles, bones and tendons. Reddish intact skin is stage 1. With skin involvement forming a shallow crater, it is at stage 2. If the crater goes deeper to involve fats and subcutaneous tissues, it is at stage 3. The client's bed sore coincides with a low Braden scale score.

30. D

The child has pediculosis capitis or head lice. The very tiny oval-shaped silvery bits attached to the hair shafts near the roots are the eggs or nits of the adult lice. Lice infestation can cause severe itching that lead to excoriation.

31. B

Spoon-shaped nails or koilonychia are characteristic of certain diseases such as iron-deficiency anemia, hemochromatosis, diabetes, lupus and Reynaud's phenomenon

32. C

Melanomas arise from the pigment-producing melanocytes in the epidermis, that which gives the skin its color. They easily and quickly metastasize and are the most lethal of all skin cancers.

33. C

The symptoms are typical of scabies. The female mite migrates and burrows its eggs into the skin. Allergic reaction to the mites causes the severe itching that is worse at night.

34. C

A macule is a small (less than 1cm) flat discoloration of the skin that is not palpable. A papule is a solid raised lesion that has defined borders and is also less than 1cm in diameter. If the solid raised lesion is bigger than 1cm, it is called a nodule. Vesicles are small fluid-filled lesions.

35. B

Patients with systemic lupus erythematosus exhibit a familiar rash that is reddish and is spread across the cheeks. The lesion crosses the bridge of the nose, giving a butterfly-like appearance.

36. D

Patients with psoriasis do not self medicate with any ointment as this may cause worsening of symptoms, or of acquiring a skin infection.

37. A

Spider angiomas are reddish with a central body and radiating legs/rays. The central part pulsates. They are seen in the upper parts of the body and accompany pregnancy, liver diseases, or could be a normal finding in some. On the other hand, spider nevi are bluish, often found in the lower extremities and are near varicose veins. There is no pulsation noted.

38. D

Petechiae are tiny (pinpoint to 3mm) deep red, purplish red lesions that may be rounded or irregular. Petechiae suggest a bleeding disorder, in this case, is apparent in dengue hemorrhagic fever.

39. C

Ecchymosis is a purple or purplish blue lesion that fades to greenish, yellowish, and brownish hue with time. It comes in variable sizes and may have a central subcutaneous nodule (hematoma).

40. A

Oral candidiasis is caused by a yeast infection and presents as white nontender patches in the mouth. It is common in those taking antibiotics and steroids and in immunocompromised clients.

41. B

The skin has many functions among which is sensing touch, pain, temperature, and pressure. Collectively, these are called sensory perception. The skin also acts as a barrier to harmful substances in the environment and acts as a thermoregulator. It synthesizes Vitamin D, gives nonverbal cues, provides identity, and allows wound healing and excretion of metabolic wastes.

42. A

The bluish discoloration of the skin is called cyanosis. It is caused by an increase in deoxyhemoglobin concentration in the cutaneous blood vessels. Central cyanosis indicates overall decreased oxygen levels in the blood. On the other hand, peripheral cyanosis is caused by slow or decreased blood flow but the rate of cellular use of oxygen remains the same. Peripheral cyanosis is caused by anxiety or a cold environment. Central cyanosis has a much greater clinical significance.

43. B

To assess for jaundice correctly, the nurse must use natural light because yellowish artificial lights can mask jaundice.

44. B

Jaundice can be difficult to assess in dark-skinned patients. Dark-skinned individuals have dirty sclerae, which appear yellowish. The nurse may check the patient's hard palate with a bright light instead.

45. A

The nurse will expect to feel a generalized coolness of the skin in patients with hypothyroidism. On the other hand, patients with fever, hyperthyroidism, cellulitis or allergic reaction of the skin will exhibit increased warmth on their skin.

46. D

In pitting edema, the interstitial water can be translocated. The nurse's fingertip, when pressed on the patient's edematous skin can create a pit. A depression of 2mm is scaled 1+. A depression of 4mm is scaled 2+. A 3+ scale means that the depression is 6mm deep and a 4+ scale means that the depression is 8mm deep.

47. B, C, D

Pressure sores develop when the compression of blood vessels caused by prolonged immobility prevents the flow of blood to the skin. Shearing forces, such as dragging and sliding movements, cause the soft tissues to break. Friction and moisture also contribute to the development of pressure sores.

48. D

A score of 10-12 on the Braden Scale indicates that the patient has a high risk of developing pressure sores. The following are the scores and their corresponding risk scale: 19-23: no risk, 15-18: mild risk, 13-14: moderate risk, 9 or lower: very high risk.

49. A

Basal carcinomas originate from the lowest level of the epidermis in areas usually exposed to the sun, such as the face and the neck. The lesion appears pearly white with some translucence, and it grows slowly.

50. B

Melanoma is a type of skin cancer that originates from the melanocytes, which are responsible for skin pigmentation. It is the most lethal type, and it metastasizes quickly. Risk factors for its development include UV rays from heavy sun exposure, severe sunburns during childhood, atypical moles, red or light hair, male gender and family history, among others.

51. B

The ABCDE-EFG method of assessing moles are strongly sensitive and specific to melanoma. A- stands for asymmetry, B- borders that are irregular, C- color change, D- diameter, E-evolving fast, and for aggressive nodular melanomas: E- elevated, F-firm when palpated and G- Growing progressively.

52. A
Erythema is the reddish hue of the skin due to increased blood flow. It is observed in inflammation, glove and stocking syndrome, and in erythema infectiosum or also known as fifth's disease or slapped cheek disease.

53. D
A yellowish hue of the skin is typical of both carotenemia and jaundice. Carotenemia is caused by the high consumption of carrots and other yellow fruits. In carotenemia, the yellowish color is very noticeable especially on the palms, but the sclerae remain white. On the other hand, jaundice is a manifestation of liver and biliary disease, and the yellowish discoloration is also noted in the sclerae.

54. C
Café-Au-Lait spots are slightly pigmented macules with irregular borders. They usually have a diameter of 0.5-1.5 cm. If the spots appear in groups and are larger than 1.5 cm, the patient should be evaluated for neurofibromatosis.

55. C
Vitiligo is a condition in which the melanocytes are impaired in some areas of the skin. Large areas of the patient's will appear depigmented or white.

56. B
The skin lesions in atopic eczema are usually found on flexor surfaces, such as behind the knees and the fold between the upper and lower arms.

57. D
Target-shaped reddish lesions are typical of Lyme disease. There is a central reddish lesion with a concentric reddish ring around the central lesion.

58. A
Annular or arciform lesions have a circular shape. The lesions of tinea faciale are annular.

59. C
Fissures are linear cracks in the skin, often seen in an overly dry skin that has been folded then stretched. A typical example of a fissure is that of the lesions caused by tinea pedis or Athlete's foot.

60. B
A spider vein is bluish in color and presents in a variety of sizes. The shapes are variable, too.

Diffuse pressure blanches the veins. They are often seen on the legs and the anterior chest. Spider angiomas are fiery red and relatively small (up to 2 cm). It has a central body that pulsates. Pressure on its body can cause blanching. Cherry angiomas, on the other hand, are bright or ruby red in color and are round and flat or slightly raised. They have no clinical significance.

61. C
    Ecchymoses are purplish or bluish discoloration of the skin caused by blood that has accumulated outside the vessels secondary to trauma or bleeding disorders. They appear in variable sizes but are usually larger than 3mm. It has no pulsations and does not blanch with pressure.

62. C
    Peripheral vascular diseases have many skin manifestations. A patient with a peripheral vascular disease would have dystrophic brittle toenails, bluish or pale extremities and hairless shins. Option A sites the signs and symptoms of Cushing's disease. Option B describes Kawasaki disease. Option D are the manifestations of liver diseases.

63. A
    Varicella lesions are generalized, vesicular and pruritic. They appear like dewdrops. The lesions start appearing in crops on the trunk.

64. D
    A patient's pressure ulcer is at Stage IV when there is full thickness skin loss, and the damage is extensive to involve also the subcutaneous tissue, muscles, and bones. Tissue necrosis is evident. Tunneling may undermine assessment, when under the seemingly small skin ulcer are tunnels of necrotic tissues.

65. B
    Clubbing of the fingers is caused by bulbous swelling of the nail base wherein the angle between the nail and proximal nail fold exceeds 180 degrees so that the nails appear to be curved downwards. It is mostly observed in patients with congenital heart disease, interstitial lung disease, lung cancer, and in inflammatory diseases of the bowels and cancers.

The Head and the Neck

Questions

1. A client comes to the clinic complaining of headache. When assessed further, the client describes the pain as viselike felt at the entire forehead and moderate in intensity lasting for hours. She confides that she had been feeling stressed out at work lately. What type of headache is the client most likely experiencing?
   a. Migraine
   b. Cluster
   c. Tension
   d. Sinus

2. A male client who has first-degree heart block returns to the clinic for a follow up checkup. He states that two days before, as he was climbing up the stairs, he felt suddenly faint, weak-kneed, and almost lost consciousness. Which condition most likely caused the client's manifestations?
   a. Presyncope
   b. Vertigo
   c. Disequilibrium
   d. Meniere's disease

3. As the nurse is assessing the client's neck, she notes two enlarged cervical lymph nodes that are fixed and immovable. Which of the following is the priority nursing action?
   a. Document accordingly
   b. Inform the physician of your findings
   c. Put some hot compress
   d. Massage gently

4. A client who has laryngeal cancer comes to the clinic for further evaluation. The nurse notes that a large tumor is evident on the right side of the throat. Which of the following assessment findings will most likely be consistent with the client's condition?
   a. Tracheal deviation to the right
   b. Tracheal deviation to the left
   c. Barking cough
   d. Enlarged immovable lymph nodes on the left base of the nec

5. A novice nurse is caring for a newborn who has just been delivered. She notes swelling on the baby's scalp. Which of the following reflects a correct concept on caput succedaneum and cephalhematoma?
   a. Cephalhematoma: soft elevated part of the scalp that does not cross the suture line
   b. Cephalhematoma: it is bleeding under the scalp that resolves within 48 hours
   c. Caput succedaneum: subperiosteal hemorrhage
   d. Caput succedaneum: takes weeks to resolve

6. A nurse is assessing the fontanels of the 1 month-old neonate who has been experiencing diarrhea for three days now. Which of the following will the nurse's UNLIKELY finding?
    a. Bulging fontanels
    b. Soft triangular posterior fontanel
    c. Soft diamond-shaped anterior fontanel
    d. Sunken fontanel

7. A mother entering the second trimester came to the clinic concerned that some discoloration on her forehead and cheeks are becoming darker and more prominent. She fears that the discoloration may signify a skin disease. What is the most appropriate response of the nurse?
    a. "I will refer you to the dermatologist"
    b. "That is called chloasma. It is caused by hyperpigmentation of skin on the forehead and cheeks that should gradually disappear after delivery."
    c. "You need to increase your intake of Vitamin A"
    d. "That is an expected sign of pregnancy called striae gravidarum."

8. An elderly client presents to the emergency room complaining of pain on both sides of the head. Upon assessments, the nurse notes that the vessels at both sides of the forehead are dilated, tortuous, hardened and tender to palpation. The nurse suspects which condition?
    a. Mumps
    b. Lymphadenopathy
    c. Grave's disease
    d. Temporal arteritis

9. A nurse is assessing several newborns and infants. Which of the following findings will warrant further evaluation?
    a. Closed posterior fontanel at 4 months of age
    b. Tonic neck reflex at 2 months of age
    c. Some head lag at 5 months of age
    d. Soft part of the scalp that does not cross the suture line right after delivery of the newborn

10. A 1-year old child is brought to the clinic for evaluation after having high-grade fever. Upon assessment, the nurse noted that there is resistance when the neck is flexed and the child becomes more distressed. Based on the client's manifestation, the nurse should create a plan of care that addresses which condition?
    a. Meningitis
    b. Hydrocephalus
    c. Torticollis
    d. Tonic neck

11. A school-aged boy had a very short haircut and the nurse noticed asymmetry of the head, wherein the back of the head looks flat. The client is performing well in school and has no known medical

condition. To which condition does the nurse associate the asymmetry of the cranium?
a. Caput succedaneum
b. Craniosynostosis
c. Plagiocephaly
d. Microcephaly

12. The nurse is caring for a 1-year old child with craniosynostosis. Which of the following information accurately describes the child's condition?
a. The posterior fontanel is still open at 1 year of age
b. One or more cranial sutures have prematurely fused
c. The cranium is symmetrically affected
d. It results to facial asymmetry

13. A 5-month old infant has been diagnosed with hydrocephalus. She has frontal bossing and sunset eyes. Which of the following correctly describes sunset eyes?
a. There is downward rhythmic movement of the eyes
b. There is apparent eye pain at sundown
c. The sclera is yellow-orange in color
d. The sclera is visible above the iris

14. A baby is born of an alcoholic mother. Which of the following is a manifestation of fetal alcohol syndrome?
a. Low set ears
b. Micrognathia
c. Sunset eyes
d. Deformed skull

15. A client has a lump in the throat later diagnosed as goiter. Which of the following client response alerts the nurse to the possible reason for the development of goiter?
a. "We live at the mountains up north. My house is about 3-hour ride away from town."
b. "I love shellfish and salty foods."
c. "I have recurrent infections in my voice box."
d. "I love to eat fried foods and pizza."

16. An elderly client has inflamed parotid glands. Which of the following alerts the nurse to the possible reason for the client's parotitis?
a. Use of diuretic
b. Intake of iodine-rich foods
c. Use of aspirin
d. Trauma

17. A client has been recently diagnosed with Grave's disease. The nurse prepares her teaching plan

to include manifestations of the condition. Which of the following are signs and symptoms of Grave's disease? Select all that apply.
a. Bradycardia
b. Loose bowel movements
c. Excessive sweating
d. Periorbital edema
e. Cold intolerance

18. A client is concerned over her weight gain in the past month. She also noticed that her face, especially her cheeks have become unusually puffy. She has also grown facial hair similar to a moustache. The nurse further assesses the client for which possible condition?
a. Acromegaly
b. Addison disease
c. Grave's disease
d. Cushing disease

19. The nurse is reviewing her concepts of Bell palsy to better care for her client who has been recently diagnosed with it. Which of the following is a sign of Bell palsy?
a. Cannot wrinkle forehead on the affected side
b. The lips on one side dip when the client frowns
c. The lips on both sides turn upward when asked to smile
d. Pain inside the ear

20. The nurse is caring for a client diagnosed with Parkinson disease. Which of the following are signs and symptoms of Parkinson disease? Select all that apply
a. Mask-like facie
b. Drooling
c. Sunken eyeballs
d. Oily skin
e. Bronze skin

21. A nurse is assessing the headache of the client who presented with a ripping pain. The nurse understands that among the types of headache, the one with the highest potential to be fatal is?
a. Tension headache
b. Cluster headache
c. Thunderclap headache
d. Migraine headache

22. Using the OLD CART pneumonic in assessing client's headache, which of the following questions coincides with the "C"?
a. How long has this been going on?
b. When did you first notice the headache?

c. What do you think triggers the headache?

d. Can you describe how it feels like?

23. A 35-year old female seeks consultation regarding her headache. The nurse asks about precipitating factors as part of her assessment of associated manifestations. Which of the following prodromal symptoms alerts the nurse to the possibility that the client is experiencing migraine headaches?

a. Dizziness

b. Aura

c. Pulsating pain

d. Watery eyes

24. The clinic nurse starts to assess a 20-year old's head and neck. The nurse notes palpable lymph nodes by the base of the nape. Which characteristic of lymph nodes in the absence of signs of infection would prompt the nurse to notify the physician immediately?

a. Painful and swollen

b. Painless and immovable

c. Barely palpable

d. Movable and enlarged

25. A nurse observes that a patient has enlarged thyroids. Which accompanying sign would make the nurse suspect that the goiter causes hyperthyroidism?

a. Protruding eyeball

b. Dry sparse hair

c. Dry skin

d. Weight gain

26. A 46-year old female client comes to the clinic and the nurse upon assessing her head and neck notes that she has round puffy cheeks and a moustache-looking hair growth above the lips. She also has striae on her nape. Which disorder would the nurse suspect the client has?

a. Cushing's disease

b. Hypothyroidism

c. Hyperthyroidism

d. Pheochromocytoma

27. When palpating for lymph nodes, the nurse is wise to use which technique to properly assess the patient?

a. Use the fingertips of the second and third fingers

b. Use the finger pads of the second and third fingers

c. Use finger pads of the thumb

d. Use the palm

28. Which of the following assessment findings of clients' head and neck will the nurse prioritize to

inform the physician?
a. Enlarged tonsillar lymph nodes
b. Dry sparse hair
c. Trachea that slightly deviates to the left
d. Prominent facial hair in the female client

29. When palpating the thyroid, the nurse notes that it is enlarged but soft. The client's eyeballs are also protruding. Which disorder is the client most likely suffering from?
a. Thyroid cancer
b. Thyroiditis
c. Grave's disease
d. Hashimoto thyroiditis

30. The community nurse is preparing her materials for health teaching on the prevention of head injuries. Which of the following objects seen in the home alerts the nurse to a potential risk for accidents?
a. Non-slip rugs near the bath tub
b. Gates on the stairs
c. Grab bars in the shower room
d. Infant walker

31. A nurse is teaching a new mother on car safety in the prevention of injury. The nurse understands that the client understood the teaching when the client makes which of the following statements?
a. "The car seat is best placed on the passenger side where I can see the baby clearly."
b. "The car seat should be positioned in the middle back seat, rear-facing."
c. "I should use a convertible car seat and position it front facing."
d. "I need to use a booster seat since my baby is too small."

32. A 4-year old child is brought by his mother to the emergency department because of fever and swelling of the right side of the cheeks up to the area below the ear. The mother is known to be against vaccination. Which of the following disorder should the nurse suspect?
a. Parotitis
b. Tooth abscess
c. Meningitis
d. Herpes simplex

33. The nurse is assessing a 5-year old boy in the outpatient department. The nurse notes that the face as well as the area around the eyes of the child are swollen. The mother states that the child's urine has become bubbly recently. The nurse needs to assess the child further for signs and symptoms of which disease?
a. Nephrotic syndrome
b. Acute glomerulonephritis

    c.   Congestive heart failure
    d.   Cushing's syndrome

34. During a complete physical examination, the nurse noticed that the patient has large hands and dry thick nails. Upon taking vital signs, the nurse notes hypertension. Which of the following head and neck assessment findings alert the nurse to the possibility that the client has acromegaly?
    a.   Protruding eye balls
    b.   Elongated head with jaw prominence
    c.   Moon facies
    d.   Hypopigmentation of the skin

35. A 37-year old client decides to seek medical help due to worsening fatigue and daytime drowsiness. She also states that she recently gained a lot of weight even without a change in diet and activity. The nurse suspects myxedema. Which of the following assessment findings of the head and neck would further support the nurses' speculation?
    a.   Enlarged supraclavicular lymph nodes
    b.   Enlarged, coarse facial features
    c.   Warm moist skin
    d.   Periorbital edema and dry course skin

36. A patient has been recently diagnosed with Grave's disease. The nurse notes upon completion of history and physical examination, that the client has fatigue, hypertension, palpitations, and thin fine hair. In the assessment of the head and neck, the nurse observes that as the client looks down, the client's lids do not follow. The nurse documents this as
    a.   Exophthalmos
    b.   Periorbital edema
    c.   Lid lag
    d.   Ptosis

37. The nurse is completing the assessment of the client's upper body. As she asks the client to perform range of motion of the neck, the client refuses to comply because of tense nape muscles and pain upon slight flexion. The patient's temperature is 39.9C. The nurse promptly institute measures to
    a.   Isolate the client
    b.   Sponge bath the client
    c.   Provide health teaching on the importance of exercise
    d.   Position the client in semi-fowler's.

38. As the nurse is assessing the client's neck, the nurse stops to check the pulse. Which pulse is the nurse palpating?
    a.   Brachial
    b.   Carotid

c. Facial
d. Apical

39. A mother of a 5-year old girl is frantic when she woke up one morning to see her child smiling on one side of the face only. The other half of the child's face seems expressionless. Upon assessment, the nurse notes that as the child raises her eyebrows, the affected side of the forehead remains flat. Which of the following disorder is the child most likely suffering from?
    a. Meningitis
    b. Temporomandibular dysfunction
    c. Stroke
    d. Schizophrenia

40. A mother of a 4-year old girl is rushing to the clinic after she noticed that her child's face has become more distorted in just a matter of hours. When the child smiles, the other half of the child's face seems expressionless. Upon assessment, the nurse notes that as the child raises her eyebrows, the affected side of the forehead remains flat. The mother is anxious to know what is wrong with her daughter. What is the best nursing response?
    a. "Your child has bell's palsy"
    b. "We will have to assess and test further and will let you know as soon as we get the results."
    c. "It might be just the cold weather"
    d. "These are signs of a potential permanent condition. The doctor needs to see her immediately."

41. A male patient is rushed to the emergency department by relatives. As the nurse examines the patient, the patient claims that he has the worst headache of his life. The patient further says that it felt like he was butted with two cymbals. Which of the following is the most immediate action that the nurse should do?
    a. Inform the physician
    b. Gather more data
    c. Administer acetaminophen
    d. Place an ice pack on the patient's forehead

42. A patient is describing their headache to the nurse. According to the patient, it happens once or twice a month, usually after a week-long overtime at the office. The pain is most severe in the temples, and it intensifies over a few hours. Which type of headache is the patient most likely experiencing?
    a. Migraine
    b. Tension
    c. Thunderclap
    d. Cluster

43. A patient tells the nurse that just before their headaches start, they see shimmering zigzags in the shape of a letter 'C'. Which of the following did the patient experience right before the headache?

a. Photophobia
b. Vertigo
c. Aura
d. Meningitis

44. A nurse is assessing several patients. In which of the following patients would the nurse most likely find enlarged lymph nodes of the neck?
    a. The patient with a tooth abscess
    b. The patient with irritable bowel syndrome
    c. The patient with congenital heart disease
    d. The patient with liver disease

45. A patient has been recently diagnosed with hypothyroidism. Which of the following would most likely characterize the patient's hair?
    a. Discolored
    b. Fine and thin
    c. Oily
    d. Dry and coarse

46. A patient is assessing a female patient with suspected Cushing's syndrome. The nurse notes that the patient has rounded cheeks and a fine, moustache-like growth of hair on the patient's face. Which of the following would be the right documentation entries for the patient's facial signs?
    a. Cheek inflammation and spider angioma
    b. Moon facies and hirsutism
    c. Obesity and alopecia
    d. Abscess formation and hair overgrowth

47. A patient with a mediastinal mass is being assessed by the nurse. Upon palpation of the patient's neck, the nurse finds that the patient has tracheal deviation. Which of the following correctly describes tracheal deviation?
    a. Trachea that not in its usual midline position
    b. Trachea that is inflamed
    c. Trachea that is painful
    d. Trachea that is enlarged

48. Which method would correctly identify the thyroid isthmus during the palpation of the thyroid gland?
    a. It feels rubbery and is the size of half the thumb in the area between the clavicles
    b. Placing the finger pads at the base of the mandible will locate the thyroid isthmus
    c. When the index fingers are just below the clavicle, the thyroid isthmus will lower down when the patient swallows
    d. When the index fingers are just below the cricoid cartilage, the thyroid isthmus will

rise when the patient swallows

49. A home health nurse is visiting the home of an older patient and is making assessments on safety, particularly identifying risk factors for falls. Which of the following suggests that the older patient and their family need further teaching on falls prevention?
    a. An extension cord is crossing the hallway
    b. Grab bars are installed in the bathroom
    c. A bath mat is near the bath tub
    d. No throw rugs on the floor

50. Which of the following patient behaviors reflects the need for more teachings on safety?
    a. Wearing a helmet when riding a motorcycle
    b. Avoiding a skirmish on the street
    c. Placing a heavy toolbox on the topmost shelf
    d. Avoiding texting when driving

51. The nurse palpates an enlarged lymph node in the area deep in the angle formed by the clavicle and the sternocleidomastoid. Which of the following nodes did the nurse found enlarged?
    a. Posterior cervical node
    b. Tonsillar node
    c. Posterior auricular node
    d. Supraclavicular node

52. A male patient is being seen by the nurse. The patient's primary complaint is a headache on one side of the head, with the pain most intense around the eye. The pain is intense and continuous. The patient describes the pain as "absent one minute and then intense in the next couple of minutes." The patient also reports thin fluid running from his nose. Which type of headache is the patient most likely experiencing?
    a. Tension
    b. Migraine
    c. Cluster
    d. Thunderclap

53. A nurse is caring for several patients who have enlarged lymph nodes. Which of the following patients would need to be referred to the physician for a thorough follow-up assessment to rule out a malignancy?
    a. The patient with tooth abscess with enlarged painful submandibular nodes
    b. The patient with pharyngitis, with enlarged inflamed tonsillar nodes
    c. The patient with a pustule in the outer ear with swollen and painful pre-auricular nodes
    d. The patient who reports recent weight loss with painless hard and immovable cervical nodes

54. Which of the following facts about an infant's anatomy and physiology increases their risk of

traumatic brain injury? Select all that apply.
a. Their skull is malleable
b. The sutures of their skull have not yet completely fused
c. They have relatively small head
d. Their neck muscles are weak
e. They still have poor sense of hearing

55. Which of the following is a trigger of migraine headaches? Select all that apply.
a. Foods that are high in monosodium glutamate or artificial flavors
b. Stress
c. Driving
d. Diarrhea
e. High-calcium diet

56. A patient is asking the nurse what they can do to relieve their headache. Which of the following activities would the nurse recommend to the patient?
a. Massage
b. Loud music
c. Large meal
d. High-fat diet

57. A patient comes to the nurse complaining of pain in and around the eyes. Upon further assessments, the nurse finds that the pain is steady, aching and severe. Which of the following conditions is consistent with the patient's symptoms?
a. Errors of refraction
b. Acute glaucoma
c. Sinusitis
d. Corneal abrasion

58. A nurse is caring for a patient with a brain tumor. Which of the following would most likely characterize the patient's headache?
a. Throbbing and persistent
b. Aching, steady and dull, worse upon waking up
c. Very severe, abrupt onset
d. Shock-like, stabbing, burning

59. Which of the following conditions has a burning-like headache as a symptom as well as pain in the cheek jaw, lips or gums?
a. Meningitis
b. Post-concussion headache
c. Trigeminal neuralgia
d. Giant cell arteritis

60. A nurse is new to the unit and is to care for several patients. Which of the following facies will suggest that the patient has nephrotic syndrome?
    a. Rounded red cheeks
    b. Red butterfly-looking rash on the cheeks and bridge of the nose
    c. Pale edematous face with slit-like eyes
    d. Dull, puffy facies with coarse and dry eyebrows

61. A patient is assessing a patient who has dull, puffy facies. Upon more careful observation, the nurse finds that the patient's eyebrows and hair are sparse, dry, coarse and thin. The patient's skin is also dry. The patient earlier reported that they feel cold even on warmer days. The nurse knows that the patient's facies is consistent with which disorder?
    a. Hyperthyroidism
    b. Myxedema
    c. Cushing's syndrome
    d. Mumps

62. Which of the following facies is characteristic of acromegaly?
    a. Flushed facial skin without periorbital edema
    b. Rounded face with small bridge of the nose, low-set ears
    c. Swollen areas anterior to the ear lobes and above the angles of the mandible
    d. Elongated head, with bony prominence of the forehead, nose and lower jaw

63. A patient is receiving treatment for Parkinson's disease. Which of the following facies is consistent with Parkinson's disease?
    a. Mask-like with decreased blinking
    b. Moon-like with blushed cheeks
    c. Coarsened and prominent
    d. Small for size

64. A nurse is assessing a patient's neck. Upon palpation of the patient's thyroid, the nurse feels a singular nodule that is hard and painless. Which of the following is the likely nature of the patient's thyroid condition?
    a. Idiopathic
    b. Infectious
    c. Neoplastic
    d. Metabolic

65. A nurse is caring for a patient who has an overactive thyroid. Which of the following will the nurse most likely note of the patient's eyes?
    a. Dull and puffy
    b. Painful

c.   Bulging or protruding
d.   Yellowish sclera

ANSWERS

1. C

   Tension headaches are described as mild to moderate pain felt as viselike or as a tight band in the frontal or occipital area. It can last anywhere from 30 minutes to days. It is associated with stress and anxiety.

2. A

   Presyncope is a state of almost losing consciousness. A client with presyncope will feel faint, lightheaded and weak with blurred vision. It is the result of decreased cardiac output.

3. B

   Enlarged cervical, axillary and inguinal lymph nodes that are fixed, immovable and matted are a cause of concern because it may suggest malignancy, such as Hodgkin lymphoma.

4. B

   There will be tracheal deviation to the unaffected side in the presence of tumors, aortic aneurysm, unilateral thyroid enlargement and pneumothorax.

5. A

   Cephalhematoma or subperiosteal hemorrhage is bleeding under the scalp within a periosteum. The newborn will have a soft elevated part on one part of the head that does not cross the suture lines. It resolves within first few weeks or months of life. Caput succedaneum is the swelling of the presenting part of the scalp that is edematous or ecchymotic. It is soft and extends across suture lines. It resolves in the next few days of life.

6. A

   Bulging fontanels is an indication of increased intracranial pressure. There may be bulging of the fontanels when the baby cries but returns to normal when at rest. Dehydration in this case will result to sunken fontanels. Both anterior and posterior fontanels are still open and soft at 1 year of age.

7. B

   Chloasma is the dark discoloration or hyperpigmentation of the face during pregnancy, especially on the forehead and cheeks that gradually disappear after delivery.

8. D

   Temporal arteritis is inflammation of the temporal arteries. The vessels appear tortuous and are dilated, hardened and tender to touch.

9. C

   Head lag after the 4th or 5th month may indicate mental or motor retardation. The client in this case needs to be evaluated further.

10. A
Bacterial meningitis is inflammation of the meninges caused by bacteria. There would be pain and resistance when the neck is flexed.

11. C
Plagiocephaly is the asymmetry of the cranium when viewed from the top. This is due to preference of only one position during the early months of life. The part of the head favored for sleep appears flat.

12. B
Craniosynostosis is the premature fusing of one or more cranial suture lines that result to deformity of the head. Surgery is indicated in extremes of cases when because of the deformity, the skull cannot contain all cranial structures.

13. D
'Sunset eyes' is common in infants with raised intracranial pressure, such as those with hydrocephalus. The infant appears to look downward and the sclera is visible above the iris, giving the eyes a sunset look.

14. B
Micrognathia means small jaw and is one of the facial features of babies born to alcoholic mothers. Other manifestations of fetal alcohol syndromes are short palpebral fissures, flat midface, absent philtrum, short nose and thin upper lips.

15. A
Goiter is enlargement of the thyroid. It is prevalent in mountainous areas where access to fish and iodized salt is scarce. Iodine is needed for the production of thyroid hormones.

16. A
Parotitis in the elderly population can be caused by a viral infection, tumor or abscess. It can also be caused by blocked ducts secondary to dehydration caused by the use of diuretics and anticholinergics.

17. B, C
Grave's disease is caused by the overproduction of the thyroid hormones. It results to increased metabolic rate. The patient exhibits hypertension, tachycardia, nervousness, shortness of breath, excessive sweating and exophthalmos, among others.

18. D
Cushing's disease is caused by overproduction of adrenocorticotropic hormones. It is manifested by moonlike facie, hirsutism, and reddish cheeks.

19. A

Bell palsy is the paralysis of the facial nerve (cranial nerve VII). There is complete paralysis of one side of the face. The patient will not be able to make movements in the affected side, including smiling, frowning and wrinkling of the forehead. The client may also complain of pain behind the ear.

20. A, B, D

In Parkinson disease, the basal ganglia do not produce enough dopamine. It is manifested by mask-like facie, drooling, oily skin and scissoring gait.

21. C

Thunderclap headache is described as sudden intense pain, thunder-like in onset and severity. The patient describes it as the worst pain ever experienced. This type of headache indicates subarachnoid hemorrhage secondary to stroke, head trauma or meningitis, and therefore has the highest potential to be fatal.

22. D

"C" in OLD CART stands for characteristic symptoms, and the nurse asks the client to describe its intensity and quality

23. B

Prodromal symptoms or early symptoms indicate the start of a disease before specific symptoms occur. They are felt or seen by people before an attack of migraine. These include an aura, or perceptual experiences (usually vision, or smell), photophobia or scintillating scotomata.

24. B

Painless and immovable enlarged lymph nodes, especially those located in the cervical and supraclavicular ones signify Hodgkin's lymphoma, a type of cancer wherein there is an abnormal proliferation of lymphatic cells.

25. A

Goiters, or enlarged thyroids can have normal, decreased or increased thyroid hormone production. Protrusion of the eyeballs called exopthalmos is a sign of Grave's disease, a type of hyperthyroidism.

26. A

In Cushing's disease, there is an increase in cortisone due to a benign tumor of the pituitary gland. It causes moon facies, hirsutism and striae on the skin.

27. B

The finger pads of the second and third fingers provide the best tactile sensation to properly assess lymph nodes

28. C

Tracheal deviation even without obvious sign of respiratory distress takes priority over the other assessment findings mentioned. It can mean a mediastinal tumor pushing the trachea out of normal anatomical position. If accompanied by respiratory distress, it could signify atelectasis, large pneumothorax. All compromise airway and breathing.

29. C

The thyroid is normal or enlarged in Grave's disease and feels soft to palpation. In Malignancies, and Hashimoto's thyroiditis, it is firm. The thyroid is painful when palpated in thyroiditis.

30. D

Infant walkers are not advisable to use because of the potential for babies to trip and fall over, roll down stairs or hurt a finger in the bendable parts.

31. B

An infant's car seat should always be positioned at the middle back seat rear-facing because this is the safest for their weight and height. If the rear facing car seat has been outgrown, preschoolers' car seat should still be positioned in the middle back seat but now front facing. For school-aged kids, belt positioning booster until they are about 4'9" in height. Older children use the lap and shoulder belt. All children younger than 13 years of age stay at the back of the car.

32. A

Parotitis or mumps is an infectious viral process that causes inflammation of the parotid or salivary glands. Patients with mumps have fever, swelling of the area around the gland, pain, dry mouth and foul mouth odors.

33. A

Nephrotic syndrome is a disorder in which the kidneys excrete protein in the urine resulting to hypoalbuminemia, and consequently, edema. The edema is first noticeable around the eyes and then the face.

34. B

The signs and symptoms of Acromegaly start when there is an abnormally high growth hormones circulating in a time when growth plates have already fused in adulthood. The client exhibits enlarged hands and feet, coarsened, enlarged facial features, coarse, oily, thickened skin, thick nails, presence of skin tags, foul body odor, fatigue, deep husky voice, headache, fatigue, headaches, enlarged internal organs, barrel chest and hypertension.

35. D

Myxedema crisis is a condition that occurs in patients with long-standing, untreated hypothyroidism and can be triggered by other accompanying pathologies such as infections, or of hypothermia. Most apparent signs and symptoms include worsening fatigue with decreasing level of consciousness, weakness, bradycardia and hypotension. There is also facial swelling and periorbital edema, neuropathies and paresthesias.

36. C
Lid lag is the static situation in which the eyelid is higher than normal with the globe in downgaze. Exopthalmos is bulging of the eyeballs. Periorbital edema is puffiness around the eyes. Ptosis is drooping of the eyelid.

37. A
High grade fever and nuchal rigidity (tense neck and nape muscles, and pain upon flexing the neck) are signs of bacterial meningitis, a highly infectious disease. The nurse promptly institutes droplet precautions.

38. B
The carotid pulse is located below the jaw, to the side of the trachea. The brachial pulse is felt on the middle of the crease above the elbow between the forearm and lower arm. The facial pulse is located on the mandible (lower jawbone) on a line with the corners of the mouth. The apical pulse is at the 5th intercostal space left midclavicular line.

39. A
Bell's palsy is paralysis of the facial nerve. The result is obvious facial asymmetry wherein the affected side seems expressionless. The paralyzed side does not move with facial expressions and there is decreased tear production on that same side, too. Sometimes, the client also complains of ear and eye pain.

40. B
The nurse informs the mother that further assessments and tests need to be performed. Although she suspects that the child has bell's palsy, it is not therapeutic to mention a medical diagnosis unless it has been confirmed to them by the physician.

41. A
A nurse must be able to make assessments and identify 'red flags' or cases that need immediate medical attention. Thunderclap headaches are an example of 'red flags'. This type of a headache is described by the patient as the worst headache of their life. It is caused by bleeding in or around the brain. The nurse must be alert to inform the physician immediately of the patient's complaint.

42. B
Tension headaches are stress-related and are caused by muscle contractions in the head and neck areas. A tension headache is felt as steady pain on both sides of the head or in the temporal regions.

43. C

An aura is any experience that precedes a headache. Auras usually signal to the patient that a migraine headache is imminent. Auras come in the form of photophobia or sensitivity to light, scintillating scotomas or C-shaped bright zigzag lines that appear in the patient's vision, or other sensory symptoms.

44. A

A nurse will most likely find enlarged lymph nodes of the neck in patients with injury, infection or tumor in the head, mouth, or neck. An infected tooth will cause enlarged, tender lymph nodes in the patient's neck.

45. D

Patients with hypothyroidism have dry, coarse hair that easily breaks and slowly grows. On the other hand, patients with hyperthyroidism will have fine, thin strands of hair. In both cases, patients may experience hair loss.

46. B

The rounded cheek appearance in Cushing's disease is also known as moon facies. The growth of hair in unlikely places, such as on the face and above the upper lips in women is called hirsutism.

47. A

Tracheal deviation refers to the trachea that is either palpated to either the right or left of the throat away from the midline where it is normally located. It is a common finding in patients with mediastinal masses, atelectasis, or large pneumothorax.

48. D

The thyroid isthmus can be palpated by placing the finger pads below the cricoid cartilage. The nurse asks the patient to swallow. As the patient swallows, the thyroid isthmus will rise.

49. A

A nurse must call the attention of the patient and their family when there is a risk for falls. Falls account for 81% of all traumatic injuries in the elderly population. Factors that can cause falls in older people are extension cords that are in corridors or those that are crossing rooms, throw rugs and non-rubber slipper or shoe soles, among others.

50. C

Examples of patient behaviors that would need more teachings on the subject of safety include, riding bicycles and motorcycles without safety gears such as a helmet, phone use while driving, placing heavy objects in high places, keeping loaded firearms in an unlocked place, and non-adherence to car seat guidelines, among others.

51. D

The supraclavicular nodes are palpated deep in the area just above the clavicle, in the angle formed by the clavicle and the sternocleidomastoid.

52. C

Cluster headaches are usually experienced by men. The pain is usually unilateral and mostly felt around the eyes or the temple. The headache is described as sharp, intense and continuous with an abrupt onset. It is accompanied by other signs and symptoms such as rhinorrhea, miosis, ptosis and eyelid edema.

53. D

Hard or fixed nodes that are non-tender suggest a malignancy. A patient with painless, hard, immovable cervical nodes must be referred to the physician because the findings suggest lymphoma.

54. A, B, D

Infants have a relatively large head in proportion to their height. Their neck muscles are still weak. Their skull is malleable, and its sutures are not yet fully fused. These are factors that increase their risk for injury, particularly traumatic brain injuries.

55. A, B

Migraine headaches are usually triggered by certain foods, such as those high in monosodium glutamate or flavor enhancers. Stress, alcohol consumption, menstruation and high altitudes also cause migraines.

56. A

If the patient would ask about activities that may help relieve headaches, the nurse may suggest massage, relaxation techniques, restful sleep in a dark, quiet room, and soft music.

57. B

In acute glaucoma, the patient will report steady, aching, often severe pain in and around the eyes. Glaucoma is caused by an increase in intraocular pressure.

58. B

The headaches experienced by patients with brain tumors are usually aching, steady and dull, and are usually worse in the morning upon awakening.

59. C

The headache caused by trigeminal neuralgia is described as shock-like, stabbing, burning. It is severe and is accompanied by pain in the cheek, jaw, lips or gums. Trigeminal neuralgia is caused by the compression of the Cranial Nerve V.

60. C

The face of the patient with nephrotic syndrome will look pale and swollen. The swelling is most evident around the eyes, called periorbital edema, in the morning. When the edema is severe, the eyes will appear slit-like.

61. B

Dull, puffy facies that is accompanied by dry, coarse, thin eyebrows and dry facial skin is consistent with myxedema. The periorbital edema in myxedema is non-pitting. The facial features in myxedema are caused by very slow body metabolism.

62. D

The facies of a patient with acromegaly appear coarsened. The head is elongated, and the bones of the forehead, nose, lips, and ears are very prominent. Acromegaly is caused by an increased growth hormone.

63. A

The facies of a patient with Parkinson's disease is described as mask-like because of decreased facial movements including blinking. The facial skin of a patient with Parkinson's disease is oily. Drooling may also be observed.

64. C

A single hard and painless nodule that is felt on the patient's thyroid suggest a growth that is neoplastic in nature. On the other hand, two or more nodules suggests a metabolic nature of the thyroid enlargement.

65. C

Patients with hyperthyroidism or overactive thyroid would have bulging or protruding eyes called exophthalmos caused by an overgrowth of connective tissues in the orbit.

The Eyes

Questions

1. A nurse is reviewing her concepts on visual reflexes. Which of the following refers to the reflex that puts an image we want to focus in in the center of the visual field, particularly in the fovea centralis?
   a. Direct light reflex
   b. Consensual light reflex
   c. Accommodation
   d. Fixation

2. The nurse wants to assess the vision of several pediatric clients. Which of the following would the nurse correctly consider before assessment?
   a. Newborns have no peripheral vision
   b. The macula is fully developed at birth
   c. Binocularity and fixation is achieved by the 4th month of life
   d. The structure of the eyeball reaches adult size by 2 years of age

3. A nurse is to care for several elderly clients in a facility. To guide her assessment of vision, she reviews her concepts on changes of vision brought about by aging. Which of the following is NOT accurate and should not be included in guiding her plan of care?
   a. 40% of elderly clients have presbyopia
   b. The lens becomes less elastic and plastic-like
   c. There is better accommodation
   d. Pupil size increases

4. The nurse is teaching safety measures to a 68-year old person who is gradually losing her central vision. Which condition related to aging causes loss of central vision due to deposition of yellow matter, and deterioration of the central portion of the retina?
   a. Cataract
   b. Glaucoma
   c. Age-related macular degeneration
   d. Diabetic retinopathy

5. A nurse wants to establish a culturally sensitive care to several clients with open-angle glaucoma. Who of her clients below has the greatest risk of having open-angle glaucoma?
   a. Black
   b. Asian
   c. Whites
   d. Native Americans

6. The nurse wants to know if an elderly client is seeing 'floaters'. Which of the following is the most appropriate question to ask the client?
   a. "Do you see halos around lights?"

b. "Do you see spots moving in your vision?"
c. "Do you see double of everything?"
d. "Do you bump into things that are at your side?"

7. A nurse is assisting an ophthalmologist assess a client. The ophthalmologist says that the client has misaligned axes of the eyes. The nurse expects the client to report:
   a. Pain when seeing in a bright room
   b. Double vision in both eyes
   c. Loss of central vision
   d. Loss of peripheral vision

8. After an eye assessment, it was determined that the client's visual acuity is 20/60. What is the most accurate interpretation of this result?
   a. The client can read at 60 feet what a person of normal vision can read at 20 feet.
   b. The client can read 20 of the 60 letters on the Snellen chart
   c. The client can see only one-third of what a person of normal vision can see.
   d. The client can read at 20 feet what a person of normal vision can read at 60 feet.

9. The nurse is reviewing the chart of a Black client who has undergone a thorough eye examination. Which of the following findings warrants additional evaluation?
   a. Yellowish deposits beneath the eyelids
   b. Dirty sclera
   c. Slight protrusion of the eyeball
   d. Bulging of the optic disc

10. A nurse plans to use a Snellen E chart to assess the visual acuity of a 5-year old child. Which of the following will alert the nurse to choose an alternative method of assessing visual acuity?
    a. The child has difficulty seeing objects from a distance
    b. The child is having difficulty identifying pictures
    c. The child does not fully know the alphabet
    d. The child is quadriplegic

11. The nurse is caring for several infants in the pediatric ward. Of her findings, which of the following will alert the nurse to a possible problem in the infant?
    a. A two-week old who cannot fixate on an object
    b. A 6-month old who cannot follow a light
    c. A 4-week old who cannot make a visual response to the nurse's face
    d. A 1-month old who cannot follow a toy in all directions

12. A nurse is performing a cover test on a child. The nurse asks the child to stare at a toy and covers one eye. She tells the child to continue to stare at the object. As she removes the cover of the tested eye, the covered eye moved to re-establish fixation. What is the most accurate interpretation of

this?
a. There is weakness of the muscles of the covered eye
b. The child is color-blind
c. The child has poor central vision
d. The child has poor peripheral vision

13. A nurse wants to inspect a newborn's ocular structures. However, the eyes of the newborn are tightly shut. Which of the following will safely open the eyes of the newborn?
a. Gently pry the lids with the thumb and forefinger of the dominant hand
b. Hold the baby in a supine position and slightly hyperextend the neck
c. Gently put the newborn in a supported sitting position
d. Startle the baby

14. A nurse is assessing the eyes and vision of a newborn. Which of the following alerts the nurse to a possible problem of the eye or vision?
a. The newborn has no tears when crying
b. The newborn eyes are tightly shut
c. The newborn cannot fixate on an object
d. The baby's eyes look in the same direction as the body is turned to one side and remains steady even after the turning halts

15. The nurse plans to assess the visual acuity of a toddler. Which of the following is the most appropriate method to use?
a. Snellen E chart
b. Standard Snellen chart
c. Cover test
d. Allen test

16. A nurse is performing screening of eye disorders on several elderly clients. Which of the following findings in considered NOT normal
a. Arcus sinilus
b. Xanthelasma
c. Opaque lens
d. Drusen

17. A nurse is screening for glaucoma in several adult and elderly clients. Which of the following findings is an accurate description of acute closed-angle glaucoma?
a. There is clogging of the canals far inside the eye that develops over time.
b. The fluid drains freely at the canals near the iris
c. There is sudden blockage over the outer edge of the iris when the pupils dilates too much or too quickly
d. There is gradual blockage over the outer edge of the iris when the pupils dilates over time

18. While assessing the eye movement of a client, the nurse performs the Diagnostic Positions Test. The nurse finds that the client cannot turn the eyes down and nasal. Which cranial nerve is most likely affected?
    a. III
    b. IV
    c. V
    d. VI

19. The nurse is assessing the structures of the eye. She notes that the lower lid of the client is exposed and rolled out. There is excess tearing. The client also complains of dryness and itchiness. Which of the following accurately describes the client's condition?
    a. Ectropion
    b. Entropion
    c. Ptosis
    d. Enophthalmos

20. A client comes to the clinic complaining of pain in his lower lid. Upon inspection of the affected eye, the nurse notes a superficial pustule, elevated from the lower lid margin. The client remembers rubbing the eyes with dirty hands. Which of the following is the client most likely suffering from?
    a. Blepharitis
    b. Chalazion
    c. Hordeolum
    d. Conjunctivitis.

21. In which of the following structures of the inner eye would the nurse find the optic nerve through an ophthalmoscope?
    a. The retina
    b. The vitreous humor
    c. The optic disc
    d. The ciliary body

22. A patient asks a nurse why we have 'blind spots'. Which of the following is the nurse's best response?
    a. "Blind spots are indicative of the beginning of the loss of normal vision, and it is caused by too much exposure to sunlight."
    b. "Blind spots are the result of an infectious process in the eyes that result to temporary loss of vision in a small part of the visual field."
    c. "Blind spots are common to elderly people, and it is caused by aging."
    d. "Normally, there is a hole in our retinas or the layer in our eyes responsible for vision; that hole is where the nerves enter the eye, and it is responsible for the blind spot."

23. Which of the following will happen if a nurse shines a light on one eye?

a. The pupils in both eyes will constrict

b. The pupil of the eye where the light was introduced will constrict, while the other pupil will not

c. The pupil in the other eye where the light was not introduced will constrict, and the other will dilate

d. The pupils in both eyes will dilate

24. A patient is having difficulty focusing on near and far objects. The patient is said to be having problems with:

a. Convergence

b. Accommodation

c. Pupillary constriction

d. Pupillary dilation

25. Which cranial nerves are responsible for eye movements?

a. CN III, IV, VI

b. CN I, II, V

c. CN VII, XI

d. CN VII, X

26. A patient reports difficulty looking at far objects. Which of the following correctly describes the patient's concern?

a. Presbyopia

b. Myopia

c. Hyperopia

d. Scotoma

27. A patient reports a loss of vision in one eye but experiences no pain in both eyes. The nurse considers several possibilities of the cause of the patient's symptoms EXCEPT:

a. Retinal detachment

b. Macular degeneration

c. Vitreous hemorrhage

d. Acute closed-angle glaucoma

28. A patient is concerned about blurred vision in both eyes. The patient reports no eye pain. Which question is most appropriate to ask the patient to determine the possible cause of the patient's symptom?

a. "Did you recently bump your head?"

b. "Did you accidentally splash any chemical in your eyes?"

c. "Have you taken any new medications?"

d. "Are you wearing contact lenses?"

29. A patient has homonymous hemianopsia caused by stroke. Which of the following correctly describes the patient's vision loss?
    a. Loss of peripheral vision
    b. Loss of central vision
    c. Loss of vision of one-half of the visual field, either the left or right side, in both eyes
    d. Gradual and progressive vision loss

30. Which of the following patient responses about their vision would warrant immediate medical attention?
    a. Inability to see far objects since childhood
    b. Inability to read a newspaper due to aging
    c. Flashing lights with floaters on one eye
    d. Seeing double since birth

31. A nurse is taking the history of a patient to assess a patient's eye and to determine vision problems. Which of the following questions will determine lifestyle habits that affect the eyes and vision?
    a. "Have you gone to the doctor before to have your eyes checked?"
    b. "Do you have double vision?"
    c. "Do you feel pain in your eyes when you bend over?"
    d. "Do you smoke?"

32. A patient's visual acuity is 20/200. Which of the following is the correct interpretation of this finding?
    a. The patient is farsighted
    b. The patient is near-sighted
    c. The patient has diplopia
    d. The patient is legally blind

33. Which of the following patient responses should alert the nurse for possible glaucoma in the patient?
    a. "My eyes hurt when I go outside in the sun."
    b. "I always bump into things that are on my side."
    c. "When I touch my eyelids while my eyes are open, I see double."
    d. "I could not read the papers unless I hold the paper away at arm's length."

34. The nurse is to perform a light reaction test. Which of the following should the nurse do first?
    a. Prepare the Snellen Chart
    b. Obtain a cotton ball
    c. Darken the room
    d. Obtain cotton buds

35. A nurse is assessing a patient's eyes and noticed that the left pupil is about 4 mm and the right

pupil is 5 mm. Which of the following correctly refers to the patient's manifestation?
a. Anisocoria
b. Mydriasis
c. Miosis
d. Blepharitis

36. The nurse is to perform the test on six extraocular movements. Which hand movement pattern should the nurse do for the patient to follow gaze?
a. H
b. C
c. A square
d. A cross

37. A patient has been having recurrent severe headaches, and the physician has suspicions that the patient may have a brain tumor. Which of the following findings is consistent with brain tumors?
a. Entropion
b. Lid lag
c. Deviations in eye movement
d. Ectropion

38. A nurse is asking the patient to follow the pencil that is moved centrally toward the bridge of the patient's nose. Which test is the nurse performing?
a. Cover-uncover test
b. Test for nystagmus
c. Corneal light reflex test
d. Test for convergence

39. The nurse is to administer mydriatic drops for an ophthalmoscopic examination. Which of the following patients should not be given mydriatic drops?
a. A patient who took thyroid medications
b. A patient with head injury
c. A patient with poor visual acuity due to myopia
d. A patient with deviations in eye movements

40. A nurse is using the ophthalmoscope to examine the patient's eyes. Which of the following findings indicates a need further assessment and eye evaluations?
a. Pigmented crescents or rings surround the disc
b. Swelling of the optic disc
c. Yellowish white color of the central physiologic cup
d. The nasal portion of the disc margin is slightly blurred

41. A patient was recently diagnosed with macular degeneration. The patient would most likely

report a loss of vision in which field?

a. Peripheral
b. Central
c. One-half
d. One-fourth

42. A patient reports eye pain on one eye. Upon careful inspection, the nurse finds that the patient's eyes are red and watery. Knowing that corneal injury, acute iritis, and glaucoma all cause red eyes and pain in the eye, which of the following findings would suggest that the patient has a corneal injury?

a. Decrease in vision
b. Pupils are normal
c. Pain is moderate to severe
d. Cloudy cornea

43. A nurse is examining a patient and finds that the patient is blind in one eye. Which of the following anatomical structures if found with lesions will cause blindness in one eye?

a. Right optic nerve
b. Right optic radiation, partial
c. Optic chiasm
d. Right optic tract

44. A nurse is assessing an 80-year old patient and notices that the patient's lower lashes are not visible because the lid margin has turned inward. How would the nurse document this finding?

a. Ectropion
b. Entropion
c. Ptosis
d. Exophthalmos

45. A nurse finds slightly raised yellowish plaques that have well-circumscribed borders above the inner canthus of the eyes. The lesions are not itchy or painful. These findings are associated with which disorder?

a. Heart disorder
b. Lipid disorders
c. Neuromuscular disorder
d. Hormonal imbalance

ANSWERS

1. D

   Fixation refers to the reflex that puts an image we want to focus in in the center of the visual field, particularly in the fovea centralis. It is affected by alcohol, drugs, fatigue and inattentiveness.

2. C

   Newborns have fully developed peripheral vision. However, the macula is non-present at birth but will gradually develop by four months until being fully developed by 8 months of age. Binocularity and fixation are achieved by the 4th month of life. The structures of the eyeball reach adult size by 8 years of age.

3. A

   At 40 years of age, half of the population had presbyopia and needs magnification to read small prints. The lenses become less elastic and glass-like. The pupils decrease in size. There is decreased accommodation and an increase need for ambient light to see more clearly.

4. C

   Age related macular degeneration condition related to aging causes loss of central vision due to deposition of yellow matter called drusen and deterioration of the macula, the central portion of the retina.

5. A

   Blacks are three times more prone to developing open-angle glaucoma than Hispanics and Whites.

6. B

   Floaters are caused by vitreous fibers that have become dense. They are seen as moving spots in the field of vision. Those with retinal detachment will report a curtain-like loss of vision or of cobwebs on the field of vision.

7. B

   Binocular diplopia is seeing double in both eyes. It is caused by misaligned exes of the eyes.

8. D

   The number on top indicates the distance in feet the client was able to read a particular line on a Snellen Chart. The lower number indicates the distance in feet a person of normal vision could have read the same line without difficulty. The correct option is therefore D.

9. D

   Bulging of the optic disc indicates papilledema, a sign of increased intracranial pressure. The client should be further evaluated. All other options are normal findings in a Black client.

10. D

In the use of a Snellen E chart, the nurse asks the child (3-6 year old) to point to the direction where the 'legs' of the letter E point. A child with all four extremities paralyzed will not be able to use the hands to point to a direction.

11. B

A 6-month old infant should be able to fixate on, follow, and reach for an object. Not being able to follow a light means a possible vision problem.

12. A

When performing a cover test and the tested eye moved to re-establish fixation after being uncovered, there is weakness of the muscles of the covered eye.

13. B

Holding the baby at a supine position, and slightly lowering the head by hyperextending the neck will have the newborn open his eyes. The nurse should not attempt to pry open the lids of the neonate, nor to put the neonate in a sitting position.

14. D

The vestibular function reflex will have the baby open his eyes and look in the same direction as he is turned, and when turning halts, the eyes will exhibit short nystagmus and then the eyes would slowly turn to the opposite side. It is normal for a newborn not to have tears and to have tightly shut eyes. The newborn will learn to fixate on an object starting at 2 weeks.

15. D

The Allen test uses picture cards familiar to the toddler (such as pictures of houses, pets, trees) and shows them at a close distance and then at a 15-feet distance. Naming 3 out of 7 pictures in 3-5 attempts is normal.

16. C

Arcus sinilus, Xanthelasma and drusen are normal age-related changes and have no effect on vision. Opaque lens indicate cataract formation that lead to decreased visual acuity.

17. C

Acute closed-angle glaucoma happens when there is sudden blockage over the outer edge of the iris when the pupils dilates too much or too quickly. It causes eye pain, headache, nausea and vomiting, blurred or loss of vision. The client may report seeing halos around lights. It is a medical emergency.

18. B

When the client cannot turn the eye downward and nasal during the Diagnostic Positions Test, consider damage to the cranial nerve IV.

19. A

In ectropion the lower lid is exposed and rolled out. Since the punta cannot reabsorb tears back, there is excessive tearing. Because of being exposed, there is also dryness and itchiness of the conjunctiva.

20. C

Hordeolum, commonly known as stye, is the infection of a hair follicle caused by staphylococcus. A superficial elevated pustule develops from the margin of the lower lid where lash protrudes. It can cause pain and swelling in the area.

21. B

The optic disc is found at the posterior of the eye and could only be seen through an ophthalmoscope. It is where the optic nerves and retinal vessels enter the eyes posteriorly.

22. D

The absence of retinal receptors at the optic disc does not complete a visual field. Thus, a small part of the visual field is blank and it is called the blind spot.

23. A

When the nurse shines a light on one eye, the pupil of that eye will constrict. This reaction is called the direct reaction to light. The light will also constrict the pupil of the other eye, and this phenomenon is called the consensual reaction to light.

24. B

Accommodation is the process of focusing on objects or making clear images of objects at different distances.

25. A

The Cranial Nerve III or the Oculomotor nerve, the Cranial nerve IV or the Trochlear nerve and the CN VI or the Abducens nerve are responsible for all ocular movements.

26. B

Myopia is difficulty looking at far objects.

27. D

Acute closed-angle glaucoma will cause intense pain and blurring of vision in the affected eye. Macular degeneration, vitreous hemorrhage, and retinal detachment will cause painless unilateral vision loss.

28. C

Blurry vision or loss of vision that is bilateral and painless suggests the use of medications that can affect refraction such as cholinergics. Cholinergic medications cause pupillary constriction. On the other hand, anticholinergics cause pupillary dilation. Steroids cause cataracts.

29. C

Homonymous hemianopsia is the loss of vision in one-half of the visual field either the left or right, in both eyes.

30. C

Seeing flashing lights with floaters, usually in one eye, suggests detachment of the vitreous from the retina. A prompt eye examination is needed.

31. D

Smoking is a lifestyle habit that needs to be evaluated when assessing the patient's eyes. Chronic and heavy smoking introduces free radicals that can cause cell damage in the eyes. Also, the vasoconstrictive effect of smoking decreases blood flow to the eye. Smoking can cause cataract formation and macular degeneration.

32. D

A 20/200 vision means that the patient can read at 20 feet what a person with normal vision could read at 200 feet. A visual acuity of 20/200 means that the person is legally blind.

33. B

Symptoms of open-angle glaucoma include gradual loss of peripheral vision. The patient may say that they bump into things that are on their sides most of the time. This is because they have started losing their sight on their periphery.

34. C

The light reaction test examines the pupils' reaction to light. A light is flashed into each pupil while the patient looks at a distance. Before doing this procedure, the nurse must darken the room first.

35. A

Anisocoria is having one pupil bigger than the other. 20% of people have anisocoria. Pupil size difference is usually between 0.5-1 mm. If pupillary reactions are normal, anisocoria is not pathological.

36. A

To perform the test on six extraocular movements, the nurse holds a pencil and asks the patient to follow gaze as the nurse makes a wide "H" pattern in the air.

37. C

Deviations in movement that are detected with the test on six extraocular movements indicate a brain tumor or injury. The deviation depends on the location of the lesion.

38. D

To perform the test for convergence, the nurse asks the patient to follow the pencil that they move toward the patient's bridge of the nose. The converging eyes would normally follow the pencil to 5 -8 cm of the nose. Poor convergence is seen in patients with hyperthyroidism.

39. B
Mydriatic drops are administered to the eye of the patient before an ophthalmoscopic examination to dilate the pupils. Dilated pupils enable the nurse to examine the posterior as well as the peripheral structures of the eyes. The use of mydriatic drops is contraindicated in patients whose pupillary reactions are critical to assessment such as in the case of head trauma or coma. It is also not given to patients with narrow-angle glaucoma because pupillary dilation will cause an increase in intraocular pressure and consequently, eye pain.

40. B
Swelling of the optic disc and the anterior bulging of the physiologic cup is called papilledema, and it necessitates further medical evaluations. Papilledema indicates many brain disorders, including meningitis, subarachnoid bleeding, trauma or brain tumor.

41. B
Macular degeneration is the loss of central vision caused by deterioration of the macula, a part of the retina. It is common in the elderly.

42. B
Corneal injury, acute iritis, and glaucoma all cause moderate to severe eye pain, red eyes, and a decrease in vision. There are also corneal changes, such as cloudiness in all three. However, in corneal injury, there is no pupillary change or abnormality. In acute iritis, the pupils may be small which may become irregular in time. In glaucoma, the pupils are fixed and dilated.

43. A
A lesion of the right optic nerve can cause right eye blindness. A lesion on the right optic radiation will cause homonymous left superior quadratic effect. Injury or tumor to the optic chiasm will cause bitemporal hemianopsia. Finally, a lesion in the right optic tract will lead to left homonymous hemianopsia.

44. B
Entropion is the turning of the lid margin inward that renders the lower lashes hidden in the folded lid. It is common in elderly patients.

45. B
Slightly raised yellowish plaques that have well-circumscribed borders, and are found above the inner canthus of the eyes describe xanthelasma. Xanthelasmas are not itchy or painful. They are associated with lipid disorders.

The Ears, Nose, Mouth and Throat

Questions

1. A nurse is assessing a patient who reports having difficulty hearing in one ear. Which of the following questions can the nurse ask the patient to know the onset of the hearing difficulty?
   a. "Did you also notice some hearing loss in the other ear?"
   b. "Do you notice any other symptoms with your hearing difficulty?"
   c. "When did you start noticing that you had difficulty hearing in that ear?"
   d. "Have you consulted any health provider for your hearing difficulty?

2. Which of the following conditions will cause sensorineural hearing loss?
   a. An infection of the tragus
   b. Increased pressure in endolymphatic system of the inner ear
   c. Blockage caused by impacted cerumen
   d. Fixation of the stapes

3. A patient reports some hearing loss in both ears. Which of the following would most likely cause bilateral hearing loss?
   a. Ear piercing
   b. Eating too many legumes
   c. Recent pharyngitis
   d. Prolonged use of aminoglycosides

4. The mother of a toddler reports that her daughter seems to have pain in the ear because she keeps on touching or pulling on her ear. After an otoscopic examination, the nurse finds that the patient's left tympanic membrane is inflamed. Which of the following details in the patient's history would be significant in determining the cause of the patient's symptoms?
   a. Breastfed since birth
   b. Recent MMR vaccination
   c. Current upper respiratory tract infection
   d. Lactose intolerance

5. A patient who reports neck pain and headaches also complains of ringing in the ears. The ringing sounds "like someone is humming." Which of the following correctly describes the patient's symptom of ringing in the ears?
   a. Nystagmus
   b. Tinnitus
   c. Vertigo
   d. Otalgia

6. A patient complains to the nurse that they have a runny nose and some nasal congestion that does not seem to go away even if they use decongestants. Which of the following questions would be significant to the determination of the patient's chronic rhinitis?
   a. "When did you last take your vitamin supplements?"

b.   "Are you drinking enough water?"
c.   "Did you get wet in the rain recently?"
d.   "How much and how long have you been using decongestants?"

7.   A nurse is assessing a patient and notices that the patient's nasal septum is perforated. The patient also has rhinorrhea and appears restless. Which of the following conditions most likely caused the patient's symptoms?
a.   Epistaxis
b.   Upper respiratory tract infection
c.   Cocaine abuse
d.   Allergies

8.   A nurse is to use an otoscope to inspect the adult patient's ears. Which of the following is the correct technique in straightening the patient's ear canal for better viewing?
a.   Pull the pinna away from the head until it is perpendicular to the head
b.   Pull the pinna upward, backward and slightly away from the head
c.   Pull the pinna downward, backward and slightly away from the head
d.   Ask the patient to lie on their side

9.   A nurse is performing a whisper test, and the patient fails the test. Which of the following results of the whisper test made the nurse conclude that the patient's hearing acuity is poor?
a.   The patient repeats the initial sequence of numbers and letters accurately
b.   The patient repeats three out of six letter-number combinations correctly
c.   The patient repeats four out of six letter-number combinations correctly
d.   The patient repeats four out of six letter-number combinations incorrectly

10. A nurse conducting the Weber test places the base of the vibrating tuning fork on top of the patient's head. The patient tells the nurse that the sound is heard in the good ear. Which type of hearing loss does the patient have?
a.   Unilateral sensorineural hearing loss
b.   Unilateral conductive hearing loss
c.   Bilateral sensorineural hearing loss
d.   Bilateral conductive hearing loss

11. Before performing an examination of the mouth, which of the following should the nurse do first?
a.   Ask the patient to brush their teeth
b.   Wear gloves
c.   Ask the patient if they have eaten or drank anything in the last 30 minutes
d.   Ask the patient to drink one glass of water

12. The nurse is examining a patient's mouth and asks the patient to say "ah." The nurse notices that the patient's uvula deviates to the right. Which of the following conditions is associated with the

patient's manifestation?
a. CN X paralysis
b. CN XI paralysis
c. Lesion on the maxillary sinuses
d. Lesion on the hard palate

13. A nurse is assessing a patient who presented with fever, malaise and throat pain. The nurse examines the patient's throat and finds the tonsils inflamed and are between the tonsillar pillars and the uvula. Which of the following is the correct tonsils grading?
a. +1
b. +2
c. +3
d. +4

14. A nurse is caring for a patient with xerostomia. The nurse wants to determine the cause of the patient's symptom. Which of the following questions is most appropriate to ask the patient to help determine the cause?
a. "Did you injure your tongue in any way?
b. "Have you had a sore throat recently?"
c. "What medications are you taking?"
d. "Are you using machinery with loud noises?"

15. An adolescent female patient is seen by the school nurse. The patient was outdoor in hot weather when she felt faint. She did not lose consciousness. Prior to the symptom, the patient claimed to have suddenly stood from a squatting position. Which of the following manifestations did the patient experience?
a. Vertigo
b. Presyncope
c. Dysequilibrium
d. Tinnitus

16. A patient experiences sudden dizziness when turning to their side or tilting their head. The dizziness lasts less than a minute, but according to the patient, they have experienced it several times in the last few days. During every episode, the patient felt slightly nauseous. Which of the following is the patient most likely experiencing?
a. Meniere Disease
b. Acoustic neuroma
c. Vestibular neuronitis
d. Benign positional vertigo

17. A patient has been recently diagnosed with Meniere Disease. Which of the following manifestations will the nurse expect the patient to report? Select all that apply.

a. Hearing loss
b. Fullness in the affected ear
c. Anisocoria
d. No nausea
e. Vertigo

18. A patient has been experiencing vertigo with variable duration. He also reported impaired hearing in one ear. The physician said that his symptoms are the result of the compression of Cranial Nerve VIII. The nurse should prepare to care for someone with:
    a. Vestibular Neuronitis
    b. Central vertigo
    c. Acoustic neuroma
    d. Dysequilibrium

19. A nurse is assessing a patient's ear and finds small lumps in the helix of the patient's ears. Upon palpation, the nurse felt the lumps to be hard and gritty. One of the lumps discharges chalky white crystals through the skin. The nurse looks at laboratory results to determine the probable cause of the patient's symptoms. The nurse would most likely find high blood levels of:
    a. Uric acid
    b. potassium
    c. bicarbonates
    d. triglycerides

20. A nurse examining a patient sees several keloid formations on a patient's ears. Which of the following questions would be relevant to determining the cause of the patient's lesions?
    a. "Do you have a cough?"
    b. "Did you go swimming recently?"
    c. "How much time do you spend outdoors?"
    d. "Did you have your ear pierced recently?"

21. A patient is currently recovering from a perforated eardrum. They ask the nurse what usually causes perforations of the tympanic membrane. Which of the following should the nurse tell the patient?
    a. Recent use of otic drops
    b. Middle ear infections
    c. Cranial nerve damage
    d. Malignancy

22. An amber-colored fluid has accumulated in the patient's middle ear. The patient reports fullness in the ear, a popping sound, and some impairment in hearing. Which of the following activities did the patient most likely performed recently?
    a. Attending a concert

b. Diving
c. Bowling
d. Gardening

23. A patient has angular cheilitis. Which of the following activities would elicit pain in the patient?
    a. Opening and closing the mouth
    b. Seeing
    c. Hearing
    d. Swallowing

24. A patient with intestinal cancer is also found to have Peutz-Jeghers Syndrome. The brown pigmented lesions in Peutz-Jeghers Syndrome will be observed in which body part?
    a. Lips
    b. Nose
    c. Eyes
    d. Ears

25. A nurse is inspecting a patient's mouth and notices white cheesy substance sticking to the patient's mucosa. The patient's history reveals that the patient has taken several types of antibiotics for recurrent tonsillitis. Which of the following accurately describes the patient's symptoms?
    a. Kaposi Sarcoma
    b. Oral candidiasis
    c. Diphtheria
    d. Torus Palatinus

26. A nurse is assessing the hearing acuity of a client. She wants to determine if the client is experiencing conductive or sensorineural hearing loss. Which of the following is an accurate information regarding hearing loss?
    a. Conductive hearing loss is caused by damage to the inner ear
    b. Damage to the cranial nerve VIII results to sensorineural hearing loss
    c. An ossified stapes will result to sensorineural hearing loss
    d. The degeneration of nerves in the inner ear will result to conductive hearing loss

27. The nurse is aware that young children aged three and below are more prone to developing ear infections. Which of the following information supports this premise? Select all that apply
    a. Their Eustachian tubes are wider
    b. Their Eustachian tubes are shorter
    c. Their Eustachian tubes are sloped
    d. Their eardrums are smaller
    e. Their Eustachian tubes are more prone to occlusion

28. A client comes to the clinic because his hearing loss according to him is strange. According to

him, he has difficulty hearing normal conversations but when people start to speaks louder to him, it hurts to hear. Which of the following conditions is the client most likely suffering from?
a. Recruitment
b. Presbycusis
c. Cholesteatoma
d. Conductive hearing loss

29. A nurse wants to assess the possible risk factors to a child's recurrent otitis media. Which of the following is appropriate to ask the child's mother?
a. "Do you have anyone in your family who also suffer from otitis media?"
b. "Does anyone in your family smoke?"
c. "Did you have otitis media when you were pregnant with your child?"
d. "Are you allergic to shellfish?"

30. A nurse is keen to observe a client for hearing loss. Which of the following are indicators that a client may have hearing loss? Select all that apply.
a. Client looks at lips instead of the eyes of the nurse
b. Client leans forward
c. Client fidgets in his seat
d. Client's speech is garbled
e. Client speaks in a loud voice

31. A client comes to the clinic to report that 3 days ago he felt himself spinning in the room. Which of the following accurately describes the client's condition?
a. Objective vertigo
b. Subjective vertigo
c. Syncope
d. Presyncope

32. A client confides to the nurse that recently she hears something weird, "a ringing, whistling sound like hearing with a big seashell near the ears." Which of the following factors most likely contributed to the client's condition?
a. Calcium deficiency
b. Inflamed tragus
c. Mumps
d. Aspirin toxicity

33. A nurse wants to assess the hearing of a 4-month old baby. Which of the following is appropriate for the nurse to do?
a. Check for the Startle reflex
b. Make a loud sound out of the child's sight and see if the child reacts to the sound by crying, getting startled or by efforts to locate sound

c. Use the audiometry
d. Check if the child responds to name

34. A nurse is observing a 7-month old baby on his crib. Which of the following observations should alert the nurse for a possible ear infection in the child?
    a. The baby cries when his toy fell out of the crib
    b. The baby frequently touches his ear
    c. The baby feeds from his bottle while sitting up
    d. The baby looks at the person calling his name

35. A mother brings her 10-month child to the clinic complaining that the child is fuzzy all day. She states that her child feels warmer than usual. According to her, her child was just given a measles vaccine 3 days ago. She also states that she gives him a lactose-free formula and that she props his bottle on a small pillow to prevent him from sucking air. Which of the responses alerts the nurse to suspect an ear infection? Select all that apply
    a. She baby feels warmer than usual
    b. The baby received the measles vaccine 3 days ago
    c. The baby takes a lactose free formula
    d. The baby is bottle-fed
    e. The bottle is propped on a small pillow

36. A client comes to the clinic complaining of pain of his ears. He states that even a slight movement of the ear causes extreme pain. Upon inspection, the nurse notes swollen red pinna and outer canal. The client states that he noticed the symptoms a few days after he went swimming in the lake. Which of the following conditions is the client most likely suffering from?
    a. Otitis media
    b. Otitis externa
    c. Cellulitis
    d. Frostbite

37. The nurse is assessing the client's external ear and notices yellowish hard nodes on the helix of the ears. The nodes are not painful. Which of the following is the most likely reason for the client's manifestations?
    a. Cellulitis
    b. Tophi
    c. Sebaceous cyst
    d. Keloid

38. A client is brought to the clinic after a minor accident, and the nurse is examining the head of the client. Which of the following findings should be immediately reported to the physician?
    a. A cut to the helix of the ear
    b. A keloid at the back of the ear lobule

c. Bruising behind the ears
d. Pain when the helix is touched

39. A nurse is reviewing her concepts on ear canal abnormalities. Which of the following accurately describes an osteoma?
    a. A protrusion of several small hypertrophied bone covered with epithelium
    b. A single nodule that is hard and non-tender obscuring the eardrum in the inner third of the canal
    c. Swollen and painful inflammation of a hair follicle anywhere on the tragus or any part where hair grows
    d. A growth in the ear canal that is redder than surrounding skin; there is foul purulent discharge

40. The nurse uses an otoscope and examines the ears of the client. The nurse notes that the eardrum's landmarks are very noticeable and that the eardrum appears retracted. Which of the following most likely caused the client's manifestations?
    a. Obstruction of the Eustachian tube that caused a vacuum-like effect
    b. Acute otitis media
    c. Chronic otitis media
    d. Fungal infection

41. The nurse caring for a client suspects that the client has acute otitis media. Which of the following are signs and symptoms of acute otitis media? Select all that apply.
    a. Fever
    b. Pain
    c. Absent light reflex of the eardrum
    d. Black oval shapes on the drum
    e. A growth in the ear canal that is redder than surrounding skin; there is foul purulent discharge

42. A client comes to the clinic because he is concerned that a tiny tube came out of his ear. The client states that he had undergone insertion of a tube one and a half year ago because of recurrent infections. Which of the following is the best nursing action?
    a. Refer the client to the physician for reinsertion of the tube
    b. Verify the client's claim by checking medical records and then document your finding
    c. Administer otic antibiotic drops
    d. Let the client lie on the bed with the affected ear elevated

43. A client is being treated in the clinic after sustaining wounds from a fistfight. Upon inspection of the ear, the nurse notes a black oval shape in the middle of the eardrum. The nurse documents her assessment findings as:
    a. Attic perforation
    b. Marginal perforation

c.   Central perforation

d.   Total perforation

44. The nurse is using an otoscope to assess the inner structures of the client's ear. She notes that the eardrums appear bluish-purple. Which of the following describes the client's condition?

a.   Otorrhea

b.   Hemotympanum

c.   Chlolesteatoma

d.   Otomycosis

45. A nurse reviews a client's records, and she reads that the client has positive Rinne test. Which of the following correctly describes the documentation entry?

a.   Bone conduction is equal air conduction

b.   Sound lateralizes to better ear

c.   Bone conduction is longer than air conduction

d.   Air conduction is longer than bone conduction

46. A pregnant client is concerned because she says she is prone to bleeding lately. As the nurse asked for clarification, the client confides that her gums bleed when she brushes her teeth and that she experiences nosebleeds. She also states that she seem to have a stuffy nose. Which of the following is the most likely reason for the client's complaints?

a.   Decreased blood viscosity

b.   Hormonal changes

c.   Decreased erythrocyte count

d.   Increased platelet activity

47. A female elderly client tells the nurse that her mouth feels dry even if she increases fluid intake. The nurse is aware that certain medications can cause dry mucosa. Which of the following medications causes dry mouth? Select all that apply.

a.   Aminoglycosides

b.   Aspirin

c.   Anticholinergics

d.   Antidepressants

e.   Bronchodilators

48. A nurse is preparing a teaching plan on the prevention of both tooth decay and ear infections to several mothers. Which of the following will contribute to both tooth decay and ear infection?

a.   Upper respiratory infection

b.   Intake of sweets

c.   Swimming

d.   Bottle-feeding

49. An elderly client tells the nurse that he has a decreased sense of smell. Which of the following should the nurse advise to ensure safety of the client at home?
    a. Install grab bars in the client's bathroom
    b. Install smoke detectors in the client's house
    c. Provide the client with emergency contact numbers
    d. Provide calcium rich meals to help re-establish sense of smell

50. A nurse is conducting a physical assessment of the mouths of several clients. Which of the following findings will warrant further evaluation?
    a. An African American with bluish lips and dark line on the gingival margin
    b. A Hispanic with coral colored gums that are with stippled or dotted surface
    c. A Caucasian with strawberry colored tongue and prominent papillae
    d. An Asian whose ventral side of the tongue is smooth and with prominent veins

51. A nurse assessing the mouth of a client notes tiny cream-colored papules on the mucosa of the cheek. The client says they are painless. What is the nurse's best action regarding her findings?
    a. Immediately notify the physician
    b. Advise the client to gargle with salt water
    c. Document her findings
    d. Advise client to increase intake of vitamin A

52. The nurse is assessing a client complaining of pain when swallowing. Upon inspection of the throat, the nurse notes that the tonsils are inflamed and swollen and are touching the uvula. How should the nurse document the grade size of the tonsils?
    a. 1+
    b. 2+
    c. 3+
    d. 4+

53. A nurse is performing a physical examination of a client. She specifically wants to assess the functions of both the glossopharyngeal (CN IX) and vagus (CN X) nerves. Which equipment/instrument should she prepare?
    a. Tongue depressor
    b. Different types of foods
    c. Cotton ball
    d. Speculum

54. A nurse is dealing with an uncooperative infant who refuses to open his mouth for inspection. Which of the following is the best technique to view the child's throat?
    a. Use a speculum
    b. Insert a tongue blade in the buccal mucosa and turn and swipe in between the back teeth and press on the back of the tongue

c. Mummy restrain the child and pry open the mouth
d. Give a sedative and then inspect the throat when the child falls asleep

55. A nurse is assessing the mouth of a newborn and she notices white pearl-like nodes on the roof of the mouth. How should the nurse document her findings?
    a. Fordyce granules are evident on the roof of the mouth
    b. Oral candidiasis patches evident on the roof of the mouth
    c. Milk residues stuck on the hard palate
    d. Epstein pearls evident on the hard palate

56. A competent nurse is aware that breath odors can help identify certain disorders. Which of the following breath characteristics suggest uremia or increased urea and other nitrogenous waste in the blood?
    a. Fruity
    b. Fetid
    c. Ammonia-like
    d. Mouse-like

57. The nurse is to care for elderly clients in a housing facility. Which of the following is NOT an age related change in the mouth of elderly clients?
    a. "varnished" look of the mucosa
    b. Yellowish teeth
    c. Receding gums
    d. A small leathery patch on the mucosa

58. The nurse is conducting health teaching to several clients on the use of smokeless tobacco. Which of the following effects of smokeless tobacco should NOT be included in her teachings?
    a. Fatal heart attack
    b. Hypoparathyroidism
    c. Decreased sperm count
    d. troke

59. It is early spring and a client is complaining of stuffy nose, itchy watery eyes and disturbed sleep. Which of the following conditions is the client most likely suffering from?
    a. Upper respiratory infection
    b. Sleep apnea
    c. Allergic rhinitis
    d. Hives

60. A client is a known addict of cocaine for years. Prior to confinement, the client confesses to having a 'snort'. Which of the following is an expected finding of the client's nose structures?
    a. Nasal polyp

b. Perforated septum
c. Rhinorrhea
d. Furuncle

61. A client is concerned to have another child with a cleft palate. She asks the nurse what should be avoided to prevent having another child with the same condition. Which of the following should NOT be included in the nurse's list?
    a. Smoking
    b. Benzodiazepenes
    c. Phenytoin
    d. Aspirin

62. A client shows the nurse several ulcer-looking ruptured pustules in the upper lip margin that are slightly painful. Which of the following would the nurse note during history taking as a precipitating factor for the development of the sores?
    a. Fever
    b. Trauma to the face
    c. Yeast infection
    d. Vitamin C deficiency

63. A nurse inspects the mouth of an HIV positive patient. She finds white cheesy patches on the tongue and the mucosa. When the nurse tries to scrape off the white substance, some came off leaving a red base that bled. Which of the following conditions is the client most likely suffering from?
    a. Candidiasis
    b. Leukoplakia
    c. Herpes Simplex I
    d. Aphthous ulcer

64. A female client is very concerned with the appearance of her tongue that blackened and became 'hairy'. It has negatively affected her social life. Which of the following most likely caused the client's condition? Select all that apply.
    a. Chronic steroid use
    b. Antibiotic use
    c. Overuse of mouthwash
    d. Heavy smoking
    e. Intake of phenytoin

65. A client has been having high-grade fever for 3 days now. She has difficulty swallowing and is complaining of sore throat. Tonsils are 3+ with yellow exudates. Which of the following is the client most likely suffering from?
    a. Acute tonsillitis

b. Sinusitis
c. Laryngitis
d. Throat cancer

ANSWERS

1. C

    To determine the onset of the patient's difficulty hearing, the nurse may ask the nurse when they started to notice the symptom.

2. B

    Injury or other problems in the inner ear can cause sensorineural hearing loss. In Meniere's disease, for example, there is high pressure in the inner ear's endolymphatic system, which leads to sensorineural hearing loss.

3. D

    Certain medications have an adverse effect of hearing loss when used in the long-term. Examples of these medications are aminoglycosides, aspirin, NSAIDS, quinine, and furosemide.

4. C

    Otalgia and an inflamed tympanic membrane are manifestations of otitis media or infection of the middle ear. Upper respiratory infections can cause inflammation of the middle ear, especially in children three years old and below because their eustachian tubes that link the nasopharynx and the middle ear are shorter and straighter.

5. B

    Tinnitus is ringing in the ears without any outside source. Patients describe tinnitus in many ways. The ringing they hear sounds like blowing, roaring, buzzing, humming, whistling, or hissing.

6. D

    When assessing a patient with signs and symptoms of rhinitis, the nurse must ask about their use of decongestants because excessive use of this medication can worsen the symptoms, a condition known as rhinitis medicamentosa.

7. C

    Perforated nasal septum and rhinorrhea are signs of cocaine abuse. Cocaine is an illicit drug that is snorted. The abuse of cocaine damages the nasal passages and affects the sense of smell. Restlessness in the patient further supports the cause.

8. B

    Before inserting the otoscope inside a patient's ear, the nurse must pull the patient's pinna upward, backward and slightly away from the head. This technique straightens the ear canal, enabling the nurse to view the inside of the patient's ear.

9. D

    If a patient incorrectly repeats 4 out of 6 letter-number combinations that the nurse would whisper, then the patient's hearing acuity is decreased. Further testing by an audiometry is necessary.

10. A

While performing the Weber test, a patient with unilateral sensorineural hearing loss will hear the sound of the vibrating tuning fork in the good ear. On the other hand, those with conductive hearing loss will hear the sound in the impaired ear.

11. B

Before examining the patient's mouth, the nurse must first put on gloves. Nurses must observe universal precaution in all client contacts. To prevent being in contact with the patient's saliva during their examination of the patient's mouth, the nurse should wear gloves.

12. A

In the paralysis of cranial nerve X or the Vagus nerve, the soft palate does not rise, and the uvula moves to the side opposite the lesion when the patient says "ah."

13. B

Tonsils are graded based on size. When tonsils are visible, the grade is +1. When they are between the tonsillar pillars and the uvula, the grade is +2. When they are already touching the uvula, the grade is +3. When the tonsils are so large that they are already touching each other, the nurse assigns a grade of +4.

14. C

People with xerostomia have dry mouth due to reduced salivation, increasing their risk for tooth decay, mucositis or gum disease. Drugs that cause dry mouths are antihistamines, decongestants, and anti-anxiety and antidepressant medications.

15. B

Presyncope is near faint or the feeling of being lightheaded. It is caused by orthostatic hypotension secondary to medication intake, arrhythmias, and vasovagal attacks. Orthostatic hypotension also occurs when suddenly standing from a sitting position.

16. D

Benign positional vertigo is experienced as the patient changes position, usually when turning to their side. An episode usually lasts less than a minute, and it can recur up to a few weeks. The patient may experience nausea, vomiting, and nystagmus with the vertigo.

17. A, B, E

A patient with Meniere's disease will have sensorineural hearing loss, sudden vertigo, tinnitus, feeling of fullness in the ears, nausea, vomiting, and nystagmus.

18. C

Acoustic neuroma is brought about by the compression of the vestibular branch of the Cranial

Nerve VIII or the vestibulocochlear nerve. A person with acoustic neuroma will experience vertigo of variable duration accompanied by tinnitus and hearing impairment in one ear.

19. A

Hard, gritty lumps in the helix and anti-helix of a patient's ears, as well as in areas near the joints and hands, are characteristic of tophi. Tophi are deposits of uric acid crystals on the skin because of high blood levels of uric acid. Some lumps will have uric acid crystals discharging through the skin.

20. D

Keloid is a firm nodular mass that is the result of hypertrophied scar that extends beyond the injury. A keloid may develop from ear piercings that have healed.

21. B

Middle ear infections, especially the purulent ones, usually cause perforations in the tympanic membrane. Discharge from the middle ear comes out through the perforation. A reddened ring of granulation tissue indicates chronic infection.

22. B

Amber-colored fluid accumulation in the middle ear, fullness and popping sensations and some hearing impairment are signs of serous effusion. Serous effusions are caused by a sudden change in air pressure, such as in diving.

23. A

Angular cheilitis is the softening of the skin at the angle of the mouth, which fissures when the mouth is opened. It may be caused by nutritional deficiency or overclosure of the mouth. With angle cheilitis, activities that involve opening and closing the mouth, such as eating or speaking will be painful. Saliva also wets and macerates the skin, making it easily damaged.

24. A

The lesions of Peutz-Jeghers Syndrome primarily appear in the dermal layers of the lips and buccal mucosa. The lesions are small but prominent, and are brown in color. Peutz-Jeghers Syndrome accompanies many types of gastrointestinal cancers.

25. B

Patient with oral candidiasis or thrush will have cheesy white substance sticking to their buccal mucosa. It is a type of yeast infection caused by Candida albicans. People with immunosuppression such as patients with AIDS, those taking steroids, and those who had prolonged use of antibiotics usually develop thrush.

26. B

Any damage to the inner ear structures, nerves (Cranial nerve VIII), and the auditory part of the cerebral cortex will result to sensorinueral hearing loss. Damage or abnormality of outer and middle ear, or obstruction in the ear canal can cause conductive hearing loss.

27. A, B, E
Young children aged three and below are more prone to infections because their Eustachian tubes are wider, shorter and horizontal than those of adults. The tube is also prone to occlusion because of the presence of lymphoid tissues in the tubes at these ages.

28. A
In recruitment, the sensory cells of the cochlea are damaged that result to limited range of hearing. A client will have difficulty hearing normal conversations but will experience discomfort when hearing higher intensity sounds.

29. B
Passive smoking and smoking during pregnancy can predispose a child to otitis media. Other factors that can contribute to the development of otitis media are attendance at Day Care centers and bottle-feeding.

30. A, B, D, E
Signs that indicate that a person has hearing loss include looking at the lips instead of the eyes of the person spoken to (because of lip reading), leaning forward to hear, garbled speech, speaking in a loud voice, and asking the person spoken to to repeat the question.

31. B
Subjective vertigo is the feeling that you are spinning in a room. On the other hand, objective vertigo is the feeling that the room is spinning around you. Syncope is the loss of consciousness and presyncope is feeling faint, the state of being almost unconscious.

32. D
The client's experience describes tinnitus, or a subjective ringing, crackling, whistling or buzzing in the ears. Factors that cause tinnitus are middle ear infections, impacted ear canal, or ototoxic medications such as aspirin and aminoglycosides.

33. B
Age appropriate test for a 4-month old is to make a loud sound out of the child's sight and see if the child reacts to the sound by crying, getting startled or by efforts to locate sound. The startle reflex may have already disappeared at this age. Audiometry is for older children who can follow simple instructions. Responding to one's name is a milestone of infants who are at least 6 months of age and therefore not reliable in assessing hearing problems in a 4-month old.

34. B
A 7-month old infant is not yet able to communicate his needs. Frequent touching or pulling of the

ears may indicate discomfort brought about by an ear infection. This warrants further evaluation.

35. A, D, E

Ear infections in infants are related to bottle-feeding practices and upper respiratory infections. Signs that an ear infection is present are low-grade fever, discomfort, fuzziness and constant pulling of the ear.

36. B

Otitis externa is the infection of the outer structures of the ear. It is sometimes referred to as swimmer's ear because it is related to recent swimming activities. The outer ear appears red, inflamed and painful. There may be scant purulent discharge coming from the outside structures.

37. B

Tophi are uric acid deposits on the skin. On the ears, these appear as superficial yellowish-node looking protrusions on the helix of the ears. They are not painful.

38. C

Ecchymosis behind the ears over the mastoid process is called the battle sign. It is an indication of basilar skull fracture. This finding should be immediately reported to the physician.

39. B

An osteoma is a single nodule that is hard and non-tender obscuring the eardrum in the inner third of the canal. Although benign, it is recommended to be removed to prevent hearing problems.

40. A

The signs are consistent with obstruction of the Eustachian tube that caused a vacuum-like effect that caused the retraction.

41. A, B, C

Acute otitis media is infection of the middle ear. It is characterized by fever, pain, absent light reflex of the eardrum because of increasing pressure. The eardrum also appears red and bulging that in the later stage can become yellowish in color because of pus behind it.

42. B

Tympanostomy tubes are inserted to prevent recurrent middle ear infections. When inflammation subsides, the tubes fall out spontaneously in 12-18 months. There is no additional care needed.

43. C

Perforation of the eardrums can be the result of trauma (e.g. slapping) or infections. When the perforation is at the pars tensa in the middle part of the eardrum, it is called central perforation.

44. B

Hemotympanum is caused by accumulated blood behind the eardrum usually caused by trauma.

It is bluish purple in color.

45. D

A positive result in a Rinne test means that air conduction is heard longer twice than bone conduction. It indicates normal hearing.

46. B

The main reason for epistaxis and bleeding gums in pregnancy is hormonal changes. It is also partly caused by hyperemia.

47. C, D, E

Certain medications can cause xerostomia or dry mouth. Examples of these medications are anticholinergics, antidepressants, bronchodilators, antihypertensives and antipsychotics.

48. D

Bottle-feeding can cause both tooth decay and ear infection. The sugar in formula milk, and the constant pressure posed by the silicone nipple on the teeth, cause tooth decay. Propping the bottle on sleeping babies cause milk to pass through the Eustachian tubes leading to middle ear infections.

49. B

Elderly clients with decreased sense of smell will not be able to smell smoke. Smoke detectors should be installed in the client's home.

50. C

Strawberry colored tongue with prominent papillae is a sign of pathology, specifically scarlet fever. This necessitates further evaluation. All other options are normal findings.

51. C

Tiny cream-colored or whitish painless papules on the mucosa of the cheeks, lips and tongue are sebaceous cysts called Fordyce granules. They have no clinical significance. The nurse duly documents her findings.

52. C

The sizes of tonsils are graded as follows:
1+ Visible
2+ Halfway between tonsillar pillars and uvula
3+ Touching the uvula
4+ Touching one another

53. A

To assess the glossopharyngeal (CN IX) and vagus (CN X) nerves that are responsible for the gag reflex, the nurse would need a tongue depressor.

54. B

The safest technique to open the mouth of an uncooperative child is to insert a tongue blade in the buccal mucosa, turn and swipe in between the back teeth, and press on the back of the tongue. The gag reflex will open the mouth of the child and the nurse should seize this opportunity to quickly inspect the child's throat.

55. D

White glistening pearl-like nodes on the hard palate are called Epstein pearls. They are a normal finding and should disappear on their own in a few weeks.

56. C

A client with uremia because of a kidney disorder will have an ammonia smelling breath. Diabetics will have sweet fruity breath. Those with infections of the teeth and mouth will have foul smelling breath. Those with diphtheria will have mouse-smelling breath.

57. D

A leathery or smooth patch on the mucosa can signify a cancerous lesion and is not an age-related change.

58. B

Smokeless tobacco can cause numerous dangerous sequelae including fatal heart attack and stroke, decreased sperm count, sterility, tooth decay, cancer and hypertension.

59. C

Allergic rhinitis is characterized by rhinorrhea, nasal congestion, itchy watery eyes and sneezing.

60. B

Perforated septum can be noted in cocaine or methamphetamine addicts who snort drugs to get high. Other causes of perforation include constant picking, trauma and surgery.

61. D

Smoking, drinking alcohol and the intake of some medications such as benzodiazepenes, phenytoin, and steroids increase the risk of having a child with cleft lip or palate. Aspirin intake is unrelated to cleft palate development.

62. A

Common precipitating factors for the development of cold sores or Herpes Simplex I are fever, allergy, colds and prolonged exposure to the sun.

63. A

People with decreased immune function such as those with HIV infection, and the chronic steroid users, and people with altered flora such as antibiotic users are prone to the development of oral candidiasis, which is characterized by cheesy white patches that when scraped, bleed easily.

64. A, B, C, D
Black hairy tongue is a temporary condition caused by altered flora on the tongue. Chronic steroid use, antibiotic use, overuse of mouthwash and heavy smoking predispose to having black and hairy tongue.

65. A
Signs and symptoms of acute tonsillitis are high-grade fever, inflamed, painful and swollen tonsils with yellow exudate. The client complains of sore throat and difficulty swallowing.

The Breasts and the Regional Lymphatics

Questions

1. A nurse is receiving endorsement from a nurse of an earlier shift who had performed a Tanner staging of breast development of several female clients. Which of the following information accurately describes Tanner stage 3?
    a. The areola and nipple form a secondary mound over the breast
    b. The breast and areola enlarge and the nipple is flush with the breast surface
    c. Only the nipple is protruding; the areola is flush with the rest of the breast
    d. A small mound of breast and nipple develops and the areola widens

2. A female client has expressed concern that she is having scant nipple discharge on both breasts that is clear and with no distinct smell. The nurse performed a urine pregnancy test and she tested negative. Which of the following factors could have contributed to her galactorrhea?
    a. Use of steroids
    b. Manual stimulation
    c. Ectopic pregnancy
    d. Chronic use of aspirin

3. The American Cancer Society has several recommendations for screening breast cancer in women. Which of the following does NOT belong to the recommendations?
    a. Breast self-examination should begin at 20 years of age
    b. From age 20 to 39 years of age, every woman should undergo clinical breast exam every 3 years
    c. By 40 years of age, should have a mammogram done every year
    d. By 40 years of age, should have clinical breast exam done every year

4. The nurse is conducting a screening for breast cancer in women. Which of the following factors when identified will have a risk factor score of >4?
    a. Never breastfed a child
    b. Dense breast on mammography
    c. Received high dose radiation to the chest
    d. Early menarche

5. A nurse is assessing the breasts of a 45-year old woman. Which of the following findings indicates a need for follow-up assessment?
    a. A ridge of compressed tissue on the lower part of both breasts
    b. A dark circular nipple-looking patch of tissue 5-6 cm below the left breast
    c. A painless fixed node on the upper left quadrant of the right breast
    d. The left breast is bigger than the right

6. When conducting a clinical breast examination, the nurse should ensure several techniques to be able to properly identify suspicious lumps. Which of the following is NOT appropriate to be done during a clinical breast exam?

a. Tuck a small pillow underside the opposite breast to be examined
b. Raise the arm to be examined over her head
c. Ask the woman to turn her hip opposite to the breast to be examined
d. Use three finger pads when palpating

7. The nurse is palpating the breasts of a woman. She is aware that most tumors are found in a particular quadrant of the breast. Which particular quadrant will the nurse pay extra attention to?
a. Upper outer quadrant
b. Upper inner quadrant
c. Lower outer quadrant
d. Lower inner quadrant

8. The nurse is aware that there are suspensory connective tissues in the breasts that support the breast. These are vertical suspensions from the chest wall that keep breast tissues in shape. What are these suspensions called?
a. Adipose tissues
b. Tail of Spence
c. Lactiferous ducts
d. Cooper ligaments

9. A nurse reads in the client's records that the client is complaining of mastalgia. Which of the following can cause mastalgia?
a. Trauma
b. Increased calcium intake
c. Use of steroids
d. Anemia

10. A nurse wants to assess the breasts of a woman who is concerned about a lump she felt while taking a bath. She hopes to assess both genetic and non-genetic factors. Which tool should the nurse to conduct the assessment?
a. Gail Model
b. Breast Cancer Risk Assessment tool
c. Tyrer-Cuzick Model
d. Asian-American Breast Cancer Study

11. A nursing mother complains to the nurse that her nipples hurt when nursing. Which of the following should the nurse instruct the mother to help speed healing of the sore nipples? Select all that apply
a. Clean the breasts with soap and water
b. Air dry the nipples
c. Apply petroleum jelly in between feedings
d. Nurse the baby more frequently

e.   Wear bras with underwires

12. A novice nurse checking the records of her client in the female cancer ward encounters the term "skin tether". Which of the following accurately describes skin tether?
    a.   Exaggeration of the hair follicles because of edema
    b.   A shallow dimple caused by skin retraction
    c.   Underlying tissue is stuck on the chest wall
    d.   Retracted nipple

13. Peau d'orange is caused by edema. Edema in the breast is caused by which process?
    a.   Fibrosis
    b.   Inflammation
    c.   Lymphatic obstruction
    d.   Thrombosis

14. A nurse plans to perform a triple test on a client to determine possible cancerous lumps on a female breast. Which of the following are included in the triple test? Select all that apply.
    a.   Needle biopsy
    b.   CT scan
    c.   Palpation
    d.   Ultrasound
    e.   Chest X-ray

15. An 18-year old female college student is concerned about a lump she has felt on her left breast. Upon assessment, the nurse notes a 3cm a hard rubbery mass at 6 o'clock location from the nipple. It is round and easily slides and moves when palpated. Which of the following is the nurse's most likely finding?
    a.   Carcinoma
    b.   Fibroadenoma
    c.   Fibrocystic breast disease
    d.   Cyst

16. A 45-year old female client seeks consultation because she is concerned about lumps she feels on her breasts. She says that they sometimes feel painful especially a week before her menses. Upon further assessment, the nurse notes several small lumps on both breasts that are movable and tender to palpation. Which of the following conditions is likely responsible for the clients manifestations?
    a.   Carcinoma
    b.   Fibroadenoma
    c.   Fibrocystic breast disease
    d.   Cyst

17. A nurse is describing a woman's breasts for documentation. What is the term used to denote asymmetrical, unilaterally distorted breast caused by fibrotic breast tissues that are pulled and stuck on the chest wall?
    a. Deviation
    b. Retraction
    c. Dimpling
    d. Fixation

18. A nurse is assessing a male client and noticed that the breasts are bilaterally enlarged. Upon palpation, the nurse notes glandular tissue under the areola. Which of the following conditions is the client most likely suffering from?
    a. Breast cancer
    b. Gynecomastia
    c. Fibrocystic disease
    d. Fibroadenoma

19. A nurse is assessing the breasts of an elderly male client. The nurse has made several findings. Which of the following findings is most significant?
    a. Presence of skin tags
    b. Nipple discharge
    c. Supernumemary nipple
    d. Lentigines

20. A nurse assessing the breasts of a female client notes that the areola of the left breast is reddened and that the nipple appears scaly and crusted. A bloody discharge is also noted. The client also claims to feel 'prickly sensations' to the area, as well as itching. Which of the following is the client most likely suffering from?
    a. Paget's disease
    b. Gynecomastia
    c. Fibrocystic disease
    d. Fibroadenoma

21. The nurse has been doing health teaching on breast self-examination. Which of the following client statement indicates correct understanding?
    a. "I begin my examination by using my palm to feel the entire left breast."
    b. "I don't like to put pressure because my breasts are painful"
    c. "I use the fingertips of middle three fingers of each hand to feel both my breasts."
    d. "I inspect the contour of my breasts while standing in front of a mirror"

22. The nurse is doing a clinical breast examination on a 45-year old woman. The nurse understands that all of the following are indicative of a normal breast EXCEPT:
    a. The surface of the areola has small, rounded elevations

b. The left breast is slightly larger than the right
c. An extra nipple 4 inches below the right breast
d. Stellate lump on the right breast

23. A nurse is doing an examination of the client's chest and breasts. Which of the following findings indicate the need to inform the physician immediately?
    a. Minimal blood-tinged discharge on the right breast
    b. Hyperpigmentation of the areola
    c. Significant fat tissues of both breasts
    d. Inverted nipple from birth

24. During health history, the nurse uses the "OLD CART" pneumonic. Which of the following questions is under the "T" category?
    a. "What does the lump feel like?"
    b. "In which breast is the lump?"
    c. "Have you done anything about the lump to make it disappear?"
    d. "When did you first notice the lump?"

25. A 35-year old mother of three came to a clinic to address a complaint of pain in the abdomen. As you examine the breasts as part of a complete physical exam, you noted a milky discharge on both breasts. The client has weaned her youngest a year before and has tested negative for pregnancy? The nurse documents this finding as
    a. High risk for malignancy
    b. Galactorrhea
    c. Normal
    d. Benign breast disorder

26. Which of the following can indicate pathologic breast changes?
    a. Inverting or retraction of a nipple from just a year ago
    b. Loss of adipose tissue since age 40
    c. Tenderness 4 days before menses
    d. Hyperpigmentation of the areolae during pregnancy

27. 27. Which of the following documentation of the client's history indicates a risk for breast malignancies?
    a. History of mastitis
    b. 2 years of breastfeeding an infant
    c. Past chest trauma
    d. Repeated chest x-rays

28. If the patient has overly large breasts, inspection for contour can be difficult. Which technique is most helpful to attain this objective?

a. Lift each breast and examine closely
b. Have the patient stand and lean forward, supported by the back of the chair
c. Have the client turn 90 degrees while standing
d. Push one breast to the side while examining the other

29. Which of the following findings suggests to the nurse that the client has mammary duct ectasia?
a. Firm nodular lumps appearing before menses
b. Irregularly shaped lump non tender and immovable
c. Unilateral tenderness and inflammation
d. Bloody nipple discharge

30. Which of the following documentation entries need to be rectified and clarified? "Breasts pendulous with diffuse fibrocystic changes. Single firm relatively small mass, mobile and nontender, with overlying peau d'orange appearance in right breast, upper outer quadrant at 11 o'clock, 2 cm from the nipple."
a. Breasts pendulous with diffuse fibrocystic changes
b. Single firm relatively small mass
c. Mobile and nontender, with overlying peau d'orange appearance
d. in right breast, upper outer quadrant at 11 o'clock, 2 cm from the nipple

31. The nurse is interviewing a patient who reports that she has some nipple discharge on both her breasts. The nurse understands that of women who report nipple discharge, what are the chances that it means breast cancer?
a. 20%
b. 15%
c. 10%
d. 5%

32. A nurse is assessing risk factors of a woman for breast cancer. Which of the following factors is modifiable?
a. Age
b. Postmenopausal obesity
c. Family history
d. Race

33. A client has just undergone mammography. What is the significance of breast density in the development of breast cancer?
a. Breast density may account for up to 30% of the risk for breast cancer and has a strong inherited component
b. The breast tissue that is predominantly fatty is considered radiologically dense
c. Low breast density is high risk for cancer
d. Breast density is not a risk factor for breast cancer

34. The nurse notes that the client's left breast is positive for retraction. She understands that which process is responsible for this?
    a. Breast tissues disintegrates
    b. It is caused fibrosis or tissue scarring
    c. Breast tissues expands
    d. Breast tissues become fatty

35. As the nurse is assessing the skin of the client's breasts, she noticed that the skin thickened and the pores have enlarged on the area. The nurse is sure to document this as
    a. Intraductal ectasia
    b. Paget's disease
    c. Peau d'orange sign
    d. Skin dimpling

36. A client comes to the outpatient department with a chief complaint of itchiness of the breast particularly the nipple and areola. Upon assessment, the nurse finds a scaly part that has excoriated. Which breast disorder is the client most likely having?
    a. Intraductal ectasia
    b. Paget's disease
    c. Fibroadenoma
    d. Mastitis

37. The nurse obtains a health history from the following clients. To which one should she give priority in teaching about breast cancer prevention?
    a. A 57-year old woman who has been using estrogen therapy for the last 10 years, and presently having dense breast tissues as seen through a mammogram
    b. A woman with menarche at 14 years, now a mother of three
    c. A 65-year old woman with large fatty breasts
    d. A 35-year old woman with a sister who has uterine cancer

38. Which of the following refers to the convexity of the breasts?
    a. Dimpling
    b. Retraction
    c. Orange peel
    d. Contour

39. A nurse is performing a clinical breast examination on a 63-year old woman. The nurse checks for lumps and palpates the group of nodes lining up towards the axilla. What is this group of nodes called?
    a. Pectoral nodes
    b. Lateral nodes

c.   Tail of spence
d.   Subscapular nodes

40. A client comes to ask physician's advice because she has milky discharge from both breasts. She is not pregnant and her youngest is now 4 years old and has fed from a bottle since age 1. Which is the most probable cause of this milky discharge?
a.   Hyperprolactinemia
b.   Breast cancer
c.   Paget's disease
d.   Increased progesterone levels

41. A nurse is examining the chest and abdomen of a female adult patient and notes the presence of a small nipple and areola on the patient's right upper quadrant. Upon palpation, the nurse did not feel any lumpy underlying tissue. Which of the following is the nurse's best action regarding the findings?
a.   Check the extra nipples for any discoloration
b.   Inform the physician immediately
c.   Document the findings
d.   Check for lymphadenopathy near the area

42. A nurse palpates a lump on the female patient's left upper outer breast. Which of the following is the best question to ask the patient to assess for the onset of the breast lump?
a.   "Does the lump change over time or does it come and go?"
b.   "What else happens when you feel the lump?"
c.   "When did you first notice the lump?"
d.   "Is the lump much bigger before your menstruation?

43. A nurse is examining a female patient's breasts. Which of the following information obtained from the patient suggests that the lumps palpated in the patient's breast are physiologic and NOT pathologic in nature?
a.   The lumps are fixed on the chest wall.
b.   The lumps increase in size two weeks before menstruation and decrease in size two weeks after
c.   The lumps are hard
d.   The lumps are small

44. A nurse is examining the breasts of a female patient who is in their early fifties. The nipple of the right breast is turned inward. The nipple of the left breast is not. The patient has noticed that the nipple inversion started four months before. Which of the following refers to the patient's manifestation?
a.   Peau d'orange
b.   Scaling

c. Nipple retraction

d. Dimpling

45. The nurse is screening a patient for breast cancer. Which of the following, if found in the patient suggests increased risk for breast malignancy? Select all that apply.
    a. Menarche after the age of 14
    b. Advanced age
    c. Personal history of fibrocystic breast changes
    d. Breast tissue density on mammogram
    e. Irregular menstruation cycle

46. Which of the following factors will have a >4.0 relative risk for breast cancer?
    a. No full-term pregnancies
    b. Biopsy-confirmed atypical hyperplasia
    c. Long-term use of hormone replacement therapy
    d. High-dose radiation to the chest

47. Which of the following autosomal dominant gene mutations, if found in a 70-year-old woman, indicates a high risk for breast cancer?
    a. CFTR gene
    b. p53
    c. io9
    d. BRCA1 and BRCA2

48. What is the current recommendation for clinical breast examination in women aged 40 and above?
    a. Annual
    b. Bi-annual
    c. Every other year
    d. Every three years

49. Which of the following prevention is the current recommendation for women with a very high genetic risk for breast cancer?
    a. Low-fat diet and annual clinical breast examination
    b. Estrogen replacement therapy
    c. Mammography every six months
    d. Prophylactic bilateral mastectomy

50. A nurse doing a clinical breast examination on a 35-year-old female patient feels a single lump in the patient's left breast. It is small, round, mobile and tender to palpation. Which of the following breast conditions would the nurse most likely consider?
    a. Cyst

b. Fibroadenoma
c. Cancer
d. Lymphedema

51. A nurse is assessing the breast of a female patient who has been recently diagnosed with breast cancer. Which of the following describes the mobility of the cancerous breast mass?
a. Changes location every month
b. Mobile
c. Fixed to the skin or underlying tissue
d. Very mobile

52. An adolescent female patient is concerned about the breast lumps she feels when she showers. During a clinical breast examination, the nurse notes lumps in both breasts. They feel firm and lobular, very mobile but nontender. Which of the following breast changes should the nurse consider?
a. Fibroadenoma
b. Cysts
c. Cancer
d. Lymphoma

53. A novice nurse asks a senior nurse what causes nipple retraction in women with breast malignancy. Which of the following mechanisms causes nipple retraction?
a. Gangrene of the underlying breast tissues
b. Thinning of the skin
c. Thickening of the skin
d. Fibrosis

54. The nurse wants to properly check for skin dimpling in the breast of a female patient. Which of the following positions should the nurse help the patient assume?
a. Supine, with the arms elevated above the head
b. Side-lying with a small pillow under the breast
c. Standing with the hands behind their back
d. Sitting up straight, with the patient's arms relaxed, and hands on their thighs

55. A nurse is examining the breasts of a female patient with advanced breast cancer. Which of the following will the nurse observe on the skin of the patient's affected breast?
a. Ecchymosis
b. Discoloration
c. Enlarged pores
d. Petechiae

56. The patient's breast with malignancy has thick skin with very visible enlarged pores. Which of the

following correctly describes this manifestation?
a.   Nipple retraction
b.   Dimpling
c.   Peau d'orange
d.   Paget's disease

57. A nurse is reviewing her concepts of breast malignancy to better care for a patient. Which of the following mechanisms causes the skin edema that leads to Peau d'orange?
a.   Accompanying general fluid accumulation
b.   Lymphatic blockage
c.   Adipose tissue malformation
d.   Uremia

58. A nurse observes that the breasts of the patient with breast cancer are asymmetrical. The affected breast would most likely deviate in which direction?
a.   Outward
b.   Inward
c.   Downward
d.   Toward the underlying mass

59. A female adult patient comes to the clinic to have her breast examined. Upon examination, the nurse notes the presence of a scaly, crusty eczema-like lesion on the nipple and areola. As the nurse palpates the affected breast, a lump is felt underneath the nipple. Which of the following conditions most likely caused the patient's manifestations?
a.   Breast cancer
b.   Paget's disease of the nipple
c.   Tuberculosis of the skin
d.   Fibroadenoma

60. Which of the following criteria for classifying breast cancer risk is considered a moderate risk?
a.   Known BRCA mutation
b.   History of chest radiation between ages 10-30 years
c.   Known first-degree relative with BRCA mutation
d.   Dense breasts on mammograms

61. A female patient has been found to have a high breast cancer risk. What is the chance that they will have breast cancer in their lifetime?
a.   20-25%
b.   15-20%
c.   10-15%
d.   5-10%

62. A nurse wants to determine a patient's risk for breast cancer. Which of the following assessment tools will help the nurse achieve this goal?
    a. Braden score
    b. CAGE
    c. The Gail Model
    d. MMSE

63. According to the recommendation of the American Cancer Society, how often should women aged 20-39 years undergo clinical breast examination?
    a. Every three years
    b. Every two years
    c. Annually
    d. Bi-annually

64. Which of the following tests involves the compression of the breasts between two metal plates, and then uses x-ray to capture images of breast tissues?
    a. MRI
    b. Mammogram
    c. Radiography
    d. CT scan

65. Which of the following is the recommendation for screening mammography in women 50 to 74 years old, according to the American Cancer Society?
    a. Annual
    b. Biennial
    c. Every two years
    d. Every three years

ANSWERS

1. B

    Tanner Breast Development staging:

    (i)   Stage I (Preadolescent) - Only the nipples are elevated above the chest wall.

    (ii) Stage II - (Breast Budding) – a small mound of breast tissue is evident and the nipples slightly protrude; the areolae has increased in diameter

    (iii) Stage III - The breast mounds becomes bigger and areolae widens even more; nipples flush with the breast

    (iv) Stage IV - The areolae and nipples form a contour above the level of the breasts that have now formed bigger mounds

    (v)   Stage V - Mature female breasts; nipples protrudes; areolae flush with the contour of the breasts

2. A

    Several medications can cause galactorrhea. These are steroids, phenothiazines, diuretics, digitalis, calcium channel blockers and methyldopa.

3. A

    Breast self-examination should start as soon as the breasts are fully developed. Although the American Cancer Society does not have any recommendations on breast self-examination, it recommends that at age 20-39, women should undergo clinical breast exam every 3 years. By 40 years, women should undergo both clinical breast exam and a mammogram.

4. B

    Risk factors that will have a score of >4.0 are age 65+ vs. <65 years, atypical hyperplasia as confirmed by biopsy, mutations of BRCA1 and/or BRCA2, localized lobular carcinoma, dense breasts on mammography, early onset breast cancer and two or more first-degree relatives with breast cancer

5. C

    Any immovable node fixed on the chest wall palpated through the breast however small should be evaluated, and the woman should undergo full screening procedure.

6. A

    A small pillow should be tucked beneath the breast to be examined to flatten the breast for easy palpation.

7. A

    Most tumors are found in the upper outer quadrant of the breasts including the Tail of Spence.

8. D

    Cooper ligaments are vertical suspensions from the chest wall that keep breast tissues in shape thereby providing support to the breasts.

9. A

Mastalgia is breast pain. Causes of mastalgia are trauma, infection, inflammation and benign breast disorders.

10. C

The Tyrer-Cuzick Model assesses both genetic and non-genetic factors of breast cancer development. It is a computer program that provides an estimate of risk. The program will ask to complete a family tree of three generations, and will ask questions regarding parity, BMI, height, age of first menstruation and cessation of menstruation, use of hormonal replacements, and the age of first live birth.

11. B, D

Air-drying the nipples and nursing frequently help heal sore nipples faster.

12. B

A skin tether is a shallow dimple caused by skin retraction secondary to fibrosis of the ducts.

13. C

Peau d'Orange is the thickened skin with prominent pores. This happens because of edema secondary to lymphatic obstruction.

14. A, C, D

The triple test consists of needle biopsy, palpation and ultrasound.

15. B

A fibroadenoma is a round or oval shaped small mass that is rubbery in texture and is well circumscribed. It is also movable. No swollen lymph nodes are evident.

16. C

Fibrocystic breast changes are several lumps that feel tender, rubbery and movable. The pain usually accompanies other symptoms. It is felt at certain days of the month.

17. D

Asymmetrical breasts with one breast looking distorted may signal breast cancer. Fibrotic breast tissues that are pulled and stuck on the chest wall is called fixation.

18. B

Gynecomastia is breast enlargement in males. It is caused by increased levels of estrogen over testosterone. The breasts feel glandular under the both areolae.

19. B

Nipple discharge in males with or without a palpable mass should be further evaluated as it can be a sign of male breast cancer.

20. A

Paget's disease or intraductal carcinoma starts with dry scaly crust from the nipple that spreads to affect the areola. The areola becomes reddened. There is also a thin yellowish discharge. Later, the nipple becomes eczematous, crusted and retracted. Discharge also becomes blood-tinged.

21. D

Breast self-examination involves standing in front of a mirror with hands pressing firmly on the hips, while looking for any changes in size, shape or contour, and for any dimpling, redness or scaliness of the nipple or breast skin.

22. D

A stellate or irregular lump on one breast that is not movable or tender is an indication of malignancy. All other options indicate normal breast tissue. The extra nipple is termed supernumerary nipples.

23. A

Bloody discharge from the nipples is always pathological and will necessitate further medical attention.

24. C

"T" in the pneumonic OLD CART means treatment. The nurse asks if the client has done anything to make the lump disappear, or if medical consultation has been done to address the concern.

25. B

Galactorrhea, or the inappropriate discharge of milk-containing fluid, is abnormal if it occurs 6 or more months after childbirth or cessation of breast-feeding. Excessive breast stimulation, medication side effects or disorders of the pituitary gland (hyperprolactnemia) all may contribute to galactorrhea. Sometimes, galactorrhea is idiopathic. The condition may resolve on its own.

26. A

Nipple retraction is when the nipple is pulled inward. This is not an indicator of a disorder if the breast has had an inverted nipple since birth; however, it necessitates further examination if this is a recent change as it could be an indicator of breast cancer or adhesions below the skin surface.

27. D

Risk factors for breast cancer include previous breast cancer, an affected mother or sister, biopsy showing atypical hyperplasia, increasing age, early menarche, late menopause, late or no pregnancies, and previous radiation to the chest wall.

28. B

In assessing the contour of large or pendulous breasts, it will help if the client leans forward while holding into the backrest or armrest of a chair.

29. C

Tender inflamed cords at one breast suggest mammary duct ectasia, a benign but sometimes painful condition of dilated ducts with surrounding inflammation. It occurs when a milk duct beneath the nipple widens, the duct walls thicken and fills with fluid which in turn become blocked or clogged with a thick, sticky substance. The condition can be asymptomatic, but some women may have nipple discharge (not bloody), breast tenderness or inflammation of the clogged duct.

30. B

In documentation, the nurse should specify the size of the lump. Using small or large to describe a lump needs to be rectified and clarified to be specific.

31. D

Breast cancer occurs in up to 4% of women with breast complaints, in approximately 5% of women reporting a nipple discharge, and in up to 11% of women specifically complaining of a breast lump or mass

32. B

Non-modifiable risk factors for breast cancer include: gender, age, family history, race, genetics, personal history of breast cancer, age at first full-term pregnancy, early menarche, late menopause, and breast density. Modifiable risk factor include: postmenopausal obesity, use of estrogen-progesterone combination HRT, alcohol use, and physical inactivity.

33. A

Mammographic breast density, although considered a strong independent risk factor for breast cancer has been identified as "the most undervalued and underused risk factor" in studies of breast cancer. It has the important attribute of "being present in the tissue from which the cancer arises." Breast density may account for up to 30% of the risk for breast cancer and has a strong inherited component.

34. B

As breast cancer advances, it causes fibrosis or tissue scarring. Shortening of this tissue produces dimpling, changes in contour, and retraction or deviation of the nipple. Other causes of retraction include fat necrosis and mammary duct ectasia.

35. C

Edema of the skin of the breast is caused by the blockage of lymph flow. It appears as thickened skin with enlarged pores—the so-called peau d'orange or orange peel sign because it resembles orange skin. It is often seen first in the lower portion of the breast or areola.

36. B

Paget disease of the nipple is a type of breast cancer that usually starts as a scaly, eczema-like lesion that may weep, crust, or erode. A breast mass may be present. Suspect Paget disease in any persisting dermatitis of the nipple and areola.

37. A

The client in option A has 2 risk factors (age and chronic use of hormonal replacement) and a strong indicator of breast cancer which is a significant density as seen in a mammography

38. D

Contour refers to the convexity of the breasts. Special positioning may be necessary to observe for any abnormal contour. A common abnormality is flattening of the outer lower quadrant of the left breast.

39. C

Nodules in the tail of the breast in the axilla (the tail of Spence) are sometimes mistaken for enlarged axillary lymph nodes. Options (A), (B) and (D) are lymph nodes near the breasts

40. A

Milky discharge unrelated to a prior pregnancy and lactation is nonpuerperal galactorrhea. It is caused by hypothyroidism, pituitary prolactinoma, and dopaminergic drugs, including many psychotropic agents and phenothiazines.

41. C

Supernumerary nipples usually appear along the 'milk line.' The extra nipple is with an areola, with or without a glandular tissue underneath. It has no clinical significance. The nurse must document her findings.

42. C

To assess for the onset of a symptom, such as a lump on the breast, the nurse asks the patient when they first notice the symptom. It is the first question to ask using the OLD CART mnemonic of assessment.

43. B

When lumps are present in the patient's breast, the nurse must ask the patient if they have noticed any change in the size of their breast that corresponds to the monthly cycle. Lumps that increase in size before the menses, and decreases in size after the menses suggest fibrocystic changes, and are considered non-pathologic.

44. C

Nipple retraction is the inversion of the nipple. If the inversion is not present since birth, it signifies breast malignancy.

45. B, D

The most significant risk factors for breast cancer are advanced age, BRCA (breast cancer gene mutation) status, and breast density on a mammogram. Other important risk factors include a personal history and family history of breast cancer.

46. B

A patient who has atypical hyperplasia of the breast confirmed through biopsy will have a >4.0 relative risk for breast cancer. If the patient never had a full-term pregnancy, or if they have undergone high-dose radiation to the chest, the relative risk is 2.1-4.0. Long-Term use of hormone therapy has a relative risk of 1.1-2.0.

47. D

Women with the BRCA1 and BRCA2 (BReast CAncer) gene mutations have 57% and 49% risk of having breast cancer by age 70.

48. A

According to the American Cancer Society, women aged 40 years and above should undergo clinical breast examination (CBE) once a year. It should be performed together with mammography.

49. D

According to the US Preventive Services Task Force, women with very high genetic risk for breast cancer should undergo a prophylactic bilateral mastectomy.

50. A

Cysts are breast lumps that are commonly palpated in the breasts of women 30-50 years old. There may be one or more round lumps that may be soft or firm. They are mobile and tender to palpation.

51. C

Cancerous breast masses are usually fixed to the skin or underlying tissues.

52. A

Fibroadenomas are benign breast masses that are very common in women aged 15-25. The fibroadenomas are round, disc-like or lobular with well-delineated borders. The lumps are mobile and usually nontender to palpation.

53. D

As breast cancer advances, scar formation or fibrosis happens in the breast. Scar tissue formation pulls the nipple inward causing nipple retraction.

54. D

Skin dimpling that is commonly observed in the breast of a patient with breast cancer will be more evident if the patient is made to sit comfortably, and with their arms relaxed, and their hands resting on their thighs.

55. C

Patients with advanced breast cancer will have edema of the skin of the breast. The edema causes the pores to enlarge.

56. C

The characteristic edematous thick skin with enlarged pores in breast cancers is called Peau d'orange. It is so called because the skin of the breast looks like an orange peel.

57. B

The obstruction of lymph flow caused by fibrosis in advanced-stage breast disease leads to the edema of the skin of the breast, which in turn results in Peau d'orange.

58. D

Fibrosis of the breast tissues in breast malignancy causes scar tissues to be shortened so that the breasts look asymmetrical. The deviation is typically toward the underlying cancer.

59. B

Paget's disease of the nipple starts as a scaly eczematous nipple lesion that may weep, crust or erode. The lesion is red, itchy and inflamed. The cancer starts in the nipple, specifically in the milk ducts, and then spreads to affect the areola. A mass may or may not be present underneath.

60. D

According to the American Cancer Society, a patient with dense breasts as seen on a mammogram has a moderate risk of developing breast cancer. The patient is encouraged to discuss advantages and disadvantages of undergoing MRI with their physicians. High-risk patients (options A, B and C), however, are encouraged to undergo MRI in conjunction with a mammogram.

61. A

Patients who are considered high risk for breast cancer development have a 20-25% lifetime risk as based on the risk assessment tool used.

62. C

The Gail Model is also known as The Breast Cancer Risk Assessment Tool. It is used by clinicians to estimate the risk of breast cancer in women.

63. A

The American Cancer Society recommends that all women who are aged 20-39 years old should undergo clinical breast examination every three years, and those aged 40 and above, annually.

64. B

A mammogram is used to screen patients for possible breast cancer. It uses x-ray to capture images of breast tissues. During the procedure, the patient's breasts are compressed by two x-ray plates in different positions.

65. B

Screening mammography is recommended for women 50-74 years of age every six months. Both screening and diagnostic mammography use low-dose x-ray to look for changes in breast tissue. Screening mammography differs from a diagnostic mammography in that it is only done in two views. This reduces exposure to x-ray than that of diagnostic mammograms which capture images in different views.

The Respiratory System

Questions
1. The nurse wants to locate the second intercostal space. Which of the following landmark would be most useful for the nurse to locate first?
   a. Trachea
   b. Angle of Louis
   c. Midclavicular line
   d. Nipple

2. A nurse is examining the chest of the client. She finds that the costal angle is more than 90 degrees. Which of the following conditions will result to increased costal angle?
   a. Lower respiratory tract infection
   b. Atelectasis
   c. Chronic obstructive pulmonary disease
   d. Malnutrition

3. The nurse is assessing a pregnant mother at 34th week gestation. The mother is having premature labor. The nurse is concerned that the fetal lungs are not yet ready for extrauterine life. Which of the following substance acts to reduce surface tension that in turn allows the alveoli to inflate and deflate to facilitate respiration in the newborn?
   a. Lanugo
   b. Vernix caseosa
   c. Primitive lung bud
   d. Surfactant

4. A nurse is caring for several elderly clients in the respiratory ward. Which of the following is NOT considered an age-related change in the respiratory function of the elderly?
   a. Decreased vital capacity
   b. Increased residual volume
   c. Increased lung elasticity
   d. Decreased number of alveoli

5. A culturally competent nurse is aware that although tuberculosis has significantly decreased in the US, there are certain groups or population that bears the burden of TB. Which of the following cultural group/race has the highest rate of TB?
   a. White non-Hispanics
   b. Hispanics
   c. Asians
   d. Blacks

6. A client in the Intensive Care Unit suddenly developed pulmonary edema and started coughing up sputum. Which of the following correctly describes the sputum of a patient with pulmonary edema?

a. Yellowish
b. Rust-colored
c. Pink frothy
d. Clear

7. A client seeks medical consultation after not being relieved of his cough that has been his problem for a long time now. Upon further assessment, the client confides that for the current year, he has been coughing up large amounts of sputum for four months now. The previous year during the winter, he also had similar manifestations that lasted 5 months. He tried taking over-the-counter cough suppressants but they did not help. Which of the following disorders is the client most likely suffering from?
a. Chronic bronchitis
b. Acute bronchitis
c. Tuberculosis
d. Pneumonia

8. An elderly client asks a nurse why he has to receive flu vaccine every year. What is the best response of the nurse to address the client's concern?
a. "The effects of the flu vaccine last one year only."
b. "The flu vaccine expires one year from production date."
c. "I understand how you feel. Let me talk to the doctor so he can discuss this better with you."
d. "The flu vaccine is given annually because they are produced according to the strain of flu virus that is prevalent in the current year."

9. The nurse is assessing the chest of a client with chronic bronchitis. Which of the following finding is consistent with the client's diagnosis?
a. Increased anteroposterior diameter
b. The spinuous processes are not in a straight line
c. Symmetric elliptical chest
d. Scoliosis

10. The nurse is aware that certain disorders can cause change in fremitus. Which of the following conditions can decrease fremitus? Select all that apply.
a. Lobar pneumonia
b. Pleural effusion
c. Pneumothorax
d. Emphysema
e. Asthma

11. A nurse is assessing the breath sounds of several clients. Which of the following sounds she heard on several clients does NOT indicate a pathology?
a. Rales

b. Atelectatic crackles
c. Wheezes
d. Rhonchi

12. A client with laryngeal cancer is being assessed by the nurse. Which of the following correctly describes forced expiratory time?
a. It is the time it takes for a person who has taken the deepest breath to exhale all the air that he can
b. The client blows as hard as he can without inhaling first
c. The normal time for exhalation is 5 seconds
d. It is a screening for cancer of the throat

13. A nurse is examining a newborn who has just been admitted to the neonatal intensive care unit. Which of the following signs, if observed by the nurse, warrants immediate medical intervention?
a. Absent adventitious sounds
b. Irregular breathing through the nose
c. Sternal and intercostal retractions
d. Bulging abdomen during inspiration

14. A nurse is practicing her physical examination skills and is trying to differentiate different types of breath sounds. Which of the following provides accurate information regarding breath sounds?
a. Vesicular sounds are those sounds heard over the trachea
b. Bronchovesicular sounds have equal length of inspiration and expiration
c. Bronchial sounds are those that are heard around the scapulae and in the first and second intercostal space
d. Bronchovesicular sounds are harsh, hallow and tubular sounds

15. A nurse observes that a client seemed to sit unevenly on a chair. The nurse wants to assess for abnormal curvature of the thoracic spine. Which of the following would the nurse have the client to do to?
a. Ask the client to sit properly
b. Ask the client to undress
c. Ask the client to turn around while standing
d. Ask the client to reach for his toes with the knees straight

16. A client is assessing the respiratory patterns of several clients. Who among the following will experience bradypnea?
a. A 15-year old client with meninggococemia
b. A 26-year old with hyperthyroidism
c. A 55-year old with alkalosis

    d.   A 33-year old in diabetic coma

17. A nurse is observing a client. She notes that her inspirations and expirations gradually decrease in depth and rate until a period of apnea is noted. After the period of apnea, there is again a gradual increase in depth and rate of respirations. Which of the following is the correct documentation entry for the nurse's observations?
    a.   Biot's respiration
    b.   Bradypnea
    c.   Cheyne-Stokes respiration
    d.   Chronic obstructive breathing

18. A 5-year old child has just been diagnosed with acute epiglottitis. The nurse is tasked with monitoring the client's respirations. During her bedside visit, she noted that the client is producing a high-pitched crow-like monophonic sound heard best over the neck. Which of the following adventitious lung sounds correctly matches the client's manifestations?
    a.   Wheeze
    b.   High-pitch wheeze
    c.   Friction rub
    d.   Stridor

19. A client with acute bacterial lobar pneumonia is being cared for by the nurse. Which of the following is NOT a manifestation of acute bacterial lobar pneumonia?
    a.   Lung consolidation
    b.   Dull on percussion
    c.   Tachypnea
    d.   Increased fremitus

20. A client suddenly sits up and leans forward. The client is manifesting severe respiratory distress. There is chest pain that worsen on inspiration. The client is coughing out blood-tinged sputum. Pulse oximeter reads 90% oxygenation saturation. A CT-scan revealed a pulmonary embolus occluding the bifurcation of the bronchi. Which of the following is the most likely cause of the client's clot formation?
    a.   Recent cesarean section due to hypertonic contractions
    b.   Acute lobar pneumonia
    c.   Diabetic coma
    d.   Hospitalization for a week due to a rickettsial disease

21. Which of the following is a normal finding when assessing the respiratory system of an emphysema client?
    a.   A increased anteroposterior diameter and low inspiratory and expiratory ratio
    b.   Audible breath sounds without auscultation
    c.   Increased chest expansion

d. Flatness on percussion

22. A community health nurse is doing her rounds in the neighborhood when she was suddenly summoned by a frantic mother whose 1-year old child appears to be in distress. The mother says that her child is making strange noises as she breathes. Upon assessment, the nurse hears a high-pitched sound during inspiration. This alerts the nurse to which finding?
    a. Wheeze
    b. Stridor
    c. Rales
    d. Ronchi

23. A nursing supervisor instructs a new nurse to watch out for intercostal retraction on a 1-year old patient. Which of the following describes intercostal retraction accurately?
    a. The muscles between the ribs are pulled inward as the client inhales
    b. The diaphragm expands during expiration
    c. The chest expands on one side only
    d. The muscles between the ribs puff as the client inhales.

24. The nurse is auscultating the lungs of a patient and hears bronchovesicular sounds at the base of the right lungs. Which of the following is an accurate interpretation of your findings?
    a. It is expected and is normal
    b. It may suggest fluid or mass in the right lower lobe
    c. It suggests atelectasis of the right lower lobe
    d. The client must be positioned on his left before auscultation

25. A nurse hears fine crackling sounds in the client's lungs upon auscultation. The client complains that he is catching up on his breaths and is feeling really tired. Which of the following clients is the nurse most probably assessing? The client with
    a. Upper respiratory tract infection
    b. Asthma
    c. Congestive heart failure
    d. Pneumothorax

26. The nurse is assessing the oxygen saturation of a woman who just underwent normal delivery. Her delivery was uneventful. Her vital signs are normal. Upon checking her pulse oximeter, she got a reading of 66%. To which factor can the nurse attribute the reading?
    a. Too much ambient light
    b. Malfunction of the oximeter
    c. Pulse oximeter has slid out of her finger
    d. Pulse oximeter is slid under her thumb

27. The nurse is auscultating the lungs of the patient. In an otherwise healthy patient, what type of

breath sounds are expected to be heard over the 3rd intercostal space and lower in the lung fields?
a.   Bronchial
b.   Bronchovesicular
c.   Vesicular
d.   Crackles

28. A new nurse is performing a complete physical examination of a client suspected of having a lung tumor. She understands that, in assessing for fremitus, the nurse's hands should be positioned
a.   Cupped over the lower back
b.   Flat and touching the lower back
c.   Fisted and touching the front of the chest
d.   Level to the heart, and finger pads touching the back

29. A client comes to the clinic with difficulty of breathing. He reports that sometimes, he wakes up at night gasping for air. He added that he has to prop himself up with 2 pillows to be able to sleep without breathing difficulty. The nurse assesses fremitus, and understands that which of the following conditions will the nurse probably feel a decrease in fremitus?
a.   Pneumonia
b.   Pleural effusion
c.   Lung tumor or mass
d.   Pulmonary fibrosis

30. The nurse is helping a community prevent an outbreak of streptococcal pneumonia. She performs vaccinations on different age groups in all walks of life. Which of the following patients is the vaccine highly recommended to be administered to?
a.   A 35-year old female teacher with hoarseness of the voice
b.   A 26-year old male soccer player with a pulled muscle
c.   A 46-year old bank executive with vitiligo
d.   A 23-year old new employee about to receive a cochlear implant

31. The nurse is assessing a client with emphysema. How would the client most likely describe his dyspnea?
a.   Slowly progressive
b.   Acute episodes, separated by symptom-free periods.
c.   Sudden onset
d.   Episodic

32. A nurse admits a client with chills, high fever and dyspnea. His blood works states that he has a high level of alcohol in his blood. He is also expectorating red, sticky and jelly-like sputum. The nurse attributes the signs and symptoms to which disorder?

a. Tuberculosis
b. Lung abscess
c. Laryngitis
d. Klebsiella pneumonia

33. The nurse admits a client with left-sided heart failure secondary to mitral stenosis in the intensive care unit. He had developed pulmonary edema and is for constant monitoring. The nurse understands that which characteristics of the client's sputum is the nurse most likely to observe?
a. Greenish, mucoid, sticky
b. Red, jelly-like
c. Pinkish tinged, frothy
d. Foul-smelling purulent

34. A client is developing complications of pneumonia. Which characteristics of chest pain would alert the nurse to the possibility of pleurisy?
a. Pressing, squeezing sensation relieved by rest
b. Burning pain and lying on the involved side relieves it
c. Sharp, knife-like, worsened by movement and inspiration
d. Pressing, squeezing sensation unrelieved by rest

35. A 65-year old patient is admitted to the emergency department with a chief complaint of ripping chest pain after accidentally being hit on the chest with a ball. His medical records show that he has chronic hypertension. The nurse is quick to institute measures to care for a patient with which condition?
a. Myocardial infarction
b. Pericarditis
c. Endocarditis
d. Dissecting aortic aneurysym.

36. A nurse admits a client in the emergency department after a vehicular accident. He complains of pain and is having difficulty in breathing. He is also diaphoretic. The nurse observes his chest and notes paradoxical chest movement. Which is an accurate description of paradoxical chest movement?
a. The chest expands on the unaffected side only
b. The flail part of the chest is sucked in on inspiration and bulges during expiration
c. The flail part of the chest bulges on inspiration and is sucked in during expiration
d. The intercostal muscles move inward during inspiration

37. A client involved in a car crash is admitted due to chest injuries. Upon auscultation, the nurse notes fine creaking sounds confined to a small area of impact and is heard on both inspiration and expiration. The sound can be sometimes heard continuously. The nurse hears which kind of

adventitious sounds?
a. Stridor
b. Ronchi
c. Crackles
d. Pleural rub

38. A nurse is caring for a client with complete atelectasis of the lower lobe of the left lung. Which assessment finding is most accurate?
a. Absent breath sounds on the left side of the chest
b. Dullness over the left lower chest on percussion
c. Bronchovesicular sounds heard over the lower chest on auscultation
d. Increased fremitus over the entire chest area

39. A client obtained a traumatic sports injury to the chest. He was admitted to be treated for pleural effusion. Which of the following assessment findings would necessitate the nurse to promptly inform the physician of the client's condition?
a. Decreased breath sounds on the affected side
b. A pleural rub on auscultation
c. Minimal tracheal deviation to the unaffected side
d. Pain on the affected side

40. A nurse assessing the client with fever notes that the client also has dry and painful non-productive cough. During the interview, the nurse notes that he has hoarseness of the voice. The nurse continues to assess the client for more signs and symptoms of which disorder?
a. Pneumonia
b. Asthma
c. Bronchiectasis
d. Laryngitis

41. A novice nurse is performing a physical examination of an obese patient and is trying to locate the 2nd intercostal space (ICS). Which anatomical location would best guide the nurse to locate the 2nd ICS?
a. Xiphoid process
b. Nipples
c. Angle of Louis
d. Clavicle

42. A patient who is very anxious restlessly paces the hall. The patient tells the nurse that they feel 'pins and needles' around their lips and in their hands and feet. Which of the following refers to the sensation of 'pin and needles'?
a. Pleurisy
b. Dyspnea

c. Wheezing

d. Paresthesias

43. A nurse is assessing a patient's cough and is asking the patient what new medications they have taken recently. The nurse knows that some medications have cough as a side effect. What is an example of a drug that can cause coughing?
   a. Metroprolol
   b. Acetaminophen
   c. Aspirin
   d. ACE inhibitors

44. A nurse is assessing a patient who is coughing up blood. Which of the following signs and symptoms will point to the origin of the bleeding as the stomach and not the lungs?
   a. It will always hurt when it comes from the lungs
   b. The patient will feel faint if bleeding comes from the lungs
   c. The coughed-out blood is darker and with food particles
   d. The coughed-out blood would be paler and thicker

45. A 50-year-old patient from South-East Asia looks underweight and tells the nurse that every night he has fever and night sweats. He is experiencing hemoptysis and chronic cough. Which of the following vaccines did the patient probably missed?
   a. BCG
   b. DPT
   c. MMR
   d. Varicella

46. A nurse is to examine the patient's posterior and lateral thorax, and their lungs. What is the best position for the patient should assume to facilitate this examination?
   a. Sitting with the arms folded across the chest and each hand touching the opposite shoulder
   b. Supine with the arms straight on their sides
   c. On their side with their arms hugging a pillow
   d. Sitting with the arms straight and each hand touching the opposite knee

47. The nurse observes a patient breathing and notices that the patient's sternocleidomastoid and scalene muscles are contracted during inhalation. Which of the following is the correct interpretation of the nurse's observation?
   a. The patient is hyperventilating
   b. The patient is breathing normally
   c. The patient has mild breathing difficulty
   d. The patient has severe breathing difficulty

48. A patient who is a chronic smoker has been recently diagnosed with chronic obstructive pulmonary disease (COPD). Which of the following findings will the nurse most likely note of the patient's thorax?
    a. Decreased AP diameter
    b. Increased AP diameter
    c. Pigeon breast
    d. Protruding ribs

49. The nurse is examining the patient's back and symmetrically places their hand in different locations on the patient's back. The nurse asks the patient to say 'ninety-nine' every time they change the placement of their hands on the back. The nurse notes that in both lung fields, the vibrations of the patient's voice are very loud. Which of the following disorders will have the same manifestation?
    a. Pleural effusion
    b. Pneumonia
    c. Emphysema
    d. Pneumothorax

50. The nurse is performing a physical examination on a patient and is percussing a patient's back. Which of the following is the right information about doing percussion?
    a. The pleximeter is the forefinger of the non-dominant hand
    b. Avoid touching the patient's skin, except with the pleximeter
    c. With a hard wrist motion, strike the pleximeter with the dominant hand's middle finger
    d. Aim at the proximal interphalangeal joint

51. A nurse who is percussing the back of a patient with a large pneumothorax hears a drum-like sound. Which of the following correctly describes the nurse's findings?
    a. Flatness on percussion
    b. Dullness on percussion
    c. Resonance on percussion
    d. Tympany on percussion

52. A nurse is auscultating the chest of a patient and hears crackles caused by chest hair. Which of the following can the nurse do that will help in the auscultation?
    a. Use the bell of the stethoscope instead
    b. Ask the patient to hold their breath for a few seconds
    c. Ask the patient to lie down
    d. Wet the chest hairs

53. The nurse is auscultating the patient's posterior chest to assess for breath sounds. While the stethoscope is placed over the right and left 4th intercostal space, the nurse hears a soft, low-

pitched sound that persists from the start of the inspiration to one-third of the way through exhalation. Which breath sound did the nurse most likely hear?
a. Bronchial
b. Tracheal
c. Vesicular
d. Bronchovesicular

54. A nurse is assessing the breath sounds of a patient with early congestive heart failure. The nurse hears soft, short, high-pitched sounds, like the sound of a lock of hair that is rubbed between two fingers and positioned near the ear. Which adventitious breath sound did the nurse most likely hear?
a. Ronchi
b. Wheezes
c. Rales
d. Stridor

55. A patient who has asthma is recovering from an acute attack. The patient asks the nurse why the sound of their breathing sound musical when they breathe out. Which of the following is the best nursing response?
a. "The musical sound is produced by collapsing lungs."
b. "The air passages are filled with fluid that makes the musical sound."
c. "Your body is trying to get in more air to the lungs."
d. "The musical sound is produced by narrowed airways."

56. A nurse is to examine the anterior chest of the patient with dyspnea. Which of the following actions indicate that the nurse needs further teaching?
a. Help the patient lie supine
b. Sit the patient up in bed
c. Elevate the head of the bed
d. Allow the patient to sit and slightly lean forward

57. Which of the following will cause inaccurate SpO2 readings using a pulse oximeter? Select all that apply.
a. Age above 60-years-old
b. Dark nail polish
c. Too much ambient light
d. Fair skin
e. Diabetes

58. A nurse who is examining a patient recovering from an acute asthma attack wants to assess the maximum volume of air that the patient expels from the lungs during a forceful expiration. Which of the following equipment is most appropriate to use for this assessment?

a. A peak flow meter
b. A stethoscope
c. A brown paper bag
d. An incentive spirometer

59. A nurse doing a health teaching on smoking cessation is explaining that the nicotine in tobacco and cigarettes cause many types of cancers. Which of the following cancers can be caused by smoking?
    a. Kidney
    b. Lungs
    c. Bladder
    d. All of the above

60. A nurse is to administer a live attenuated flu vaccine on a preschool child. Which route will this vaccine be administered?
    a. IM
    b. SQ
    c. Intra-nasal
    d. Oral

61. A female post-partum patient suddenly developed tachypnea and severe dyspnea and is looking very distressed. Which of the following factors could be a cause of sudden severe dyspnea?
    a. Chronic bronchitis
    b. Pulmonary embolism
    c. Anxiety with hyperventilation
    d. Lung cancer

62. A patient who presented to the emergency department with high-grade fever and cough has been diagnosed with bacterial pneumonia. What would be characteristic of the sputum of a patient with bacterial pneumonia?
    a. Clear
    b. Frothy
    c. Dry
    d. Rusty

63. A novice nurse is distinguishing whether the patient's chest pain is angina or myocardial infarction (MI). Which of the following factors will alert the nurse that the patient has MI and NOT angina?
    a. May occur at rest
    b. Pressing, squeezing pain
    c. The pain is retrosternal

d.   Chest pain is not relieved by rest or nitroglycerin

64. A nurse is looking at the breathing of a patient who suffered brain trauma. The nurse observes that the patient has periods of deep breathing followed by apnea. Which of the following refers to the rhythmic waxing and waning of respiration?
    a.   Biot breathing
    b.   Obstructive breathing
    c.   Cheyne-Stokes breathing
    d.   Bradypnea

65. A patient is examining a patient diagnosed with a large pneumothorax. Which of the following will the nurse most likely observe of the patient's trachea?
    a.   Midline
    b.   Collapsed
    c.   Shifted toward the affected side
    d.   Shifted toward the unaffected side

ANSWERS

1. B

    The angle of Louis is a slightly protruding fused connection between the manubrium and the sternum. It coincides with the 2nd rib. Sliding downward and sideward will locate the second intercostal space.

2. C

    Conditions that result to hyperaerated overdistended lungs such as emphysema or chronic obstructive pulmonary disease will increase the costal angle.

3. D

    Surfactants act to reduce surface tension in the lungs. It allows the alveoli to inflate and deflate to facilitate respiration in the newborn.

4. C

    After age 50, there are significant changes to the respiratory system. These include a decreased vital capacity, increased residual volume, decreased lung elasticity, and number of alveoli, and a gradual loss of intra-alveolar septa.

5. D

    The blacks have the highest rate of TB, 7.3 times non-Hispanic Whites.

6. C

    The sputum of a client with pulmonary edema is pink-tinged and frothy. This is because of minute capillaries that rupture and become leaky. It is frothy because it is fluid with trapped air.

7. A

    Chronic bronchitis is inflammation of the bronchus that lasts for more than three months for at least two years in a row. It is characterized by productive cough.

8. D

    The flu vaccine is given annually because they are produced according to the strain of flu virus that is prevalent in the current year. They are modified annually.

9. A

    People with COPD or chronic obstructive pulmonary disease such as chronic bronchitis have increased anteroposterior diameter, making the chest look as if it is in constant chest expansion or inspiration.

10. B, C, D

    Any barrier present between the palpating hands and the client's lung decreases fremitus. Such conditions are pleural effusion, pneumothorax and emphysema. Lobar pneumonia, on the other hand, increases fremitus

11. B

Atelectatic crackles are heard over deep breaths. Because deep breaths are not continuous in the respiratory cycle, these sounds disappear after a few breaths. Atelectatic crackles are fine popping sounds that are produced by air trapped in scant secretions in older adults and sleepers.

12. A

Forced expiratory time is the time it takes for a person who has taken the deepest breath to exhale all the air that he can. It usually takes four seconds to do the exhalation this way. It helps to assess airway obstruction.

13. C

Nasal flaring and sternal and intercostal retractions are signs of severe respiratory distress. The neonate would need immediate medical attention.

14. B

Bronchovesicular sounds are heard around the scapulae and in the first and second intercostal space. They are of moderate intensity and harshness. They also have equal length of inspiration and expiration.

15. D

Asking the client to reach down towards his toes will expose the back and the nurse will have a good view of any abnormality in spine curvature.

16. D

People in diabetic coma, those with depressed respiratory center and those with increased intracranial pressure will experience bradypnea.

17. C

Cheyne-Stokes respiration is the waxing and waning of respiration. Inspirations and expirations gradually decrease in depth and rate until a period of apnea is noted. After the period of apnea, there is again a gradual increase in depth and rate of respirations.

18. D

A stridor is a high-pitched crow-like monophonic sound heard best over the neck. It is usually manifested in acute epiglottitis.

19. D

In acute bacterial lobar pneumonia, the nurse will note dullness on percussion, a decrease in fremitus, and tachypnea. Lung consolidation will also be evident in chest x-rays.

20. A

Pulmonary embolism is caused by any large obstruction to the larger airways like the bronchi. The obstruction can be a thrombus, fat, air or amniotic fluid as a result of conditions such as hypertonic uterine and deep vein thrombosis, to name a few.

21. A

Emphysema is a chronic obstructive pulmonary disease characterized by an increased in anteroposterior diameter caused by permanent enlargement of the airspaces distal to the bronchioles secondary to decreased elastin in the lungs. With decreased elasticity, the lungs are in constant hyper aerated state, accumulating carbon dioxide. In an attempt to excrete the carbon dioxide, the patent exhales longer than normal, accounting for the lower I:E ratio.

22. B

Stridor is a loud, harsh, high pitched respiratory sound caused by obstruction of the larger airways (trachea, larynx or pharynx). A wheeze is a coarse whistling sound heard during expiration. Rales are small clicking, bubbling, or rattling sounds in the lungs heard during inhalation. Ronchi are low pitched, snore-like sounds and are caused by airway secretions and airway narrowing.

23. A

Intercostal retractions are the inward movement of the intercostal muscles, the muscles between the ribs during inhalation. These are caused by blockage of the airways.

24. B

Bronchovesicular sounds are breath sounds heard best in the first and second intercostal space anteriorly and between the scapulae. In these locations, the inspiration and expiration sounds are about equal. If heard in the lower areas, it may indicate fluid or mass occupying the lobe/s.

25. C

Rales are fine non-musical crackling sounds when small airways blocked by fluid open as one inhales. It is heard in pneumonia, fibrosis, early congestive heart failure, bronchitis, bronchiectasis and pulmonary edema.

26. A

Certain factors affect pulse oximeter readings such as ambient light, hemoglobin and blood volume deficiencies, patient movement, strong electromagnetic fields, irregular heartbeats, nail polish, dark skin pigmentation and intravenous dyes.

27. C

Vesicular breath sounds are soft, relatively low-pitched sounds heard over most of the lung fields lower than the 2nd intercostal space.

28. B

    In assessing for fremitus, the both hands should be flat on the back or front of the chest to efficiently feel vibrations as the client speaks.

29. B

    In cases where the lungs are filled with fluid (e.g. pleural effusion) or air or are vacant, the fremitus is decreased. The signs and symptoms of the client are characteristic of pleural effusion. Fremitus is increased in conditions that will have consolidations in the lungs such as pneumonia or in lung tumor and fibrosis.

30. D

    The pneumococcal vaccine is highly recommended for the following risk groups: 65 years old and older, those with chronic illnesses aged 2-64, anyone about to receive a cochlear implant, the immunocompromised, and healthy children older than 6 months.

31. A

    Emphysema is a progressive disease wherein symptoms gradually worsen over time. The nurse expects that the client will report difficulty breathing that worsens over months or years.

32. D

    Klebsiella pneumonia is a bacterial infection of the lungs that typically manifest in people with compromised immune systems or those with accompanying morbidity, especially chronic ones. It is also common among alcoholics. Aside from the typical signs and symptoms of pneumonia such as high-grade fever, malaise, and dyspnea, the client expectorates red, sticky and jelly-like sputum.

33. C

    The client with pulmonary edema will have pink frothy sputum. The pinkish tinge is due blood coming from minute capillaries erupting, and the fine bubbles that makes it frothy is created by air trying to escape from the fluid-filled alveolar bed.

34. C

    Chest pain in pleurisy is described as a sharp and knife-like and is worsened by movement and inspiration. Burning pain and the consequent relief when lying on the affected side describe chest pain in tracheobronchitis. Pain that is pressing, squeezing is of cardiac origin. If the chest pain is relieved by rest it is caused by angina pectoris. If the pain persists and unrelieved by rest, it is caused by myocardial infarction.

35. D

    In a dissecting aortic aneurysm, the aorta (usually the thoracic artery) gets torn from the inside. The tear allows blood to seep between the layers of the aorta causing it to bulge and most likely rupture. It causes decreased blood flow to the lower parts of the body and produces severe ripping pain. It is considered a medical emergency.

36. B
Paradoxical chest movement happens when the flail part of the chest is sucked in on inspiration and bulges during expiration. This happens when fractured ribs cannot simultaneously move with the rest of the chest.

37. D
A pleural rub is a fine creaking sound heard over a small area of the lungs and is heard on both inspiration and expiration, and sometimes heard continuously in both phases of respiration. It is produced by the inflamed and roughened pleura rubbing against each other.

38. B
Atelectasis is collapse of the lung or part of the lungs due to obstruction or a mucus plug in the airways. There is dullness on the airless area, absent breath sounds on the affected part (with the exception of the right upper lobe where tracheal sounds are still apparent) and absent fremitus (increased in upper right lobar atelectasis).

39. C
Tracheal deviation in a client with pleural effusion is a medical emergency. It signifies that the effusion has gotten so large that it pushes the lungs and mediastinal organs to the unaffected side. All other assessment findings in A, B and D are expected.

40. D
Laryngitis is inflammation of the vocal cords caused by infection, overuse or of irritating substances such as smoke. In addition to fever, the client exhibits hoarseness of the voice and has dry painful non-productive cough.

41. C
The angle of Louis or the sternal angle is approximately 5cm below the suprasternal notch or the hollow curve between the two clavicles. The sternal angle is the bony ridge where the manubrium connects to the body of the sternum. Moving horizontally to either side, the nurse will feel the second rib, and exactly below the rib, the firm musculature is the second intercostal space.

42. D
Patients who are hyperventilating, such as those who are overly anxious, would usually report tingling sensations that most people describe as 'pins and needles'. The tingling sensations are called paresthesias and are commonly felt around the lips, and in the hands and feet.

43. D
ACE inhibitors are antihypertensive medications that can cause coughing. When a patient has a

cough, the nurse must also determine the medications the patient is taking to rule out cough as a medication side-effect.

44. C

The coughing out of blood is called hemoptysis. Blood or blood-streaked mucus may originate either from the mouth, the pharynx or the stomach. If the source of bleeding is in the gastrointestinal tract, the coughed-out blood would be a darker red or coffee-ground in color, and it would usually be mixed with regurgitated food particles.

45. A

Some countries administer the BCG (Bacillus Calmette-Guerin) vaccine to their newborns to reduce the risk of contracting tuberculosis. The manifestations of tuberculosis include cough, hemoptysis, fever, night sweats and weight loss, among others.

46. A

When the nurse is to examine the posterior and lateral thorax, the patient should be sitting up with their arms across their chest, and each hand is touching the opposite shoulder. This position increases the area between the scapulae that can be examined.

47. D

A patient is breathing with effort if their sternocleidomastoid and scalene muscles contract whenever they inhale. This breathing effort is called supraclavicular retraction, and it signals that the patient is having severe breathing difficulty. In this case, the physician must be notified immediately.

48. B

Older patients or those with chronic obstructive pulmonary disease (COPD) will have increased anteroposterior diameter (AP diameter). A chest with increased AP diameter is shaped like a barrel. It is caused by the hyperinflation of the lungs.

49. B

When the nurse assesses for fremitus, they place their hands on the patient's back in different locations. As the nurse's hands change locations, the patient says 'ninety-nine.' When the vibration of the patient's voice is loud, then the fremitus is increased. The fremitus is increased in pneumonia or malignancy. It is decreased or absent in COPD, pneumothorax, pleural effusion, and emphysema.

50. B

When performing percussion, the nurse uses the middle finger of the non-dominant hand as the pleximeter. Only the pleximeter should be touching the patient's skin. The nurse aims at their distal interphalangeal joint and strikes it with a quick, sharp but relaxed wrist motion.

51. D

A tympanic percussion sound is drum-like, loud, and high-pitched. It is also of longer duration. Percussing over the gastric air bubble, or over a large pneumothorax will elicit a tympanic sound.

52. D

When auscultating a hairy chest, the nurse may hear crackles as the diaphragm of the stethoscope is placed on the chest. To prevent hearing the crackles, the nurse may press the stethoscope harder on the patient's chest, or wet the patient's hair.

53. C

Vesicular breath sounds are heard over most of the lung fields. They are soft and low-pitched, with inspiratory sounds longer than that of expiratory sounds.

54. C

Rales are soft, high-pitched non-musical sounds that are short and discontinuous. The nurse will most likely note rales in patients with early congestive heart failure, pneumonia, fibrosis, bronchitis or bronchiectasis.

55. D

Patients with asthma will have musical sounding expiration during an acute attack. The musical sound is called wheezing, and it is caused by narrowed airways.

56. A

Patients with breathing difficulty will be very uncomfortable when they are to be examined on their back. The supine position can worsen the breathing problem. The nurse may sit the patient up or elevate the head of the bed before examining the patient's anterior chest.

57. B, C

A pulse oximeter measures the arterial oxygen saturation or SpO2. The normal SpO2 is 95-100%. Dyes in some nail polish, too much ambient light, hypotension and poor perfusion, among others, will yield inaccurate readings.

58. A

A peak flow meter is a device that measures the maximum volume of air that the patient can expel from their lungs during a vigorous expiration. The peak flow decreases during an acute asthma attack.

59. D

Smoking can cause many types of cancers especially that of the respiratory system. Smoking can also contribute to cancers of the bladder, cervix, colon, rectum, kidney, and many others.

60. C

Live attenuated flu vaccines are available as nasal sprays and are to be administered to healthy people only between the ages of 2 and 49. Inactivated flu vaccines are administered intramuscularly (IM).

61. B

A sudden manifestation of severe dyspnea and tachypnea in a post-partum client highly suggest acute pulmonary embolism, which is a medical emergency.

62. D

Patients with bacterial pneumonia will have consolidation of the lung tissues. When they cough, their sputum is mucoid or purulent and is rusty-looking, blood-streaked or diffusely pinkish.

63. D

The chest pain of angina pectoris and myocardial infarction are similar in many ways. The pain is retrosternal or across the chest and is described as pressing, squeezing, vise-like, heavy or even burning. One major difference is that angina is relieved by rest or nitroglycerin, and myocardial infarction is not.

64. C

Cheyne-Stokes breathing is described as the rhythmic waxing and waning of respiration. The patient has periods of deep breathing, followed by episodes of apnea. It is commonly observed in patients with uremia, heart failure, drug-induced respiratory depression, and brain trauma.

65. D

A patient with a large pneumothorax will have a big volume of air in the pleura of the of the affected side. The accumulated air collapses the lungs in the affected side and pushes mediastinal organs toward the unaffected side. The trachea of the patient with a large pneumothorax will, therefore, be shifted toward the unaffected side.

The Cardiovascular System

Questions
1. A nurse is assessing a 10-year old child. She auscultates for heart sounds and hears an extra sound just after S2. It is low-pitched, dull and soft. It sounds like thunder heard from a distance. Which heart sound did the nurse hear?
    a. S4
    b. Ejection click
    c. S3
    d. Atrial gallop

2. A client diagnosed with pericarditis is being cared for by the nurse. As she auscultates the heart, she hears a scratching sound like two rough sheets being rubbed together. The sound is high-pitched. Which heart sound did the nurse hear?
    a. aS3
    b. Atrial gallop
    c. Split S2
    d. Pericardial friction rub

3. The nurse is assessing a client who is on a treadmill. After the use of the treadmill, which of the following will be true of the client's status?
    a. Increased preload
    b. Decreased afterload
    c. Decreased preload
    d. Decreased heart rate

4. The nurse wants to understand how pregnancy can affect heart work. Which of the following conditions happens during pregnancy?
    a. Cardiac output decreases
    b. Pulse rate decreases
    c. Blood volume decreases
    d. Arterial BP decreases

5. The nurse wants to assess the apical heart rate, and extra heart sounds of a 2-year old child. Where should the nurse place the diaphragm of the stethoscope to hear it best?
    a. 3rd intercostal space left sternal border
    b. 4th intercostal space left of the left midclavicular line
    c. 5th intercostal space left midclavicular line
    d. 5th intercostal space left sternal border

6. An elderly client asks the nurse why the aged have higher systolic BP than young adults. Which of the following is the best reply of the nurse?
    a. "Blood volume is increased in the elderly."
    b. "Blood vessels are stiffer and have smaller lumens because of fat and calcium deposits inside

the vessels."
   c. "The elderly have higher body metabolism than those of young adults and the increase in systolic BP is needed to meet the demand."
   d. "The heart is starting to fail and the increase in systolic BP is the first manifestation."

7. The nurse wants to know how gender can be a factor in developing hypertension. Which of the following concepts is accurate information on the prevalence of hypertension according to gender?
   a. A higher percentage of women have hypertension until 45 years of life than men
   b. Both men and women have the same prevalence of hypertension from 65 years and above.
   c. From 45 years to 60 years, men have higher percentage of having hypertension than women
   d. From 65 years and beyond, females have higher percentage than men in having hypertension

8. The nurse received instructions to note any pulse deficits in a client with atrial fibrillation. Which of the following nursing actions will correctly assess for the pulse deficit?
   a. Assess both apical and radial pulse simultaneously
   b. Assess first the apical and then the carotid pulse next
   c. Assess the radial pulses of both arms simultaneously
   d. Assess the carotid pulse first before the apical pulse

9. The nurse is reviewing the medical records of a client with hypertrophic cardiomyopathy. She learned that the client has a grade 6 murmur. Which of the following correctly describes a grade 6 murmur?
   a. Barely audible by stethoscope and heard only if the room is quiet
   b. Faint sound by stethoscope but clearly audible
   c. Loud by stethoscope with a palpable thrill
   d. Loudest, heard even without a stethoscope, with palpable thrill and visible heave

10. A newborn is being cared for by the nurse. Upon auscultation of the chest, the nurse hears a machinery sounding murmur that disappeared after 3 days. Which of the following is the most likely condition of the newborn?
   a. Pericarditis
   b. Ventricular fibrillation
   c. Patent ductus arteriosus
   d. Atrial gallop

11. A mother has just delivered her newborn. The newborn is having respiratory distress as she cries. Upon auscultation of the newborn's chest, the nurse hears a loud murmur during the entire systole. Which of the following conditions is the newborn most likely suffering from?

a. Atrial septal defect
b. Ventricular septal defect
c. Patent ductus arteriosus
d. S2 split

12. A client comes to the clinic because of complaints of chest heaviness and tightness that morning. According to the client, he felt really close to losing consciousness and he was sweating profusely. Upon further assessment, the nurse learned that the client was just lying on the bed when the chest pain occurred. Which of the following type of chest pain did the client most likely experienced?
    a. Angina pectoris
    b. Prinzmetal angina
    c. Myocardial infarction
    d. Acute coronary syndrome

13. A client who just suffered myocardial infarction several days ago complained of sharp stabbing pain to the chest. According to the client, it worsens when he inhales, especially of taking a deep breath. When he tried lying down, he also reports more pain. However, as he sat right up and reached forward to fix his blanket, he experienced some relief. Which of the following conditions most likely is causing the client's chest pain?
    a. Pericarditis
    b. Myocarditis
    c. Gastroesophageal reflux
    d. Prinzmetal angina

14. An elderly client with aortic aneurysm has been instructed by his physician to refrain from heavy lifting. However, when his granddaughter came to visit, he carried her. The client then experienced severe and sudden chest pain, which he described as 'like something was torn inside'. Within a few minutes, he was rushed to the hospital. He lost consciousness on the way. Which of the following most likely caused the client's chest pain?
    a. Pericarditis
    b. Aortic dissection
    c. Mitral valve prolapse
    d. Pulmonary embolism

15. A nurse is assessing a client who has been recently been diagnosed with heart failure. Which of the following is NOT a manifestation of heart failure?
    a. Cough with pink and frothy sputum
    b. Nausea and vomiting
    c. Dependent non-pitting edema
    d. Ronchi

16. A client with mitral stenosis asks the nurse to explain what his condition is. Which of the following

is the correct response of the nurse?

a. "There is obstruction of blood flow going to the left lower chamber of your heart because the valve that allows blood to flow through has hardened."

b. "The blood going to the lungs is obstructed by a blood clot."

c. "The blood vessel connecting the right side of the heart to the left is damaged causing obstruction."

d. "There is increased blood flow to the rest of the body because the valve that allows blood to flow through becomes flaccid."

17. A client who has been chronically taking steroids came to the clinic because of pain on the chest. Upon careful assessment, the nurse notes vesicular lesions on one area of the chest that is painful to palpation. The client refuses to wear a shirt because of the pain. Which of the following conditions will have manifestations such as the above?

a. Varicella zoster

b. Herpes zoster

c. Herpes Simplex I

d. Pleurisy

18. The nurse is assessing a client with pulmonic valve stenosis. Upon examination of the chest, the nurse observes that there is a diffuse lifting beat by the left lower sternal border. Which of the following will the nurse write on her documentation to describe the client's manifestation?

a. Bruit

b. Thrill

c. Heave

d. Pressure overload

19. The nurse is looking at the ECG patterns on the monitor. She counts the QRS complexes and notes that there are 4-5 of them every 10 seconds. Which of the following conditions may cause this manifestation?

a. Pneumonia

b. Pulmonary valve stenosis

c. Angina pectoris

d. Second degree heart block

20. A child with tetralogy of fallot is seen sitting on the floor of the playroom. The nurse knows that the condition is a combination of four heart disorders. Which of the following does not accurately describe tetralogy of Fallot?

a. Hardened pulmonary valve

b. Open communication between ventricles

c. Overriding aorta

d. Left ventricular enlargement

21. The nurse is assessing the cardiovascular system of several patients. Who of the patients will the nurse have the most challenging attempt to palpate for the apical impulse?
    a. A pre-school child
    b. A frail 22-year old male
    c. A 56-year old with aortic insufficiency
    d. A patient with an increased anteroposterior chest diameter

22. In which of the following clients will the nurse expect the apical impulse to be displaced laterally?
    a. A COPD client with barrel chest
    b. A client with hypotension
    c. A client with hypothyroidism
    d. A client with endocarditis

23. Which of the following is accurate with ventricular pressures?
    a. Systole is the period of ventricular contraction
    b. In systole, the aortic valve is closed
    c. In diastole, the mitral valve is closed
    d. Systole is the period of atrial contraction

24. The nurse is performing a complete physical examination on a hypertensive client. In auscultating the chest, which of the following nursing technique needs further evaluation?
    a. Auscultates for the pulmonic sounds at the 2nd and 3rd intercostal space at the sternal boarder
    b. Auscultates for the mitral sounds at the point of maximal impulse
    c. Auscultates for the aortic sounds at the 5th intercostal space midclavicular line
    d. Auscultates for the tricuspid sounds at the left lower sternal border

25. Which of the following components of a normal ECG is correct?
    a. QRS complex corresponds to ventricular repolarization
    b. P wave corresponds to atrial depolarization
    c. T wave coincides with ventricular depolarization
    d. R wave is the downward deflection from ventricular depolarization

26. The new nurse wants to understand how the heart works as a pump. In her review, which of the following describes the load that stretches the cardiac muscle before contraction?
    a. Stroke volume
    b. Preload
    c. Afterload
    d. Myocardial contractility

27. A client with difficulty breathing also states that sometimes at night, he wakes up gasping for air. The nurse is sure to document this night time episode as

a.   Orthopnea
b.   Tachypnea
c.   Paroxysmal nocturnal dyspnea
d.   Cheyne-Stokes respiration

28. A nurse is assessing a mother breastfeeding her newborn. Which of the following observation of the newborn would prompt the nurse to refer them to a physician?
a.   Presence of white spots on the tip of the baby's nose
b.   The areas around the mouth of the baby turns bluish while feeding
c.   The arms and legs looks bluish
d.   The baby has a good suck

29. A nurse is assessing a pregnant client and wants to hear a possible S3. Which of the following auscultatory technique will help the nurse attain her objective?
a.   Places the diaphragm of the stethoscope over the apex of the heart and applies very slight pressure
b.   Places the bell of the stethoscope over the apex of the heart and applies very light pressure
c.   Positions the client on his left side and places the diaphragm over the 3rd ICS right sternal border
d.   Positions the client on his right and places the diaphragm over the 3rd ICS left sternal border

30. The nurse is reviewing the conduction system of the heart because she is to be assigned to the care of a patient with atrioventricular block. The nurse knows that the part of the heart anatomy that acts as the heart's pacemaker is the
a.   Atrioventricular node
b.   Sinoatrial node
c.   Bundle of His
d.   Bundle of His branches

31. A client has been admitted due to trauma sustained from a vehicular accident. The client has lost a significant amount of blood but is still conscious and coherent. What changes in the heart is true?
a.   Higher blood pressure
b.   Low jugular vein pressure
c.   Bounding carotid pulse
d.   High right ventricular pressure

32. The nurse notes that there are 7 QRS complexes in a 6-second ECG strip. What is the nurse's interpretation of this?
a.   It is a sign of an atrioventricular block

b. The client has normal heart rate
c. It is a sign of tachycardia
d. The client has hypertension

33. On a very rare occasion, the nurse was surprised to note the client's point of maximal impulse is at the 5th ICS on the midclavicular line of the right side instead of the left. The nurse knows to document this condition as
a. Right sided hypertrophy
b. Cardiomyopathy
c. Situs inversus
d. Dextrocardia

34. A nurse from the afternoon shift reviews the client's chart as endorsed by the nurse from an earlier shift. The chart read " Grade 6 murmur." The nurse knows that the meaning of grade 6 murmur is
a. Moderately loud
b. Loud, with palpable thrill
c. Very loud, with thrill. May be heard when the stethoscope is partly off the chest
d. Very loud, with thrill. May be heard with stethoscope entirely off the chest

35. It is defined as an abnormal backflow of blood from the left ventricle (LV) to the left atrium (LA).
a. Tricuspid Regurgitation
b. Ventricular Septal Defect
c. Mitral Regurgitation
d. Aortic insufficiency

36. Which assessment finding will alert the nurse for a possibility of abdominal aortic aneurysm?
a. Pain in the costovertebral angle
b. Pulsatile mass in the abdomen
c. Unequal pulse between apical and radial pulses
d. Board-like abdomen

37. Which of the following findings indicates right ventricular failure in a 66-year old client?
a. Pinkish sputum with very fine bubbles
b. Cough
c. Orthopnea
d. Elevated jugular vein pressure

38. Which of the following statements of a client can signal the nurse that the client has a risk for developing coronary artery disease?
a. "My mother died of cancer"
b. "I jog around 2 blocks every other day."
c. "I have difficulty breathing when the pollen count is high."

d. "I just like fast food so much."

39. Which of the following is an abnormal finding when auscultating the chest for heart sounds?
    a. S1 heard at the 4th-5th ICS in a 36-year old male
    b. S2 heard at the 2nd to 3rd ICS in a 40 year old woman
    c. S4 heard at the apex in an 81-year old male
    d. S3 heard at the apex in a teenager

40. The nurse is assessing the ECG strip of a client and notes that there are 11 QRS complexes in a 6-second strip. What is the client's heart rate?
    a. 70
    b. 80
    c. 90
    d. 110

41. A nurse wants to assess for a person's apical pulse. In which of the following anatomical location will the nurse be able to palpate for the apical pulse in a healthy adult?
    a. In the 5th intercostal space left midclavicular line
    b. In the 5th intercostal space right midclavicular line
    c. In the 5th intercostal space left anterior axillary line
    d. Near the xiphoid process

42. Which of the following happens during diastole?
    a. The aortic valve opens
    b. The aortic valve closes
    c. The mitral valve closes
    d. The ventricles contracts

43. In which of the following patients will an S3 heart sound be non-pathologic?
    a. In a 55-year-old worker
    b. in a 61-year old retired teacher
    c. In a diabetic 78-year-old adult patient
    d. In a 5-year-old school girl

44. The normal heart's sinus node will produce how many impulses in a minute?
    a. 40-80
    b. 50-70
    c. 60-100
    d. 100-120

45. A novice nurse is trying to understand an ECG strip. Which of the following ECG component corresponds to atrial contraction?

a. P wave
b. QRS complex
c. T wave
d. S wave

46. A nurse takes a patient's blood pressure measurements and obtains a reading of 160/100 mm Hg. Which of the following is true regarding the patient's condition?
    a. Decreased preload
    b. Decreased myocardial contractility
    c. Increased afterload
    d. decreased afterload

47. The nurse takes the vital signs of a patient and obtains the following results: T= 37 °C; RR= 16/min, PR= 77 bpm, BP= 130/70. What is the patient's pulse pressure?
    a. 16
    b. 50
    c. 77
    d. 60

48. The nurse is to measure jugular vein pressure. To start the procedure, how should the nurse position the patient?
    a. supine, HOB 30°
    b. supine, HOB 60°
    c. Supine, flat
    d. Side-lying

49. A nurse is assessing a female patient who is showing signs of myocardial infarction. Which of the following symptoms of myocardial infarction is usually manifested by women?
    a. Indigestion
    b. Vise-like chest pain
    c. Pressure on the chest
    d. Shortness of breath

50. The nurse wants to assess a patient for orthopnea. Which of the following questions is best to ask the patient?
    a. "Do you see halos when you experience shortness of breath?"
    b. "What activities are you performing when you feel short of breath?"
    c. "Did you ever wake up gasping for air?"
    d. "How many pillows do you use when sleeping?"

51. A nurse is asking the patient if their shoes, rings or belts ever felt tighter than usual. Which of the following problems of the cardiovascular system is the nurse trying to determine?

a. Nocturia
b. Edema
c. Cyanosis
d. Paroxysmal nocturnal dyspnea

52. A patient is diagnosed with cardiogenic shock. Which of the following will the nurse note when palpating the pulse of this patient?
    a. Weak and thready pulse
    b. Bounding pulse
    c. Regularly irregular
    d. Irregularly irregular

53. A novice nurse is locating for the jugular vein to measure the jugular vein pressure. Which of the following when observed or noted confirms that the nurse is indeed assessing the jugular vein and NOT the carotid pulse?
    a. The soft beating sensation is eliminated by light pressure on the vein
    b. It is easily palpable
    c. The height of pulsations is unchanged by position
    d. The height of pulsations not affected by inspiration

54. A nurse wants to know if a patient has thrills. Which of the following should the nurse perform?
    a. Percussion
    b. Palpation
    c. Auscultation
    d. Observation

55. The nurse is auscultating a patient's heart sounds and notices that the point of maximal impulse (PMI) is near the xiphoid process. Which of the following conditions can move the PMI lower and laterally?
    a. Dextrocardia
    b. Hypotension
    c. Bruit
    d. Ventricular hypertrophy

56. The novice nurse is trying to locate the Erb's point on the patient's chest. The Erb's point is located at the:
    a. 2nd intercostal space right sternal border
    b. 2nd intercostal space left sternal border
    c. 4th intercostal space left sternal border
    d. 3rd intercostal space left sternal border

57. The nurse is assessing the heart sounds of a patient and wants to know if the patient has left-

sided S3, S4 sounds, and mitral murmurs. How should the nurse position the patient to facilitate this examination and best hear these heart sounds?
a. Left lateral decubitus
b. Right lateral decubitus
c. Semi-fowlers
d. Fowler's

58. As the nurse is auscultating for heart sounds, they note a murmur. The murmur starts with S1 and ends at S2 without a gap. Which type of murmur did the nurse hear?
a. A midsystolic murmur
b. A pansystolic murmur
c. A late systolic murmur
d. An early diastolic murmur

59. Which of the following findings if present in a person increases their risk for cardiovascular diseases? Choose at least three.
a. Waist circumference of 40 or more in men
b. High triglycerides – 150 mg/dL or higher
c. Low blood pressure - < 120/80
d. Low high-density lipoprotein
e. High fasting blood sugar- fasting glucose of 100mg/dL or higher

60. The nurse is determining the hypertension risk factors of a patient. Which of the following factors is non-modifiable?
a. Obesity
b. Smoking
c. Age
d. Sedentary lifestyle

61. The nurse is teaching a patient how to choose healthy fats for cardiovascular health. Which of the following, if selected by the patient indicates a correct understanding of the teachings?
a. Shortening
b. Pumpkin seeds
c. Bologna
d. Cream

62. A nurse hears a heart murmur and says that the murmur is Grade 6. Which of the following is the correct interpretation of the nurse's findings?
a. The murmur is moderately loud
b. The murmur is loud, with thrill
c. The murmur is loud with palpable thrill
d. The murmur is loud, with thrill; heard with the stethoscope entirely off the chest

63. A patient has just been found to have dextrocardia. In which of the following position will the nurse most likely note the apical pulse?
    a. 5th intercostal space left midclavicular line
    b. 4th intercostal space right midclavicular line
    c. 2nd intercostal space left sternal border
    d. 3rd intercostal space left sternal border

64. A nurse is caring for a patient with heart failure. The patient has a pulse that has alternating strong and weak beats. Which of the following correctly describes the nurse's findings?
    a. Atrial flutter
    b. Bradycardia
    c. Pulsus alternans
    d. Bigeminal pulse

65. A patient is experiencing chest pain. As the nurse further examines the patient, the patient tells the nurse that the pain is worse when leaning forward and every time they breathe out. The nurse asks the patient to hold their breath, and the pain persists. Upon auscultation, the nurse hears a scratchy high-pitched heart sound that is heard intermittently in several parts of the cardiac cycle. The nurse should prepare to care for a patient with which condition?
    a. Venous hum
    b. Pericardial friction rub
    c. Patent ductus arteriosus
    d. Pleural rub

ANSWERS

1. C

    S3 is heard as a low-pitched , dull and soft. It sounds like thunder heard from a distance. Since it is soft, the room must be quiet to hear it. It is low-pitched and therefore it is best heard by the bell over the apex of the heart.

2. D

    A pericardial friction rub is a scratching sound like two rough sheets being rubbed together. The sound is high-pitched. People with pericarditis manifest this heart sound. To hear it best, have the client sit up and slightly lean forward, then ask the client to hold his breath during exhalation and listen over the apex near the sternal border.

3. A

    During exercise, the ventricles fill with more blood to meet metabolic demands. This stretches the ventricles and therefore preload is increased.

4. D

    During pregnancy, especially in the second trimester, arterial BP decreases. This is because of peripheral vasodilation. The cardiac output, pulse rate and blood volume increases when a woman becomes pregnant.

5. B

    Because the heart of children younger than 7 years of age is more horizontal, the apex is located on the 4th intercostal space left of the left midclavicular line.

6. B

    The elderly have higher systolic BP because the blood vessels are less elastic and because there are calcium and fat deposits inside the vessels that increase peripheral vascular resistance.

7. D

    For the 65-year-old and older population, there are more hypertensive females than males.

8. A

    To check for pulse deficit, the nurse and a colleague assess both the apical pulse and the radial pulse simultaneously and they note any unidentical beats. The count difference between the apical pulse and the peripheral pulse is the pulse deficit. It is calculated by subtracting the peripheral pulse count from the number of apical beats.

9. D

    Grade 1—Barely audible; heard only in a quiet room and then with difficulty
    Grade 2—Clearly audible but faint
    Grade 3—Moderately loud; easy to hear

Grade 4—Loud; associated with a thrill palpable on the chest wall

Grade 5—Very loud; heard with one corner of the stethoscope lifted off the chest wall; associated thrill

Grade 6—Loudest; still heard with entire stethoscope lifted just off the chest wall; associated thrill

10. C

Patent ductus arteriosus (PDA) causes a murmur that sounds like a machine that is continuously running. This is caused by passing of the blood through the ductus arteriosis that failed to immediately close. When the PDA closes and resolves, the murmurs disappear.

11. B

When there is communication between the two ventricles, it allows for blood to pass through from ventricle to ventricle. This movement causes the harsh sounds that can be heard at the entire cardiac event, called holosystolic murmur.

12. D

Prinzmetal angina or variant angina is described as heaviness or tightness of the chest that may be felt also on the jaw, neck, left arm or shoulder. The chest pain is felt when at rest and even in the early morning. It can be accompanied by other symptoms like palpitations, diaphoresis and syncope.

13. A

Chest pain caused by pericarditis is described as sharp and stabbing that worsens on inspiration and lying down. It improves however if the client sits up and slightly leans forward. Pericarditis can be a sequelae of myocardial infarction.

14. B

The chest pain caused by aortic dissection is described as sudden intense pain that feels like torn flesh from the inside. It happens when the aortic aneurysm starts to rupture and tear from the inside.

15. D

A client with heart failure will have the following manifestations if the left side of the heart is mostly affected: cough with pink frothy sputum, dyspnea, orthopnea and crackles. If the right side is damaged, the client will have a big waist because of ascites. He will also have edematous legs. Ronchi is produced by air passing through accumulated secretions in the trachea and the larger airways.

16. A

Mitral stenosis is the hardening of the mitral valve because of calcification that prevents the flow of blood from the left atrium to the left ventricles. Manifestations include fatigue, dyspnea on exertion, orthopnea, paroxysmal nocturnal dyspnea and coughing of pink-tinged sputum.

17. B

Herpes zoster is caused by the reactivation of dormant varicella. Unlike chickenpox, the vesicular lesions are found on one dermatome only and there is characteristic pain when the lesions are touched. It can also be accompanied by itchiness.

18. C

In right ventricular hypertrophy, such as that which is caused by pulmonary valve stenosis, the nurse may note a diffuse lifting beat by the left lower sternal border. This is called a heave.

19. D

QRS complexes reflect ventricular depolarizations or contractions. 4-5 QRS complexes every 10 seconds means that the apical rate is 24-30 per minute. Bradycardia is evident in heart blocks.

20. D

Tetralogy of Fallot is a combination of four heart abnormalities namely, pulmonary stenosis, ventricular septal defect, overriding aorta and right ventricular hypertrophy.

21. D

The apical impulse is easily palpated in children and adults with a thin frame. Challenges palpating the apical impulse include increased anteroposterior chest diameter, obesity or a thick chest.

22. A

In patients with chronic obstructive pulmonary disease, the most prominent palpable impulse or PMI may be in the xiphoid or epigastric area as a result of right ventricular hypertrophy.

23. A

Systole is the period of ventricular contraction while diastole is the period of ventricular relaxation. During systole the aortic valve is open, allowing pumping of blood from the left ventricle into the aorta. The mitral valve is closed, thereby preventing backflow of blood to the left atrium. In contrast, during diastole the aortic valve is closed, preventing regurgitation of blood from the aorta back into the left ventricle. The mitral valve is open, allowing blood to flow from the left atrium into the relaxed left ventricle.

24. C

Sounds and murmurs arising from the mitral valve are best heard at or near the cardiac apex. Tricuspid sounds are heard best at or near the lower left sternal border. Murmurs arising from the pulmonic valve are usually heard best in the 2nd and 3rd ICS at the sternal border. Murmurs originating in the aortic valve may be heard anywhere from the right 2nd intercostal space to the apex.

25. B

The P wave of an ECG component corresponds to the atrial depolarization. The QRS complex represents ventricular depolarization. The Q wave is a downward deflection from septal depolarization and followed by the R wave which is an upward deflection from ventricular depolarization. The S wave is a downward deflection following an R wave. The T wave coincides with ventricular repolarization.

26. B

Preload refers to the amount of blood that stretches the cardiac muscle before contraction, or the volume of blood in the right ventricle at the end of diastole. Stroke volume refers to the volume of blood ejected with each heartbeat. Afterload is the degree of vascular resistance to ventricular contraction. Myocardial contractility is the ability of the cardiac muscle to contract.

27. C

Paroxysmal nocturnal dyspnea describes episodes of sudden dyspnea that awaken the patient from sleep, around an hour or two after reclining on the bed. The patient wakes up, suddenly sits, stands or goes to a window for air. There may be associated wheezing and coughing.

28. B

Circumoral cyanosis while feeding in the newborn, especially if accompanied by diaphoresis signifies poor perfusion caused by a possible cardiac problem.

29. B

The bell of the stethoscope is more sensitive to the low-pitched sounds of S3 and S4 and the murmur of mitral stenosis. Apply the bell on the apex with very light pressure to produce an air seal with its full rim. Use the bell at the apex to auscultate, and then move medially along the left lower sternal border.

30. B

Each electrical impulse in the heart is initiated in the sinus node, a group of specialized cardiac cells found in the right atrium near the junction of the vena cava. It acts as the cardiac pacemaker and automatically discharges an impulse about 60 to 100 times a minute.

31. B

The jugular vein pressure (JVP) provides valuable information about the patient's volume status and cardiac function. In patients who are hypovolemic, the JVP may be low, necessitating lowering the head of the bed, sometimes even to 0°.

32. B

The QRS complex corresponds to ventricular depolarization or contraction and is therefore also indicative of ventricular rate if counted in an ECG strip. If there are 10 6-seconds in a minute, we multiply 7 QRS's to 10 to get a ventricular (heart) rate of 70, which is within normal range.

33. D

On rare occasions, a patient has dextrocardia—a heart situated on the right side. The apical impulse will then be found on the right side of the chest. In situs inversus, the liver, the stomach and the heart are on the opposite side. A right-sided heart with the liver and stomach in their right anatomical location is usually associated with congenital heart disease.

34. D

Using the 6-point scale of a murmur, a grade 6 is a very loud murmur with a thrill that may be audible even when the stethoscope is entirely off the chest.

35. C

When the mitral valve fails to close fully in systole, blood regurgitates from left ventricle to left atrium, causing a murmur. This leakage creates volume overload on the left ventricle, with subsequent dilatation.

36. B

Abdominal aortic aneurysm is the abnormal dilatation and weakening of the abdominal aorta. A pulsating abdominal mass is a common finding.

37. D

Jugular venous distention is observed in right ventricular failure as volume overload happens. This overload is reflected upwards into the jugular veins.

38. D

Unhealthy eating habits, consuming foods that are high in saturated fats and simple sugars, are risk factors for developing coronary artery disease.

39. C

S4 is an abnormal heart sound. It is indicative of decreased ventricular compliance.

40. D

A regular heart rate is calculated by multiplying the number of QRS complexes in a 6-second strip to 10. You multiply it by 10 because there are 10 6-seconds in a minute. 11 QRS's x 10 = 110

41. A

The cardiac apex is where the apical pulse is best palpated. It is also the point of maximal impulse or PMI. The apical pulse is best palpated at the 5th intercostal space, left midclavicular line, in the healthy adult.

42. B

During diastole, the aortic valve closes, preventing the backflow of blood to the left ventricles. The mitral valve opens to allow the left ventricle to be filled with blood. In systole, on the other hand, the aortic valve opens to allow the pumping of blood out of the left ventricles into the aorta. The mitral valve closes to prevent backflow of blood to the left atrium.

43. D

In young patients, an S3 heart sound is normally caused by the rapid deceleration of blood against the wall of the ventricles. It does not indicate any pathology. In older adults, the S3 heart sound, or the S3 gallop usually indicate altered ventricular compliance.

44. C

The sinus node of a normal heart will produce 60-100 impulses in a minute, corresponding to the number of times the ventricles will eject blood. Every impulse will create one beat in a normal heart so that the number of sinus impulses equals the heart rate.

45. A

The P wave is produced by atrial depolarization. The atria contracts and ejects blood at this time. The QRS wave corresponds to ventricular depolarization or contraction. The T wave is produced when the ventricles recover or repolarize.

46. C

Afterload refers to the degree of vascular resistance to ventricular contraction. Causes of increased resistance to ventricular contraction include a poor vascular tone and hypertension. In both cases, the afterload is increased.

47. D

The pulse pressure is the difference between the systolic and diastolic pressure. 130-70=60.

48. A

The usual starting point when taking the jugular vein pressure (JVP) is to position the patient with the head of the bed elevated 30°. The nurse then identifies the external jugular vein on both sides and notes the undulations. The JVP is the highest point of the vein undulation that is observed in patients with normal blood volume.

49. A

Women sometimes experience myocardial infarction differently. Instead of chest pain, they may experience pain in their upper body, indigestion, nausea and cold sweats.

50. D

Orthopnea is difficulty breathing that is experienced when the patient is lying supine but improves when the patient sits up. If the nurse wants to assess the severity of the orthopnea, they should ask how many pillows the patient is using to sleep comfortably. The more pillows used to prop themselves up, the more severe the orthopnea.

51. B

Edema refers to the accumulation of fluids in the interstitial spaces. To assess for edema which may not be so obvious, the nurse asks if the patient has noticed their shoes, rings or belt getting tighter recently.

52. A

Patients with cardiogenic shock will have decreased circulating blood volume as the heart fails to pump blood to different body parts. The patient will have a weak and thready pulse as a way of compensating for the decreased circulating blood volume.

53. A

Jugular undulations differ from carotid pulsations in several ways. It is rarely palpable. Every beat has two elevations and two troughs. The soft beating sensation, called undulations temporary disappear as pressure is applied to the vein. With every inspiration, the height of undulations usually falls.

54. B

When a nurse wants to assess for a thrill, they have to palpate the patient's chest. A thrill is a vibration caused by the turbulence of an underlying cardiac murmur. The nurse uses the ball of their hand placed firmly on the chest to check for thrills. People with aortic stenosis, patent ductus arteriosus, and ventricular septal defects will manifest thrills.

55. D

In left ventricular hypertrophy, the left ventricle becomes enlarged and thickened, usually as compensation for a more effortful pumping action caused by increased preload and afterload.

56. D

The Erb's point is located at the 3rd intercostal space, left sternal border. It is a good location for auscultation because it is the point between the apex and the base of the heart.

57. A

The left lateral decubitus position brings the ventricles closer to the chest wall so that left-sided S3, S4 sounds, and mitral murmurs are accentuated.

58. B

A pansystolic murmur is heard from the beginning of S1 until the end of S2, without a gap. Pansystolic murmurs are the result of backflow of blood across the atrioventricular valves.

59. A, B, E

People with a large waist circumference, high blood pressure, high fasting blood sugar, high triglycerides, high low-density lipoproteins are prone to developing cardiovascular problems.

Three or more of these findings indicate metabolic syndrome.

60. C

Non-modifiable risk factors are factors that can never be changed. Examples of non-modifiable risk factors for hypertension is age and family history of hypertension.

61. B

For cardiovascular health, the patient should take healthy sources of fat such as those high in mono- and polyunsaturated fats, and those with high omega-3 fatty acids. Examples of these fats are almonds, pumpkin seeds, and mackerel, respectively.

62. D

Murmurs are graded using a 6-point scale. A grade 6 murmur is the loudest and with a palpable thrill. The sound is heard even when the stethoscope is entirely off the chest.

63. B

People with dextrocardia have their heart positioned on their right instead of their left chest. The apex of the heart where the point of maximal impulse is located will be on the right side.

64. C

Pulsus alternans is alternating strong and weak arterial beats. It is a common finding in patients with severe left ventricular failure.

65. B

A pericardial friction rub is heard in people with pericarditis or the inflammation of the pericardial sac. The sound is scratchy or scraping, high-pitched and heard in both atrial and ventricular systole, and in ventricular diastole. The sound is produced by two surfaces of the pericardial sac rubbing against each other.

The Peripheral Vascular System

Questions

1. A student nurse asks her mentor why veins have valves and arteries do not. Which of the following is the best response of the nurse to answer the student's query?

    a. "The veins do not have enough pressure unlike arteries to push the blood back to the heart so the valves act to prevent backflow of blood."

    b. "The veins have valves because they are more elastic than arteries that allow the blood to pool"

    c. "The valves of the vein open and close simultaneously with the pulse and allow flow of blood back to the heart."

    d. "The veins have valves because they act as small pumps that push blood back to the heart."

2. The nurse is asked to palpate the inguinal lymph nodes of a client to assess for lumps and swelling. Which of the following locations will the nurse palpate?

    a. Antecubital fossa

    b. Popliteal area

    c. Groin area

    d. Axillary area

3. The nurse wants to determine the client's claudication distance. Which of the following should the nurse ask the client?

    a. "How many blocks would it take before you experience pain in your calf when walking?"

    b. "How long does it take before you experience pain while climbing up stairs?"

    c. "How many steps would it take before you feel numbness in your arms?"

    d. "How far can you walk before you experience chest pain?"

4. A client has peripheral arterial disease. Which of the following manifestation is consistent with the client's diagnosis?

    a. Hyperglycemia

    b. Erectile dysfunction

    c. Dilated tortuous veins in the legs

    d. Warmth in the lower extremities

5. The right leg of the client is swollen, warm and tender. The client has just undergone abdominal surgery. Which of the following conditions cause unilateral leg edema as manifested by the client?

    a. Heart failure

    b. Varicose veins

    c. Deep vein thrombosis

    d. Peripheral arterial disease

6. The nurse is to assess capillary refill of the client. Which of the following can affect the results of the assessment, and can render the findings unreliable?

    a. Cold room

b.   Use of gloves
c.   Use of a wrist watch
d.   Fever

7.   Several elderly clients ask a nurse what causes peripheral arterial disease. Which of the following factors has the greatest risk of causing peripheral arterial disease?
a.   Increased intake of high-cholesterol foods
b.   Smoking
c.   Lack of exercise
d.   Malnutrition

8.   A nurse admits a client who complains of pain in the lower extremities. She wants to determine if the problem is arterial or venous in nature. Which of the following concepts will correctly guide the nurse in her examination?
a.   Venous: brown discoloration in the upper thigh
b.   Venous: edema and claudication
c.   Arterial: cool hairless extremity
d.   Arterial: warm with dilated tortuous vessels more evident when standing

9.   A nurse is assessing the peripheral pulses of a client. She finds that the pulses are full and bounding. Which of the following conditions can cause pulses to feel full and bounding?
a.   Decreased cardiac output
b.   Aortic stenosis
c.   Hemorrhage
d.   Polycythemia vera

10. The nurse is to perform the Allen test before cannulation. Which of the following is NOT part of the procedure?
a.   Ask the client to occlude the ulnar artery first and then the radial artery
b.   Instruct the client to make a fist of the hand to be cannulated several times
c.   Ask the client to open the hand and release the ulnar artery
d.   Observe for return of color of the palms

11. A client's legs are extremely swollen and they look distorted. When pressed by the examining fingers, it causes very deep indentations that do not rebound easily. Which of the following should be the documentation entry of the nurse?
a.   Bilateral pitting edema of the lower extremities grade 4+
b.   Bilateral non-pitting edema of the lower extremities grade 4+
c.   Unilateral non-pitting edema of the lower extremities grade 2+
d.   Bilateral pitting edema of the lower extremities grade 2+

12. The nurse is having difficulty assessing the peripheral pulses of a client of a client who is

hemorrhaging. Which equipment should the nurse obtain to facilitate her assessment?
a.   Stethoscope
b.   Doppler ultrasonic probe
c.   CT scan
d.   DEXA scan

13. The nurse is to assess the Brachial-Ankle Index in a client. Which of the following situations may render the test to be delayed?
a.   Drinking a standard measure of alcohol prior to the test
b.   Smoking 1 hour before the test
c.   Dizziness of the client
d.   Hypotension

14. A nurse is talking to several clients. Which of the following client response will alert the nurse to the possibility of a vascular problem?
a.   "My belt is one size loose this month."
b.   "My shoes feel tighter than usual."
c.   "I feel pain in my abdomen when I get hungry."
d.   "I seem to forget more things lately."

15. A client lost a lot of blood due to a laceration on the arm. When palpating for the client's peripheral pulses, the nurse expects the pulses to be:
a.   Full and bounding
b.   Slow and of moderate amplitude
c.   Fast and full
d.   Weak and thread

16. A nurse is counting the pulse rate of the client with mitral stenosis. She notes that the heart rate is 60 but the beats have alternating strong and weak amplitude. Which of the following is the correct interpretation of the nurse's finding?
a.   Pulsus bigeminus
b.   Pulsus paradoxus
c.   Pulsus alternans
d.   Water Hammer pulse

17. A client asks the nurse about Reynaud's phenomenon. The nurse plans to conduct a health teaching to discuss her concerns. Which of the following should be included in her teaching plan? Select all that apply.
a.   It is a disease of the lower extremities
b.   The affected extremity may appear red, blue or pale.
c.   It can be triggered by exposure to cold
d.   It is caused by spasms of the arterioles of the hand

e. It is caused by decreased venous return to the heart

18. A female client has just undergone radiation therapy as treatment for left breast cancer. The following day, she reports that her arm on the same side of the radiation treatment feels thicker and heavier than usual, and that her wedding ring seems stuck on the finger. To which condition should the nurse attribute the client's manifestations?
    a. Lymphedema
    b. Reynaud's phenomenon
    c. Lymphoma
    d. Heart failure

19. A nurse examines a client's feet and she noticed that the right toe has a 1 cm ulcer at the tip. The feet appear callused and the patient is unaware of the wound. The blood sugar of the client is high. Which type of ulcer does the client most probably have?
    a. Venous stasis ulcer
    b. Arterial ulcer
    c. Neuropathic ulcer
    d. Pressure ulcer

20. A client has venous stasis ulcer. Which of the following findings is consistent with this disorder?
    a. Brownish leathery discoloration around the ankle
    b. Pale-looking extremity with painful abraded skin
    c. Distal gangrene
    d. Not painful

21. A man recovering from a major abdominal surgery reports pain in his calf. Upon assessment the nurse notes that the calf is warm to touch. The nurse suspects he developed deep vein thrombosis. Which manifestation is consistent of DVT?
    a. Diminished pulse distal to the clot
    b. Cyanosis distal to the clot
    c. Calf pain on dorsiflexion
    d. Pallor of the calf

22. The nurse is assessing a client suspected of having venous insufficiency. He has deep, draining foul-smelling ulcers near the ankles. The client asks how he got the ulcers. What is the best nursing response?
    a. "Your calf muscles have become so enlarged due to an infection"
    b. "There is decreased blood flow to your legs"
    c. "The ulcer is the result of pooling of blood in your legs. Blood pools because your veins are not competent to return the blood back to the heart"
    d. "Your blood sugar is high and you lack exercise. This is the reason why a small wound has become large"

23. Which of the following should the nurse include in the plan of care of a client who has undergone coronary arteriogram, a process where an artery is accessed to deliver a contrast media for x-rays?
    a. Assess abdominal sounds
    b. Assess distal pulses
    c. Monitor vital signs every 8 hours
    d. Put the client on complete bed rest with no bathroom privileges

24. The nurse is caring for a client with deep vein thrombosis and is to assess respiratory functions constantly. What is the most accurate rationale for the nurse's actions?
    a. The pain in DVT is so severe that vital signs are affected especially the respiration
    b. Elevating the legs as intervention for DVT can increase pressure in the upper body and can cause pulmonary edema
    c. Pain in the legs radiates to the chest that compromises lung compliance
    d. Thrombus from the legs may dislodge and travel to the lungs and cause occlusion of blood flow to the lungs.

25. The nurse is assessing a client with pitting edema. The client depresses the skin with one finger and notes a 6mm 'pit'. The nurse is sure to document the degree of pitting as
    a. 1+
    b. 2+
    c. 3+
    d. 4+

26. Which of the following questions if asked by the nurse, assesses for arterial insufficiency in the lower extremities?
    a. "Do you have coldness, numbness, or pallor in the legs or feet?"
    b. "Is the pain in your leg alleviated by elevating your leg on a pillow?"
    c. "Is the pain worse with prolonged standing?"
    d. "Is the calf painful to touch?"

27. A 65-year old woman complains of small ulcers in her fingertips. She says that some of her fingers turn blue, especially when reaching inside the freezer. Which test is most appropriate to perform to assess for arterial insufficiency in the hands?
    a. Deep tendon reflexes
    b. Range of motion exercises of the wrist
    c. Allen test
    d. Rhine test

28. Which of the following assessment findings in the client's history is most significant in caring for a client with deep vein thrombosis?

a. Coronary artery disease
b. Recent caesarean section
c. Use of Coumadin
d. Use of aspirin

29. A nurse is assessing the lower limbs of a client who has just climbed 2 flights of stairs. She noticed that the veins on the lower legs are dilated and tortuous. The client reports that he experiences a dull ache in the legs after prolonged standing. The nurse documents the dilated tortuous veins as
a. Deep vein thrombosis
b. Spider angioma
c. Spider veins
d. Varicose veins

30. A female client has just undergone mastectomy. After 8 hours post-op, the arm of the client on the operative side has swollen. What is the most likely cause of the swelling?
a. Serous edema
b. Lymphedema
c. Infection
d. Hypoalbuminemia

31. A client has been diagnosed to have deep vein thrombosis. Which of the following nursing actions needs further intervention?
a. Performs deep palpation of the affected extremity
b. Helps administer anticoagulants
c. Assists the client to wear compression stockings
d. Performs health teaching on the use of medications

32. A client with arterial insufficiency at the lower extremities asks the nurse what intermittent claudication is. Which of the following nursing response is most accurate?
a. "Prolonged standing causes pooling of blood in your legs and the pressure build up which in turn causes the pain"
b. "Your muscles get tired easily because they lack protein"
c. "The valves of your veins are incompetent and prevent blood from returning to the heart."
d. "The pain is caused by lactic acid irritating your muscles. The lactic acid is brought about by decreased blood flow to your legs."

33. A client was involved in a vehicular accident and complains of sudden bursting pain in the right leg as a result of blunt trauma to the calf. The area appears dusky red. What condition is the client most likely suffering from?
a. Thrombophlebitis
b. Compartment syndrome
c. Fracture

d. Intermittent claudication

34. A client presents to the clinic complaining of pain in the lower extremities. The nurse wants to know if the symptoms are of arterial or venous cause. Which of the following is an accurate differentiation of the two?
   a. Arterial: due to ischemia; venous: due to venous hypertension
   b. Arterial: bluish when dependent; venous: pale on elevation
   c. Arterial: normal; venous: cool
   d. Arterial: thick skin; venous: thin hairless

35. A nurse is assessing a client's pulse and notes that in every beat, the amplitude of the pulse differs. The nurse documents this abnormality as
   a. Pulsus paradoxus
   b. Pulsus alternans
   c. Bisferiens
   d. Bigeminal pulse

36. A nurse is reading a client's chart and noted that he has bisferiens pulse. The nurse consults literature and finds that the main cause of bisferiens pulse is
   a. Mitral regurgitation
   b. Patent ductus arteriosus
   c. Coarctation of the aorta
   d. Aortic regurgitation

37. A nurse is examining a client's edema in both lower extremities and notes that it is hard, indurated and non-pitting on palpation. The skin also looks thickened. Which process is the most probable cause for the client's symptoms?
   a. Arterial insufficiency
   b. Venous insufficiency
   c. Lymphedema
   d. Hypoalbuminemia

38. The nurse is examining the skin of legs of a client with arterial insufficiency. Which of the following assessment findings is not consistent with the client's diagnosis?
   a. Cold skin
   b. Pallor
   c. Hairless
   d. With brownish pigments around the ankles

39. A 33-year old man attends a health fair and is being interviewed by the nurse. Which of the following alerts the nurse for the presence of risk factor for peripheral arterial disease?
   a. Smoking one pack of cigarettes a day

b.   Use of anticoagulants
c.   Chronic use of aspirin
d.   Of middle socio-economic class

40.   A client who just delivered a baby through caesarean section is being assessed for the prevention and early identification of DVT. Which of the following is not a parameter of the Virchow triad?
a.   Venous stasis
b.   Hypercoagulability
c.   Hydration status
d.   Vessel wall damage

41.   A nurse is caring for a hypertensive older patient who is also a chronic smoker. The nurse wants to determine if the patient is experiencing intermittent claudication. Which of the following questions should the nurse ask the patient to assess for intermittent claudication?
a.   "Do you feel pain in your calf when you walk a certain distance?"
b.   "Are your shoes feeling tighter these days?"
c.   "Do you have wounds in your leg that would not heal?"
d.   "Do you notice a color change in your hands or fingertips?"

42.   Which of the following patient complaints will alert the nurse to the possibility of Reynaud disease?
a.   "My hands look pale."
b.   "When I reach inside the freezer, my hands become blue and purple, and sometimes red."
c.   "My stomach hurts after I eat."
d.   "I have wounds around my ankles that do not seem to heal."

43.   A nurse is examining a patient. Which of the following techniques will determine the brachial pulse?
a.   Flex the patient's elbows 90 degrees, feel the groove between the biceps and the triceps nearest the elbow in the inner upper arm
b.   Slightly flex the patient's knees and palpate in the popliteal fossa
c.   Slightly flex the patient's elbow and place the finger pads at the middle of the antecubital crease
d.   Palpate along the medial edge of the sternocleidomastoid below the angle of the jaw

44.   A nurse is assessing the peripheral circulation of a patient with right-sided heart failure. As the nurse examines the lower legs, some brownish discoloration, and several shallow ulcers are noted around the ankles. Which of the following is the most probable nature of the patient's manifestations?
a.   Arterial blood flow impairment
b.   Venous blood flow impairment
c.   Lymphatic flow impairment

d.   Musculoskeletal impairment

45. A student nurse asks a senior nurse how blood flows back to the heart when there is no pressure such as the contraction of the heart to propel the blood back to the heart. Which of the following responses correctly answers the student nurse's question?
   a.   "The venous blood returns to the heart when muscles contract."
   b.   "Veins contract on their own."
   c.   "The pressure in the heart acts as a siphon that pulls blood to the heart."
   d.   "The veins have valves that propel the blood back to the heart."

46. A nurse is reviewing a patient's records and notes that the previous shift nurse had a documentation entry indicating that the patient has a grade 3+ pulse. Which of the following is the correct interpretation of a grade 3+ pulse?
   a.   The patient's pulse is absent
   b.   The patient's pulse is weak or diminished
   c.   The patient's pulse is brisk
   d.   The patient's pulse is bounding

47. A novice nurse is assessing the legs of a patient with arterial insufficiency. The nurse asks the senior nurse why the patient's legs appear hairless and shiny. Which of the following is the correct rationale for the patient's manifestation?
   a.   Lack of hair on the legs is a congenital condition in those with arterial insufficiency
   b.   The legs of the patient with arterial insufficiency is inflamed so that no hair will grow on it
   c.   Lack of arterial blood supply to the legs could not sustain the growth of the hairs on the legs
   d.   Patients with arterial insufficiency will feel itch in their legs so the patient would shave the hairs off

48. A nurse is assessing the legs of a patient with arterial insufficiency. How will the skin of the patient's leg most likely feel during the nurse's examination?
   a.   Lumpy
   b.   Warm
   c.   Moist
   d.   Cool

49. A patient has a unilateral edema in the lower extremities. The nurse is trying to determine the probable cause of the edema. Which of the following conditions would the nurse NOT consider as the cause of the patient's edema?
   a.   Deep vein thrombosis
   b.   Right-sided heart failure
   c.   Chronic venous insufficiency
   d.   Incompetent venous valve

50. A patient has been recently diagnosed with deep vein thrombosis. Which of the following nursing actions indicates that the nurse needs further teachings?
    a. Using a tape measure to measure the patient's calf circumference
    b. Gently palpating the patient's groin for tenderness
    c. Gently compressing the patient's calf muscles against the tibia for tenderness
    d. Firmly massaging the patient's calf to relieve pain and improve circulation

51. A patient comes into the clinic with ulcers on the legs and toes. Which of the following will alert the nurse that the patient's ulcers are arterial and NOT venous in nature?
    a. The ulcers are slow-healing
    b. There is pain in the calf during movement
    c. The surrounding skin is discolored
    d. The distal pulses are absent or diminished

52. The nurse is to perform the Allen test before obtaining a sample of arterial blood. Which pulses should the nurse locate and palpate to perform this test?
    a. The facial and carotid pulses
    b. The carotid and brachial pulses
    c. The femoral and popliteal pulses
    d. The radial and ulnar pulses

53. A bedridden patient's right leg has suddenly become cold and pale. The patient tells the nurse that they feel 'pins and needles' and numbness in the right leg. Which of the following when noted in the affected extremity indicates that an emergency treatment is necessary?
    a. 1+ popliteal pulse
    b. Absent dorsalis pedis pulse
    c. Pulse rate of 87 bpm taken from the radial artery
    d. There is edema and tenderness of the right leg

54. A nurse is assessing the lower legs of a patient and notes that the patient has varicose veins. Which of the following manifestations is consistent with varicose veins?
    a. The feet are edematous and tender to touch
    b. The feet feel hot
    c. The veins look dilated and tortuous
    d. The feet look flushed

55. A patient has arterial insufficiency of the lower extremities. The nurse wants to check for postural color changes. Which of the following should the nurse do to perform the assessment?
    a. Put the patient in a supine position and raise both legs
    b. Ask the patient to make a fist
    c. Ask the patient to dorsiflex both feet
    d. Put the patient on their side and ask them to keep the legs straight

56. The nurse is to perform the Ankle-Brachial Index (ABI) screening. Which of the following values will the nurse need? Select all that apply.
    a. Pulse pressure
    b. The systolic blood pressure in the ankle
    c. The systolic blood pressure in the arm
    d. The diastolic blood pressure in the ankle
    e. The diastolic blood pressure in the arm

57. A nurse is about to perform the Ankle-Brachial Index screening. Which of the following patient responses should alert the nurse that the procedure must be delayed for at least an hour?
    a. "I just went to the bathroom to urinate."
    b. "I want a warmer room."
    c. "It's good that I had time for coffee before this procedure."
    d. "Will it hurt?"

58. A nurse has just performed the Ankle-Brachial Index screening and obtained the result of 0.7. Which of the following is the correct interpretation of the nurse's finding?
    a. Normal
    b. Lower extremity arterial disease
    c. Borderline perfusion
    d. Severe ischemia

59. The nurse performs the Trendelenburg Test on a patient and obtains a negative-negative result. Which of the following should the nurse do after obtaining this result?
    a. Perform the Allen Test instead
    b. Elevate the patient's legs
    c. Inform the physician immediately
    d. Document the findings and continue assessing the patient

60. The nurse wants to determine if the patient has a paradoxical pulse. Which of the following is a must for the nurse to do before the procedure?
    a. Obtain a tourniquet
    b. Obtain a sphygmomanometer and a stethoscope
    c. Feel for the radial pulse
    d. Count the patient's respiratory rate

61. A nurse is assessing a patient who reports sudden unilateral limb pain. After further assessments and tests, the patient has been diagnosed with acute arterial occlusion. The nurse knows that the primary cause of an acute arterial occlusion is:
    a. Embolism or thrombosis
    b. Congenital arterial malformation

c.   Left-sided heart failure
d.   Malignancy

62. The nurse is mastering the technique of differentiating arterial insufficiency from venous insufficiency of the lower extremities. Which of the following will correctly guide the nurse in her mastery?
a.   Arterial – cool to touch; venous – normal temperature
b.   Arterial – cyanotic on dependency; venous – rubor on dependency
c.   Arterial – gangrene does not develop; venous – gangrene may develop
d.   Arterial – pulses normal but difficult to palpate; venous – absent or diminished

63. In which location are the ulcers of venous insufficiency most commonly noted?
a.   At the knees
b.   At the calf
c.   Around the ankles
d.   On the toes

64. A nurse is assessing the ulcers of the patient's legs and feet. Which factors would make the nurse consider the ulcers as neuropathic?
a.   The patient has left-sided heart disease
b.   The patient has right sided heart disease
c.   The patient has diabetes
d.   The patient is bedridden

65. A nurse is caring for a patient with leg edema. Which of the following factors would suggest that the edema is caused by lymphedema?
a.   Cirrhosis
b.   Immobility
c.   Recent node dissection
d.   Congestive heart failure

ANSWERS

1. A

   The valves of the veins are important because veins do not have the pressure that pumps blood coming from the heart as with arteries. The valves prevent the backflow of blood, and this will help the blood to return to the heart and prevent pooling in the lower extremities.

2. C

   Inguinal nodes are located in the groin area. They drain lymph from the legs, the genitals and the anterior part of the abdomen.

3. A

   Asking how far a client walks before he experiences pain in the calf assesses claudication distance.

4. B

   Occlusion of the aortoiliac artery can cause erectile dysfunction. There is not enough blood flow to the penis to cause an erection.

5. C

   Deep vein thrombosis can cause unilateral leg edema. Other manifestations of deep vein thrombosis are swelling, warmth and tenderness of the leg where occlusion is present in the deep veins.

6. A

   An extremely cold room will affect capillary refill because of peripheral vasoconstriction in response to the low environmental temperature.

7. B

   Smoking is one of the factors that pose a great risk for the development of peripheral arterial disease. Nicotine in cigarettes can cause vasoconstriction. It decreases vessel elasticity that lead to decreased arterial blood flow to the extremities.

8. C

   If the vascular problem is arterial in nature, the lower extremities will be cool to touch and hairless. This is because there is not enough circulation in the leg to make it warm and to nourish hair roots.

9. D

   Polycythemia vera is overproduction of RBCs that cause hyperviscosity of and increased volume the blood which can manifest as full bounding pulse.

10. A

   In performing the Allen test, the nurse first occludes both the ulnar and radial pulses using thumbs of both hands. Then the nurse instructs the client to open and close the palms several times and then to keep the hand open. The nurse then releases one of the pulses and observes for the return of the reddish color of the palm. Consistent paleness even after the release indicates an occlusion in the artery.

11. A

When the edema of the lower extremities shows indentation marks when pressed, it is termed 'pitting'. Since both legs are affected, it is bilateral. The edema is Grade 4+ edema if the swelling is so severe that the leg looks taut and distorted. When pressed by the examining fingers, it causes very deep indentations that do not rebound easily.

12. B

The Doppler ultrasonic probe can help detect weak pulses, and monitor low blood pressure in infants and in those with hemorrhage.

13. B

The Brachial-Ankle Index can give a good assessment of the severity of peripheral arterial disease. Smoking within two hours prior to the test may render the results unreliable so that the test needs to be delayed or rescheduled.

14. B

Shoes that feel tighter than usual may indicate peripheral vascular disease that cause edema of the extremities that make the feet larger.

15. D

Clients with decreased blood volume or cardiac output manifest weak and thready pulse. The nurse may have a hard time palpating for it. The rate may be fast but the amplitude is low and may even fade during palpation.

16. C

Pulsus alternans is caused by left sided heart failure, ischemic heart diseases, damaged heart valves, increased blood pressure and cardiomyopathies. There is normal rhythm and rate but the beats have alternating strong and weak amplitude.

17. B, C, D

Reynaud's phenomenon is a vascular disease that is arterial in nature. It is caused by spasms of the arterioles of the hand usually triggered by exposure to cold. The hand appears red, blue or pale.

18. A

Lymphedema is the leakage of fluid into the interstitial spaces because of injury or removal of lymph nodes for cancer treatment. In this case, the radiation therapy damaged lymph nodes, and edema ensues. The arm affected swells and feels heavier and thicker.

19. C

Neuropathic ulcers are caused by decreased sensation and circulation to the area of the ulcer. An example of this is a diabetic wound in the feet.

20. A

Venous stasis ulcers are usually seen around the ankles. They are brown in color and thick looking. The brown discoloration is due to blood that leaked from damaged venules. The client experiences dull ache in the extremity.

21. C

Pain on dorsiflexion and warmth of the affected leg are common manifestations of deep vein thrombosis. It is caused by the pooling of blood in the lower extremities due to blockage of the deep veins with a clot.

22. C

Venous insufficiency is stasis of venous blood in the dependent areas of the body caused by incompetent valves of the veins. The stasis causes small venuoles in the lower extremities, especially around the ankles to break and spill blood into the tissues, causing ulcerations in time.

23. B

Assessment of distal pulses after any procedure that accesses an artery is important because a clot may have formed in the area that would cause an occlusion of the artery.

24. D

Dislodgement of the thrombus produces an embolus that can travel to the lungs, causing pulmonary embolism and possible death.

25. C

Edema may be pitting or nonpitting. In pitting edema the interstitial fluid can be translocated with the pressure exerted by a finger. A "pit" or depression is left for 5 to 30 seconds. The degree of pitting is measured on a 1 to 4 scale: 1+ (2 mm); 2+ (4 mm); 3+ (6mm); 4+ (8 mm)

26. A

In arterial insufficiency, the lower extremities are cold, numb and pale due to decreased perfusion. Options (B) and (C) describe venous stasis and (D) describes thrombophebitis.

27. C

The Allen test is a test of patency of the ulnar and brachial artery. The nurse asks the client to make a tight fist and compresses the ulnar and radial artery. Then the nurse asks the client to open the palm. Paleness should be observed. Then the nurse releases compression and normally, flushing should occur in less than 5 seconds. If flushing takes longer than 5 seconds, then there is arterial insufficiency.

28. B
Pregnancy, recent childbirth, intake of medications, especially oral contraceptives or hormone replacement therapy, and inflammatory diseases such as lupus, rheumatoid arthritis, or irritable bowel disease all contribute to clot formation that lead to deep vein thrombosis.

29. D
Varicose veins are dilated tortuous veins of the legs that have been distended by the stasis of venous blood caused by incompetent valves of the veins of the lower extremities.

30. B
Lymphedema of the arm and hand may follow axillary node dissection, mastectomy and radiation therapy. The nurse cares for the client by encouraging lymph flow. Keeping the arms in 'liberty' position (elevated to the side of the head) helps in draining lymph from the affected part.

31. A
Firm palpation or massage over a DVT may dislodge the clot, causing a pulmonary embolus and consequently death.

32. D
Pain felt in the calf when walking is called intermittent claudication and it indicates arterial insufficiency in the lower extremities. The pain is caused by lactic acid build up as a result of anaerobic metabolism.

33. B
Compartment syndrome is caused by pressure build up from trauma or bleeding into one of the four major muscle compartments between the knee and ankle. As each compartment is enclosed by fascia, it cannot expand to accommodate increasing pressure caused by the internal bleeding.

34. A
Arterial insufficiency is caused by decreased perfusion to distal sites and venous insufficiency is due to venous hypertension caused by pooling of blood in the dependent parts caused by incompetent valves.

35. B
The pulse differs in amplitude from beat to beat even though the rhythm is regular. When the difference between stronger and weaker beats is slight, it can be detected only by sphygmomanometry. Pulsus alternans is an indicator of left ventricular failure and is usually accompanied by a left-sided S3

36. D

    A bisferiens pulse is an increased arterial pulse with two systolic peaks. It is caused by pure aortic regurgitation and aortic stenosis with regurgitation.

37. C

    In lymphedema, the edema is soft in the early stages, then becomes indurated, hard, and nonpitting. Skin is markedly thickened; ulceration is rare. There is no pigmentation. Edema is usually noted bilaterally. Lymphedema develops when lymph channels are obstructed by tumor, fibrosis, or inflammation, and in cases of axillary node dissection and radiation.

38. D

    Brownish pigmentation around the ankles is caused by venous stasis that causes rupture of tiny venuoles that spills blood into the interstitial spaces.

39. A

    Smoking is one great contributor to peripheral vascular disease, especially arterial disorders. Smoking causes vasoconstriction and intimal changes in the arteries that compromise perfusion to the distal parts of the body.

40. C

    Prevention and early identification of DVT are critical nursing tasks, especially in the care of hospitalized patients and patients with reduced mobility. The Virchow triad—venous stasis, hypercoagulability, and vessel wall damage—set the stage for the development of a DVT.

41. A

    When a patient reports pain in their calves after they walk a certain distance, the patient is experiencing intermittent claudication.

42. B

    When a patient tells the nurse that portions of their hands, especially the fingertips change color, to usually blue, purple or red when in a cold environment, the patient may have Reynaud disease. Reynaud disease is caused by the spasms of the smaller arteries that supply blood to the hands.

43. C

    The brachial pulse can be palpated at the middle of the antecubital fossa, or the crease between the upper and lower arm. To be able to feel for the pulse easily, the nurse slightly flexes the patient's elbow and uses the finger pads of the forefinger and the middle finger to palpate for the pulse.

44. B

    Venous blood flow impairments are the result of right-sided heart failure, prolonged immobility, or valvular defects of the veins. Venous blood pools in the lower extremities and small venules rupture and release venous blood to the interstitial spaces causing the brown discoloration of the skin around the ankles, and the shallow ulcers.

45. A
Venous blood returns to the heart with muscle contractions. Veins have valves that prevent backflow of blood.

46. D
A grade 3+ pulse is bounding. Patients with aortic insufficiency or those with fluid volume excess will have bounding carotid, radial, and femoral pulses.

47. C
A patient with arterial insufficiency will have hairless shiny skin on their legs. This is due to the lack of blood supply that brings oxygen and nutrients to nourish the skin and the roots of the hair.

48. D
Due to lack of arterial blood flow to the legs, the patient's legs would feel cool to touch. It will also feel smooth because of the hairless, thin skin.

49. B
Deep vein thrombosis, chronic venous insufficiency, and incompetent venous valves will all have manifestations of unilateral calf edema and ankle swelling. On the other hand, right-sided heart failure, cirrhosis, and nephrotic syndrome will cause bilateral pitting edema.

50. D
A firm massage or palpation of a leg with a deep vein thrombosis is avoided because doing so can dislodge the clots in the leg and cause an embolism, and possibly death.

51. D
Absent or diminished distal pulses indicate that the ulcers in the patient's leg are due to an arterial problem. When the blood supply to the distal areas are diminished or absent, the cells in those areas die, leading to ulcer formation and gangrene in the digits.

52. D
The Allen test checks for the patency of both the radial and ulnar arteries. It determines arterial insufficiency in the hands. The Allen test is done prior to accessing the radial artery for starting arterial lines and obtaining blood samples. The patient makes a fist, and the nurse presses firmly on both arteries. The nurse then releases the pressure on the artery to check for its patency.

53. B
Sudden pain, numbness or tingling sensation in one leg indicates possible arterial occlusion from an embolus. The patient's leg becomes cold and pale, and pain will ensue. The pain is caused by lactic acid buildup secondary to anaerobic metabolism in the affected leg. The absence of pulses distal to the occlusion is an ominous sign that the artery has been completely occluded. Without

immediate medical treatment, the cells in the patient's most distal parts will start to die, and gangrene will ensue.

54. C

Varicose veins look dilated and tortuous. They are caused by the pooling of venous blood in the lower extremities secondary to the incompetence of the valves.

55. A

To check for postural color changes when assessing for arterial insufficiency, the nurse first helps the patient to assume a supine position and then instructs the patient to raise both legs to about 60 degrees until the feet have become pale. Next, the nurse helps the patient to sit up by the side of the bed and to dangle their feet. If the pinkness of the extremities does not return within 10 seconds, and if after a minute, the extremities become dusky (rubor), then the patient has arterial insufficiency and without collateral circulation.

56. B, C

The Ankle-Brachial Index (ABI) screening is done to assess the arterial blood flow to the extremities. It is a comparison of the systolic blood pressure in the patient's arm and ankle.

57. C

When the nurse is to perform the Ankle-Brachial Index screening, they must ensure that the patient has not eaten any food, drank any beverages, or performed any activity that can affect the blood pressure. Drinking caffeinated beverages, smoking, and engaging in strenuous activity are avoided at least one hour prior to the procedure.

58. C

To get the Ankle-Brachial Index, the nurse obtains the higher value of the systolic pressure from both ankles and divides it by the higher value of the systolic pressure from the patient's arm. A value of 1.0 is normal, meaning that the systolic pressure obtained in the arms and legs are equal. A score of 0.7 indicates borderline perfusion.

59. D

Getting a negative-negative result in a Trendelenburg Test means that the patient has no venous insufficiency. It reflects the competence of the valves of the veins. The nurse documents their findings and continues with their assessment.

60. B

Paradoxical pulse means that the pulsation is stronger during expiration and weaker during inspiration. To check for the presence of a paradoxical pulse, the nurse will need a sphygmomanometer and a stethoscope. Normally, there is a 3-4 mmHg drop in systolic pressure during inspiration. In pulsus paradoxus, the pressure difference is 10mmHg or more. Paradoxical pulse is noted in patients with cardiac tamponade, pericarditis, and obstructive airway diseases.

61. A

The manifestation of an acute arterial occlusion is very sudden. The patient would usually report pain in the foot or the leg. The pain is caused by lactic acid buildup secondary to the occlusion of an artery by an emboli or thrombus.

62. A

The legs of the patient with arterial insufficiency will be cool to touch, dusky red when in the dependent position, and with diminished or absent pulses. Gangrene may develop. On the other hand, in venous insufficiency, the patient's leg will have a normal temperature, cyanosis on dependency, and a normal pulse. Gangrene does not develop.

63. C

The ulcers formed because of venous insufficiency will be most commonly noted over the medial and sometimes lateral malleolus.

64. C

Neuropathic ulcers develop in areas of diminished sensation caused by neuropathy, such as the neuropathy of diabetes. Because of damaged nerves to the area, the patient feels no pain at the ulcer sites.

65. C

Lymphedema is caused by the accumulation of protein-rich lymph fluid when lymph channels are obstructed or disrupted, such as in a node dissection procedure.

The Gastrointestinal System

Questions

1. The nurse wants to assess for flank pain caused by inflamed kidneys. Which anatomical landmark should she use to locate the kidneys?
   a. Hypogastric area
   b. Costovertebral angle
   c. Costal margin
   d. Suprapubic area

2. The nurse wants to assess the abdomen of a client with splenomegaly. Which part of the abdomen will she particularly focus on?
   a. Upper right quadrant
   b. Upper left quadrant
   c. Lower left quadrant
   d. Midline

3. A nurse is preparing to be assigned to an aged home care. She understands that there are several age-related changes as a person ages. Which of the following are normal age-related changes in a client's gastrointestinal functions? Select all that apply.
   a. Decreased liver size
   b. Gastric emptying time increases
   c. Constipation becomes common
   d. Incidence of dry mouth increases
   e. Incidence of gallstone formation increases

4. A nurse is conducting an interview of a client and she wants to know if the client is experiencing dysphagia. Which of the following is most appropriate to ask to assess for dysphagia?
   a. "Do you have difficulty swallowing?"
   b. "Is there any pain when you swallow?"
   c. "Do you have difficulty chewing your food?"
   d. "Is there any pain in your abdomen after eating?"

5. A client reports burning midsternal pain especially after eating and after drinking alcohol. Which of the following conditions is the client most likely experiencing?
   a. Lactose intolerance
   b. Colic
   c. Angina pectoris
   d. Pyrosis

6. A nurse is assessing a client with complete obstruction of the bile duct caused by gallstones. Which of the following is characteristic of the client's stool?
   a. Fatty and frothy
   b. Acolic or clay-colored

   c.   Black and tarry
   d.   Foul smelling and frequent

7.   A nurse is assessing an infant, and she wants to know if the child is exhibiting pica behavior. Which of the following is an appropriate question to ask the mother of the child?
   a.   "Does your child enjoy eating one type of food only?"
   b.   "Does your child prefer to eat meat only?"
   c.   "Does your child regurgitate food after swallowing?"
   d.   "Does your child eat dirt, paint, plastic or any non-edible items?"

8.   A client is complaining of pain in the abdomen, and the nurse suspects ulcer. Which of the following is best to ask the client to distinguish duodenal ulcer pain from gastric ulcer pain?
   a.   "How long does your pain last?"
   b.   "How frequent do you feel pain in a day?"
   c.   "When does the pain occur, after eating or in between meals?"
   d.   "Is your pain colicky or constant and dull?"

9.   A nurse is to perform examination of a client's abdomen. Which of the following sequence should the nurse employ to assess the client's abdomen?
   a.   Inspection, auscultation, percussion, palpation
   b.   Inspection, percussion, palpation, auscultation
   c.   Inspection, palpation, percussion auscultation
   d.   Auscultation, palpation, percussion, inspection

10.   A nurse wants to assess a client for liver enlargement. She stands by the client's right side of the bed, and faces the client's feet. She then feels for the liver below the costal margin with fingers in a clawing position. Which of the following assessment procedure did the nurse perform?
   a.   Costovertebral punch
   b.   Leopold's maneuver
   c.   Duck bill positioning
   d.   Hooking technique

11.   A client complaints of abdominal tenderness and the nurse suspects that the client has appendicitis. The nurse assesses for tenderness, and chooses a site away from the painful area. She then pushes down her extended fingers deep into the abdomen and releases quickly. The client reports severe pain. The nurse documents this finding as
   a.   Murphy sign
   b.   Blumberg sign
   c.   Battle sign
   d.   Iliopsoas Muscle sign

12.   A nurse admits a client presenting with abdominal pain in the right lower quadrant, and abdominal

guarding. The client is running a fever. When the nurse palpates the abdomen, there is rebound tenderness. Her laboratory results show that her WBC count is 20,000 u/L. Other than that, there are no more signs and symptoms. She uses the Alvarado Score to determine the probability of appendicitis. Which of the following is the client's score?

a. 5
b. 8
c. 3
d. 10

13. A nurse is examining the abdomen of a 3-month old infant. Which of the following findings needs to be reported to the physician?
    a. Audible vascular turbulent sounds
    b. Visible bulge along the middle of the abdomen without distress
    c. Protuberant abdomen
    d. Palpable liver below the right costal margin

14. A client reports gnawing abdominal pain that awakens him from sleep. It is sometimes dull and aching and worsens 2-3 hours after meals. The client also claims that eating crackers gives some relief. In which of the following organs would the nurse suspect the injury is coming from?
    a. Duodenum
    b. Stomach
    c. Pancreas
    d. Spleen

15. A nurse is assessing a client suspected of having complete intestinal obstruction. Which of the following signs and symptoms is an UNLIKELY to be manifested by the client?
    a. Flatulence
    b. No passage of stool
    c. Fever
    d. Colicky pain

16. A client reports sudden onset of severe colicky flank and lower abdominal pain that made the client unable to walk. Prior to the pain, he did not eat nor had any intense activity. He also reports sweating profusely. Which of the following most probably caused the client's manifestations?
    a. Gallstones
    b. Kidney stones
    c. Appendicitis
    d. Pancreatitis

17. The nurse is auscultating the client's abdomen and hears a vascular turbulent sound. Upon palpation, the nurse feels a pulsating mass in the left of the midline of the upper abdomen. Which of the following client activity should the nurse advise the client against?

a. Wearing a tight belt
b. Wearing a wired bra
c. Taking antacids
d. Eating spicy foods

18. The nurse is palpating the right upper quadrant of the client's abdomen who is complaining of pain that worsens after eating fried foods. The client was soon diagnosed with cholecystitis. What finding would be consistent with the client's diagnosis?
    a. Hard lumps 2 cm along the costal margin
    b. Rebound tenderness
    c. borborygmus
    d. Sausage shaped mass

19. The nurse is assessing for splenomegaly. Which of the following will be true when the spleen is enlarged?
    a. Dullness on percussion on the 9th to 11th intercostal space
    b. Sausage-shaped mass on the left upper quadrant
    c. Fluid shifts on the abdomen
    d. Big hard lumps on the right lower quadrant

20. A 1-week old neonate frantically feeds but vomits with force every after feeding. Upon assessment of the client's abdomen, the nurse notes marked peristalsis and a palpable olive shaped mass on the right upper quadrant. The nurse should prepare to care for a client with which condition?
    a. Umbilical hernia
    b. Diastasis recti
    c. Pyloric stenosis
    d. Pulmonary stenosis

21. The nurse admits a client with intermittent colicky pain at the left lower quadrant of the abdomen. Which type of pain is the client referring to?
    a. Muscular pain
    b. Visceral pain
    c. Referred pain
    d. Parietal pain

22. A client with chest pain tells the nurse that he also feels the pain on the jaw and the shoulder. The nurse understands that this type of pain is called
    a. Referred pain
    b. Parietal pain
    c. Muscular pain
    d. Visceral pain

23. The nurse is doing the history of a patient with pain that ifs felt in the epigastric area. Which of the following cluster of client manifestations are considered "alarm symptoms" for gastric cancer?
    a. Dysphagia, odynophagia, coffee ground emesis
    b. Weight loss, diarrhea, dehydration
    c. Recurrent vomiting, 2cm x 2cm lump on the upper right quadrant, fever
    d. Hematochezia, hematemesis, epistaxis

24. A 21-year old woman is being seen at the emergency department due to right lower abdominal pain. She has missed her period for two consecutive months. She feels weak and dizzy. The nurse knows to prioritize which of the following nursing actions?
    a. Continue assessing by palpating the abdomen
    b. Perform a pregnancy test
    c. Apply hot compress to the affected area.
    d. Inspect the abdomen for ascites

25. A nurse is reviewing the client's records from an earlier shift and notes that the result of the barium enema revealed "apple core" lesions on the sigmoid colon. The client is passing pencil-like stools. Which disorder is the nurse most likely considering?
    a. Gastric cancer
    b. Colon cancer
    c. Diverticulitis
    d. Chron disease

26. The nurse is doing a health teaching on a client with colon cancer. She is explaining the different types of bleeding manifestations. Of particular interest to her is the type of bleeding associated with colon cancer and that is passing of fresh blood or maroon-colored stool. The client understands the teaching if he replies with which answer?
    a. Hematemesis
    b. Steatorrhea
    c. Hematochezia
    d. Melena

27. A client with hepatitis is asking the nurse why his skin turned yellow. Which response is the most accurate to explain why jaundice happens?
    a. Decreased production of bilirubin
    b. Increased uptake of bilirubin by the hepatocytes
    c. Increased ability of the liver to conjugate bilirubin
    d. Decreased excretion of bilirubin into the bile, resulting in absorption of conjugated bilirubin back into the blood

28. A client presenting with upper right quadrant steady pain is getting frantic about his stools that has turned grey. Which of the following nursing response will correctly address the client's concern?
    a. "Your body cannot digest food properly because it lacks the enzymes that turn stools brownish or greenish"
    b. "Bile, the substance in your gallbladder that gives color to the stool, has been totally blocked from flowing to your intestines"
    c. "The bacteria that are causing your infection have spread to affect your bowels as well."
    d. "You are deficient in an important mineral that is affected by your disorder."

29. The nurse is asking this series of questions to assess a client: "Do you have trouble starting your stream? Do you have to stand closer to the toilet to void? Is there a change in the force or size of your stream, or straining to void? Do you hesitate or stop in the middle of voiding?" The nurse is eliciting information about which disorder?
    a. Pyelonephritis
    b. Colon cancer
    c. Benign prostatic hypertrophy
    d. Urethritis

30. The nurse is examining a patient who reported dull pain in the upper right quadrant of the abdomen. The nurse also notes that the client has an enlarged abdomen and does percussion if the enlargement is due to ascites or to bloating. Which of the following assessment findings are true?
    a. If the client sits upright, percussion reveals tympany over the entire upper abdomen and dullness on the lower abdomen
    b. If the client turns to the left while lying on the examining table, dullness shifts to the more dependent side, and tympany shifts to the top.
    c. If the patient lies prone on the table, the tympany is noted on the client's right side only
    d. If the patient lies prone, the dullness is felt over the entire back

31. A patient comes to the emergency department in a wheelchair because of pain in the abdomen. He is bent down with arms hugging his abdomen. The nurse suspects appendicitis. Which of the following is an accurate manifestation of appendicitis?
    a.   (+) Rovsing sign – increased abdominal pain when the patient is asked to raise his thigh against the nurse's hand positioned above the knee
    b.   (+) psoas sign - Pain in the right lower quadrant during left-sided pressure
    c.   (+) obturator sign – pain in the right hypogastric area when the client is asked to flex thigh at the hip and the knee bent and rotated internally
    d.   (-) cutaneous hyperesthesia – localized pain as the nurse pinches the abdomen

32. A patient with acute cholecystitis has just been admitted to the unit. The nurse wants to assess the client for murphy sign. Which of the following maneuver is correct in eliciting murphy sign?

a.   the patient is asked to raise his thigh against the nurse's hand positioned above the knee

b.   the nurse exerts downward pressure on the lower left quadrant of the abdomen

c.   the client is asked to flex thigh at the hip and the knee bent and rotated internally

d.   hooking the fingers of the right hand on the client's right costal margin and asking him to breathe deeply

33. The nurse is taking the history of a client with suspected colorectal cancer. Which of the following is NOT an indication of high risk for colorectal cancer?
a.   History of appendicitis in the recent 3 years
b.   History of inflammatory bowel disease
c.   Single small adenoma (<1 cm): 3 to 6 years after initial polypectomy
d.   Single large adenoma (>1 cm), multiple adenomas, adenoma with highgrade dysplasia or villous change: within 3 years of initial polypectomy

34. A 56-year old client comes to the clinic complaining of abdominal pain. Upon assessment by the nurse, the client reports that the pain is gnawing in quality especially right after meals. Sometimes the pain is also felt at the back. Palpation and percussion of the abdomen reveals no abnormalities. The assessment findings are consistent with which disorder?
a.   Chron disease
b.   Irritable bowel syndrome
c.   Peptic ulcer
d.   Diverticulitis

35. The nurse is reviewing literature on a client's symptoms known as biliary colic. Which of the following is not consistent with biliary colic?
a.   Poorly localized periumbilical pain, followed usually by right lower quadrant pain
b.   Steady, aching; not colicky pain
c.   Sudden obstruction of the cystic duct or common bile duct by a gallstone
d.   Epigastric or right upper quadrant, may radiate to the right scapula and shoulder

36. A client is being seen by the nurse in the out-patient department. The client states that he has long been suffering from acid reflux and recently has started regurgitating partly digested solid food. The client does not report any chest or abdominal pain and denies any weight loss. The nurse suspects which of the following disorders?
a.   Peptic ulcer
b.   Cholecystitis
c.   Esophageal stricture
d.   Esophageal cancer

37. A mother takes her 2 year old child to the emergency department after the child suddenly lets out a loud cry and saying that her tummy hurt. The nurse notes "currant jelly" looking stools on the child's diaper. Diagnostic tests reveal telescoping of the bowel into itself. The nurse suspects

which condition?
a.   Biliary colic
b.   Intussusception
c.   Protrusion of an hernia
d.   Fecal impaction

38. A nurse in a hospice care facility is caring for a 70-year old coherent bedridden client who reports abdominal fullness and discomfort. Upon digital rectal examination, the nurse notes fecal mass that is large, firm and immovable. Which of the following questions asked by the nurse should take priority?
a.   "When was the last time you had a bowel movement?"
b.   "When was your last meal?"
c.   "What did you eat in the last 24 hours?"
d.   "When was the last time you took your medication for hypertension?

39. A patient has been found to have pancreatic insufficiency and is showing signs of malabsorption. The client reports passing stools that are "fatty, frothy, foul-smelling and floating." The nurse is sure to document this subjective finding as
a.   Melena
b.   Steatorrhea
c.   Acholic stools
d.   Hematochezia

40. A woman with a history of 3 normal deliveries and one caesarian section that are all uneventful is being seen by the nurse on the examining table. When assessing her abdomen, the nurse asks the client to raise her head while lying down. She notes a vertical ridge in the abdomen of the client that seems to separate the abdomen into left and right portions. Auscultation, percussion and palpation did not reveal any abnormality. The client denies any pain or discomfort. What is the best nursing action?
a.   Document the findings
b.   Inform the physician immediately
c.   Put the client on NPO
d.   Administer an enema

41. A patient with a history of chronic and heavy alcoholism is complaining of pain in the right upper quadrant. Which type of pain is the patient experiencing?
a.   Somatic pain
b.   Visceral pain
c.   Pleuritic pain
d.   Parietal pain

42. A patient is complaining of colicky pain in the middle of the abdomen, around the umbilicus. The patient is curled up with their hands across their abdomen. According to the patient, they vomited once. Which of the following conditions would the nurse most likely consider as the cause of the patient's manifestations?
    a. Early acute appendicitis
    b. Gastroenteritis
    c. Renal colic
    d. Biliary obstruction

43. A patient suspected of having acute appendicitis suddenly reports relief of abdominal pain. A few minutes later, the patient complains of very intense abdominal pain which is of a different quality than previously felt. The pain is very severe and steady, and the abdomen is tensed and the patient screams in pain even with the slightest of movement. Which of the following pain is the patient currently experiencing?
    a. Visceral pain
    b. Referred pain
    c. Parietal pain
    d. Pleuritic pain

44. A patient who has angina pectoris tells the nurse that as they experience the crushing chest pain, they also feel pain in their jaw. Which of the following refers to the pain felt on the jaw?
    a. Bone pain
    b. Trigeminal neuralgia
    c. Referred pain
    d. Visceral pain

45. A patient who is experiencing gnawing abdominal pain in the epigastric area is also vomiting. According to the patient, the pain started early in the morning and had intensified since then. The pain is also felt on the right shoulders. Using the OLD CART mnemonic, which of the following findings will the nurse document under the category associated manifestations?
    a. Gnawing
    b. Vomiting
    c. Pain that started early morning
    d. Pain in the epigastric area

46. A patient tells the nurse that many times during the week, they feel a burning pain in their throat at the center of the chest. The pain is triggered when the patient bends over to reach for something on the floor, or after drinking coffee and other caffeinated drinks. Which of the following is the patient most likely experiencing?
    a. Epigastric pain
    b. Parietal pain
    c. Dysphagia

    d.   Heartburn

47. Which of the following when noted on abdominal palpation will suggest to the nurse that the patient has diverticulitis?
    a.   Tensed abdominal muscles, nausea
    b.   RLQ colicky pain
    c.   LLQ pain with palpable mass, fever
    d.   Tender abdominal muscles, cramping pain

48. A patient tells the nurse that, at times, an acidic fluid backs up to their throat, and is sometimes accompanied by undigested food particles. The patient says that "it just happens" even if they are not feeling sick. Which of the following manifestation is the patient most likely experiencing?
    a.   Regurgitation
    b.   Nausea
    c.   Vomiting
    d.   Retching

49. A patient who is recovering from bacterial gastroenteritis is concerned about their stools that had become oily, bubbly and floating. The patient tells the nurse that their stools "stinks bigtime." How would the nurse document the patient's concern?
    a.   Diarrhea
    b.   Steatorrhea
    c.   Melena
    d.   Hematemesis

50. Which position is best for the patient to assume when their abdomen is to be examined?
    a.   Supine, with the arms resting above the head
    b.   Supine, with a pillow under the head and the knees slightly flexed
    c.   Supine, HOB 60° with the legs kept straight
    d.   Left lateral with a pillow between the legs

51. A nurse is examining the patient's abdomen and is doing an inspection while standing at the foot of the bed. The nurse notices bulging flanks. Percussion of the bulge reveals tympany over the umbilicus and dullness at the laterals. Which of the following correctly describes the patient's symptom?
    a.   Pregnancy
    b.   Bladder malignancy
    c.   Ascites
    d.   Hernia

52. A nurse is assessing a patient with suspected intestinal obstruction. Which of the following is the correct auscultation technique to use when examining the patient's abdomen?
    a.   Use the diaphragm of the stethoscope to auscultate on one quadrant, while pressing deeply with hand on the opposite quadrant
    b.   Use the bell of the stethoscope and press deeply in different locations
    c.   Auscultate from each side alternately every one minute.
    d.   Auscultate in each quadrant for 5 minutes

53. A nurse is examining the abdomen of an obese patient with visceral pain in the right upper quadrant. The nurse is trying to trace the liver borders laterally and medially but is having a hard time because of increased abdominal fat in the patient. Which of the following can help the nurse perform this examination?
    a.   The hooking technique
    b.   Percussion
    c.   Pressing the diaphragm of the stethoscope firmly on the left upper quadrant
    d.   Asking the patient to turn to their right side

54. The nurse is assessing for the presence of the psoas sign in the patient with suspected appendicitis. Which of the following is the correct technique of eliciting the psoas sign?
    a.   Place one hand above the patient's right knee to act as resistance, and tell the patient to raise that thigh against the hand
    b.   Place one hand above the patient's left knee and tell the patient to raise that thigh as high as they can
    c.   Flex the patient's right hips and knees, and rotate the leg internally at the hip
    d.   Press deeply in the lower left quadrant

55. A nurse is conducting a health teaching regarding the transmission of Hepatitis A virus. Which of the following indicates a correct understanding of the spread of Hepatitis A?
    a.   Sterilize all clothing when coming from countries with high prevalence of Hepatitis A
    b.   Do not share a bed
    c.   Avoid undercooked shellfish
    d.   Do not engage in unprotected sex

56. A nurse is screening several patients for colorectal cancer. Which of the following patients has the highest risk for developing colorectal cancer?
    a.   68-years old patient, with presence of adenomatous polyps, with a first cousin diagnosed with colorectal neoplasia
    b.   45-years old patient, single, smoking 5-6 cigarette per day
    c.   38-year old Black American female, with a history of alcoholism
    d.   55-year old American male who is obese and whose diet is mostly meat and fish

57. A nurse is conducting health teachings on how to prevent and manage incontinence. Which of the following will the nurse include in her teaching?
    a. Pelvic muscle exercises
    b. Low-fat diet
    c. Decreased fluid intake
    d. Increased daytime nap

58. A nurse is caring for a patient with acute pancreatitis. Which of the following correctly describes the abdominal pain of patients with acute pancreatitis?
    a. Left lower quadrant cramping pain
    b. Mild periumbilical pain at the early stage and concentrates on the right lower quadrant as the condition advances
    c. Steady epigastric pain that may radiate to the back or other parts of the abdomen
    d. Colicky pain in the right upper quadrant

59. A nurse is assessing a female patient who is a mother of three. The nurse is examining her abdomen and notes the distinct separation of the rectus abdominis muscles. The midline ridge of the abdomen bulges. The patient feels no pain. Which of the following should the nurse do at this time?
    a. Ask the patient to avoid high-fat diets
    b. Document the findings
    c. Inform the physician immediately
    d. Apply hot compress to the abdomen

60. How should the examination of the abdomen proceed?
    a. Inspection, auscultation, percussion, palpation
    b. Inspection, percussion, palpation, auscultation
    c. Inspection, palpation, auscultation, percussion
    d. Inspection, percussion, auscultation, palpation

ANSWERS

1. B

    The kidneys lie behind the abdominal organs and are found behind the 11th and 12th ribs. To assess the kidneys, the nurse locates the costovertebral angle, or the angle formed between the spine and the 12th rib.

2. B

    The spleen is located at the left posterolateral wall of the abdominal cavity, just below the diaphragm. To assess for splenomegaly, the nurse palpates the left upper quadrant of the abdomen.

3. A, C, D, E

    As a person ages, the liver decreases in size, gastric emptying time increases and peristalsis slows which lead to constipation. There is also an increase in gallstone formation. The mouth becomes dry.

4. A

    Dysphagia is difficulty swallowing. Painful swallowing is called odynophagia.

5. D

    Pyrosis is the burning sensation in the chest caused by reflux of acid to the esophagus. It is brought about by eating, or by intake of alcohol and caffeinated beverages.

6. B

    A client with completely obstructed bile ducts will have acolic or clay-colored stools because bile, which gives the usual brown or greenish color of the stool, does not flow to the small intestines.

7. D

    Pica behavior is the eating of non-edible items such as dirt, plastic or paint. It becomes apparent by 18-24 months of age.

8. C

    Pain caused by gastric ulcer is experienced right after eating. This is because of increased secretion of gastric acid, and mechanical irritation caused by food in the stomach. It can also be apparent when the stomach is empty because gastric secretions are triggered by hunger pangs. Duodenal ulcer pain is felt 2-3 hours after meals, and coincides with gastric emptying. This happens when the duodenal ulcer becomes irritated with food and gastric secretions from the stomach.

9. A

    In the assessment of the abdomen, the nurse inspects the abdomen first and then proceeds to do auscultation because percussion and palpation can alter bowel sounds.

10. D

The hooking technique is used to palpate the liver. The nurse stands by the client's right side of the bed and faces the client's feet. She then hooks her fingers and traces the borders of the liver below the right costal margin.

11. B

Blumberg sign or rebound tenderness is pain that is felt after the nurse quickly releases her fingers that press deep on a site away from the source of pain.

12. A

The Alvarado Scoring system determines the probability of Appendicitis. The following signs and symptoms are assigned a score if present. The client gets a score of 5, 2 for tenderness at RLQ, 1 for rebound tenderness, 1 for fever, and 1 for leukocytosis.
Symptoms
Migration to right iliac fossa1
Anorexia*1
Nausea and vomiting1
Signs
Tenderness, RLQ2
Rebound tenderness1
Elevation of temperature (oral ≥37.3°C)1
Laboratory Findings
Leukocytosis (white blood cell count >10,000/μL)2
Shift to the left (>75% neutrophils)1
Total Possible Points10

13. A

Peristaltic sounds are normally heard over the abdomen. There should be no vascular sounds or bruit heard during auscultation of the abdomen. All other options are normal or non-pathologic in a 3-month old child.

14. A

Duodenal ulcers produce gnawing dull aching pain in the abdomen that is worse or felt 2-3 hours after meals. The pain may awaken him from sleep. Eating food provides relief.

15. A

In complete intestinal obstruction, the client cannot pass gas and stool. The client complains of colicky pain. In early obstruction, the client will have hyperactive bowel sounds that become less and absent in the later part.

16. B

Kidney stones that pass through the ureters produce severe sudden colicky pain in the flank and lower abdomen that render a person unable to walk. There may also be diaphoresis.

17. A

The manifestations of the client are characteristic of abdominal aortic aneurysm. Care should be taken to maintain the integrity of the vessel that is prone to rupture. Wearing a tight belt can increase abdominal pressure that can rupture the aneurysm.

18. D

When the gallbladder is filled with stones, its shape becomes sausage like. All options are not characteristic of cholecystitis.

19. A

The spleen is located above the diaphragm protected by the 9th to 11th rib. The nurse will note dullness on percussion of the 9th to 12th intercostal space.

20. D

Pyrolic stenosis is the enlargement and hardening of the pyloric sphincter that causes obstruction that prevents gastric emptying. Upon palpation, the nurse feels an olive-shaped mass at the right upper quadrant. It is manifested by peristaltic waves, frantic feeding and projectile vomiting.

21. B

Visceral pain occurs when hollow abdominal organs such as the intestine or biliary tree contract unusually forcefully or are distended or stretched. Solid organs such as the liver can also become painful when their capsules are stretched. Visceral pain may be difficult to localize. It is typically palpable near the midline at levels that vary according to the structure involved. Visceral pain varies in quality and may be gnawing, burning, cramping, or aching. When it becomes severe, it may be associated with sweating, pallor, nausea, vomiting, and restlessness.

22. A

Referred pain is felt in more distant sites that share the same innervations as the source of pain. Referred pain often develops as the initial pain becomes more intense and thus seems to radiate or travel from the initial site. It may be felt superficially or deeply but is usually well localized.

23. A

Red flags or alarm symptoms for gastric cancer include: difficulty swallowing (dysphagia), pain with swallowing (odynophagia), recurrent vomiting, and evidence of gastrointestinal bleeding (coffee ground emesis), weight loss and anemia.

24. B

With the given findings of lower abdominal pain and missed periods, the nurse suspects ectopic pregnancy especially if accompanied by other symptoms like rigidity of abdominal muscles, weakness and dizziness. Palpating the abdomen is contraindicated as the risk of rupturing the fallopian tube is high.

25. B

Thin, pencil-like stool occurs in an obstructing "apple core" lesion of the sigmoid colon. The nurse considers colon cancer if the above are accompanied by the following: melena, hematochezia, diarrhea, constipation, feeling of incomplete bowel emptying, bloating, cramps weight loss and fatigue.

26. C

Hematochezia is passing of blood-streaked stools, stools that are bright or dark red in color. This is caused by lower gastrointestinal bleeding. Hematemesis is vomiting of fresh blood or of occult blood of 'coffee-grounds' consistency. Steatorrhea is passing of fatty malodorous stools. Melena is presence of occult blood in the stool.

27. D

Jaundice or the yellowing of the skin is caused by several factors: increased production of bilirubin, decreased uptake of bilirubin by the hepatocytes, decreased ability of the liver to conjugate bilirubin, decreased excretion of bilirubin into the bile, resulting in absorption of conjugated bilirubin back into the blood

28. B

When excretion of bile into the intestine is completely obstructed, the stools become gray or light colored, or acholic, without bile.

29. C

Benign prostatic hypertrophy is the enlargement of the prostrate that surrounds the urethra that results to hesitancy in urination, decrease in size and force of urine, and dribbling urine.

30. B

Ascitic fluid characteristically sinks with gravity, whereas gas-filled loops of bowel float to the top. Percussion gives a dull note in dependent areas of the abdomen. In a person without ascites, the borders between tympany and dullness usually stay relatively constant.

31. C

In appendicitis, pain in the right lower quadrant during left-sided pressure suggests appendicitis (a positive Rovsing sign). There is also – increased abdominal pain when the patient is asked to raise his thigh against the nurse's hand positioned above the knee (psoas sign). If the client is asked to flex thigh at the hip and bend the knee and rotate it internally, and pain is felt in the hypogastric are, the client is positive for obturator sign. The client should also be able to localize pain over the lower left quadrant if the nurse pinches skin in different areas of the abdomen (cutaneous hyperesthesia).

32. D

The nurse hooks her left thumb or the fingers of her right hand under the costal margin at the point where the lateral border of the rectus muscle intersects with the costal margin. Or if the liver is enlarged, the nurse hooks thumb or fingers under the liver edge at a comparable point below then asks the patient to take a deep breath. A sharp increase in tenderness with a sudden stop in inspiratory effort constitutes a positive Murphy sign of acute cholecystitis.

33. A

Colonoscopy is indicated for the following increased risk factors: single small adenoma <1 cm): 3 to 6 years after initial polypectomy, single large adenoma (>1 cm), multiple adenomas, adenoma with highgrade dysplasia or villous change: within 3 years of initial polypectomy, history of resection of colorectal cancer: within 1 year after resection, any first-degree relative younger than 60 years, two or more first degree, relatives with either colorectal cancer or adenomatous polyps: at age 40 or 10 years before youngest case in immediate family, whichever is earlier, familial adenomatous polyposis or nonpolyposis colon cancer, and history of inflammatory bowel disease, chronic ulcerative colitis, or Crohn disease.

34. C

Peptic ulcer refers to a mucosal ulceration, usually in the duodenum or stomach. Dyspepsia causes similar symptoms but no ulceration. Infection by Helicobacter pylori is often present. The pain experienced by the client is described as gnawing, burning, boring, aching, pressing, or hunger-like, and may radiate to the back.

35. A

Biliary colic is caused by sudden obstruction of the cystic duct or common bile duct by a gallstone. The pain in biliary colic is steady and aching but not colicky and is felt in the epigastric or right upper quadrant that may radiate to the right scapula and shoulder.

36. C

Esophageal stricture is a kind of mechanical narrowing of the esophagus that is largely caused by repeated irritation by acid reflux. The narrowing of the passageway causes swallowed solid food to be regurgitated. If the symptoms are associated with chest pain or back pain with accompanying weight loss, the nurse suspects esophageal cancer.

37. B

Intussusception is the telescoping of the bowel into itself. The client reports colicky abdominal pain, abdominal distention, and often "currant jelly" looking stools (red blood and mucus).

38. A

Fecal impaction is characterized by the presence of a large, firm and immovable fecal mass in rectum. It is characterized by rectal fullness, abdominal pain, and diarrhea around the impaction. It is common in debilitated, bedridden, and elderly patients. It would be pertinent to ask about last bowel movement in this case.

39. B

In pancreatic insufficiency, there is defective absorption of fat, including fat-soluble vitamins, with steatorrhea (excessive excretion of fat). The stools are typically bulky, soft, light yellow to gray, mushy, greasy or oily, and sometimes frothy; particularly foul smelling and usually floats in the toilet.

40. A

Separation of the two rectus abdominis muscles, through which abdominal contents form a midline ridge when the patient raises head and shoulder, is called diastasis recti. It is often observed in repeated pregnancies, obesity, and chronic lung disease and it has no clinical significance.

41. B

Visceral pain is felt when abdominal organs such as the intestines or the bile duct get distended or stretched, or contract more forcefully than normal. The pain is described as gnawing, cramping, aching, or burning. The abdominal pain felt by patients with advanced liver diseases is visceral.

42. A

The pain in early acute appendicitis is felt in the periumbilical area. Patients often describe it as colicky, and it intensifies as the inflammation of the appendix worsens. The pain may concentrate in the right lower quadrant in its later stage.

43. C

Parietal pain is caused by an inflamed parietal peritoneum. It is described as very intense, aching and steady. The pain is worsened by movement or by coughing so that the patient refrains from moving.

44. C

Referred pain is felt not on the original location but on a distal site that has the same innervation as the source.

45. B

Associated manifestations are other symptoms that the patient is experiencing together with the primary complaint. Vomiting is the associated manifestation of the main complaint, which is the gnawing abdominal pain.

46. D

Heartburn is retrosternal pain that is described as rising to the throat. It is triggered or aggravated by certain foods and drinks, such spicy foods, chocolates, citrus fruits, coffee or tea. Activities that require the patient to bend over, lift or jump also starts the pain.

47. C

When a nurse notes a palpable mass in the patient's left lower abdomen, especially when accompanied by other symptoms such as fever, chills, and in some cases, fresh blood in the stool, the nurse should anticipate caring for a patient with diverticulitis. Diverticulitis is the inflammation of a diverticulum, which is a pouch that has formed in the wall of the colon.

48. A
Regurgitation is the raising or backing up of gastric contents to the esophagus or throat. There is an acidic sensation with or without undigested food particles. The patient will not feel sick to the stomach and will not have the forceful, involuntary spasm of the stomach as is evident in retching.

49. B
Oily or greasy stools that are frothy and floating are characteristic of steatorrhea. They are also foul-smelling. Steatorrhea is the result of undigested and unabsorbed fats.

50. B
Before examining a patient's abdomen, the nurse must put them in a supine position, with a pillow under the head and one under the knees to keep the knees slightly flexed. This position relaxes the abdominal muscles and will make the examination easier. An arched back or a stretched abdominal skin will tighten the abdominal muscles.

51. C
Ascites is the abnormal accumulation of fluid in the peritoneal cavity. It is caused by liver diseases and some kidney conditions such as nephrotic syndrome. When the ascites is large, the abdomen will appear to bulge at the sides and at the flank area, especially when seen from the foot of the bed. The umbilical area will be tympanic on percussion, and the lateral and flank area will be dull.

52. D
A nurse who is to auscultate the abdomen of a patient suspected of having intestinal obstruction should hear for bowel sounds for 5 minutes in one quadrant. The bowel sounds coming from an obstructed colon will have rushes of high-pitched sounds. If there is a complete obstruction, no bowel sounds will be heard below the obstruction.

53. A
The hooking technique is useful when tracing the liver edge, especially in obese patients. To do the hooking technique, the nurse places both hands side by side below the liver dullness and presses with their fingers in and up toward the costal margin. The nurse asks the patient to take a deep breath. At this time, the liver edge becomes palpable.

54. A
To elicit the psoas sign, the nurse places one hand above the patient's right knee to act as resistance and then tells the patient to raise that thigh against the hand. Alternatively, the nurse can turn the patient to their left and extend the patient's legs at the hip. There is positive psoas

sign when pain is worsened or felt in the abdomen.

55. C

Hepatitis A is transmitted through the fecal-oral route. It is contracted by ingesting contaminated food and water. The nurse should teach the patient how to perform thorough handwashing to prevent contracting the disease. Furthermore, the nurse should teach the patient to avoid eating raw or undercooked food, especially seafood.

56. A

The strongest risk factors for colorectal cancer are increasing age, personal history of colorectal malignancy, polyps or inflammatory bowel conditions and having a family history of colorectal neoplastic growth in the immediate family up to the first-degree.

57. A

Pelvic muscle exercises strengthen the pelvic floor muscles which control urination and defecation. It is sometimes referred to as Kegal exercises. The patient consciously squeezes and relaxes the pelvic floor muscles much like stopping and continuing the flow of urine.

58. C

Acute pancreatitis is the autodigestion of the pancreas. Enzymes are released precociously and affect the pancreas itself, causing inflammation. The pain of acute pancreatitis is steady and epigastric, may be referred to the back or other parts of the abdomen.

59. B

When the nurse notes a distinct separation of the two rectus abdominis muscles so that the patient's abdomen has a vertical bulge in the abdomen without any other symptom, the nurse must consider diastasis recti. It is common in multiparous women, in obese individuals, and those with chronic lung disease. It is benign. It is unrelated to the lung disease. The nurse should duly document the finding.

60. A

During the examination of the abdomen, the nurse should proceed in this sequence: inspection, auscultation, percussion, palpation. Auscultation should follow inspection because percussion and especially palpation can affect the bowel sounds and will make the assessments inaccurate.

The Muskuloskeletal System

Questions

1. A nurse is doing a physical examination of the client. She asked the client who is lying supine on the examination table to move the ankles, and turn the feet inwards and then outwards. Which of the following did the nurse make the client do?
   a. Abduction and adduction
   b. Inversion and eversion
   c. Pronation and supination
   d. Retraction and protraction

2. A nurse is conducting physical examination of several clients. In which situation is lordosis non-pathologic? Select all that apply.
   a. Pregnancy
   b. Elderly
   c. Infancy
   d. Post spinal surgery
   e. Adolescence

3. A client is complaining of joint pains of the knees and the hips that is felt late in the afternoon, especially after carrying heavy items during the day. The client has no fever and there are no other significant signs and symptoms. Which of the following conditions most likely causes the client's manifestations?
   a. Rheumatoid arthritis
   b. Osteoarthritis
   c. Tendinitis
   d. Reynaud phenomenon

4. A client experiencing joint pains has been recently diagnosed with rheumatic fever. Which of the following will the nurse note in the client's history that caused the rheumatic fever?
   a. Strep throat
   b. Palpitations
   c. Constipation
   d. Intestinal infection

5. The nurse is conducting a thorough musculoskeletal assessment. She hopes to assess passive joint movements in a client. What would she ask the client do?
   a. Rotate the shoulders
   b. Kick the pillow
   c. Relax as the nurse extends the elbow
   d. Tense the muscles of the upper arm

6. The nurse is assessing range of motion (ROM). Which of the following is an abnormal finding?
   a. Hyperextension of the wrist at 70 degrees

b. Palmar flexion at 90 degrees
c. Ulnar deviation 50 degrees
d. Radial deviation 5 degrees

7. The nurse instructed a client to flex the elbows, and lift the arms 90 degrees. She then asked the client to have the backs of the hand touch each other in front at the level of the upper chest, and maintain that position for a minute. Which test did the nurse ask the client to perform?
    a. Tinel Test
    b. Rinne test
    c. Phalen test
    d. Blumberg test

8. The nurse assessing a client who is suspected to have carpal tunnel syndrome wants to know if the client is exhibiting the Tinel sign. Which of the following should the nurse perform?
    a. Ask the client to flex the elbows
    b. Percuss the median nerve
    c. Ask the client to flex and hyperextend the wrist
    d. Use forefinger and thumb to palpate for any swelling of the elbow joint

9. A nurse is reviewing the medical record of a client. She reads that the client has osteoarthritis, and has Bouchards and Haberden's nodes. To validate the entries, she will have to inspect which anatomical part of the client?
    a. Feet
    b. Elbows
    c. Hips
    d. Hands

10. A nurse assessing the spine of the client asked the client to bend and reach his toes. She notes a deformity in the lumbar area. The client tests positive for which sign?
    a. Tinel sign
    b. Phalen sign
    c. Thomas sign
    d. Murphy sign

11. A nurse working in an elderly facility wants to identify who is at risk for falls. Which tool is most appropriate to use?
    a. Functional assessment for ADLs
    b. Get Up and Go Test
    c. ROM tests
    d. Cognitive test

12. A nurse is conducting health teachings on the prevention of osteoporosis. Which of the following preventive measures should be included in her teaching plan? Select all that apply.
    a. Increase milk and milk products
    b. Avoid bearing weight
    c. Increase exposure to the sun early in the morning
    d. Quit/refrain from smoking
    e. Avoid strenuous activities

13. The nurse is trying to assess the damage to the joint of a client who experiences pain upon awaking in the morning. Accompanying symptoms are fever and lymphadenopathy. Which type of process is involved that cause the client's manifestations?
    a. Inflammatory
    b. Degenerative
    c. Resorption
    d. Trauma

14. A nurse is caring for a client with ankylosing spondylitis. Which of the following information is true regarding this condition?
    a. It is a form of osteoarthritis
    b. Chronic progressive inflammation of sacroiliac joints and the spine
    c. There is spasm of the abdominal muscles
    d. There is limited movements of the knees

15. A nurse wants to identify who among her clients is at risk for developing osteoporosis. Which of the following clients is at greatest risk for developing osteoporosis?
    a. A middle aged woman of African descent who is overweight
    b. An elderly White woman who is thin and frail
    c. A 30-year old woman who is taking oral contraceptives
    d. An elderly woman who is obese and suffering from chronic fatigue

16. A male client who fell in a football game comes to the clinic hunched and in severe pain. As the nurse attempts to abduct the shoulder, the client could not maintain the position. He tries to move the shoulder forward to compensate. Which of the following conditions is responsible for the client's manifestations?
    a. Dislocated shoulder
    b. Torn rotator cuff
    c. Joint effusion
    d. Atrophy

17. An elderly bedridden client complains of limited mobility of the shoulders over time. She said she has been having trouble reaching for things that are above her head. Recently the shoulder started to hurt. Which of the following is the client most likely experiencing?

a. Bursitis
b. Tendinitis
c. Adhesive capsulitis
d. Rheumatoid arthritis

18. A client has a swollen big toe that has grown big as a potato. The client reports severe pain even with the smallest of toe or feet movement. The area is hot to touch and is red and swollen. Which of the following conditions is the client most likely suffering from?
    a. Rheumatoid arthritis
    b. Osteoarthritis
    c. Gouty arthritis
    d. Epicondylitis

19. A client with long-standing rheumatoid arthritis has deformed hands. The proximal joints of his fingers are overstretched while the distal joints are constantly flexed. It makes fine motor movements of the hands really challenging. Which of the following terms should the nurse expect to be written on the client's record to refer to her findings? Select all that apply.
    a. Swan's neck deformity
    b. Tophi
    c. Boutonnière deformity
    d. Ulnar deviation
    e. Haberden nodes

20. A 56-year old female client who is suffering from rheumatoid arthritis is admitted to the hospital. Upon examination, which of the following assessment findings does the nurse expect to find?
    a. Asymmetric joint involvement
    b. Bouchard's nodes
    c. Obesity
    d. Small joint involvement

21. In assessing a client with osteomyelitis, the nurse expects to find which finding as indicative of the diagnosis?
    a. Warm erythematous tender skin at the site
    b. Decreased white blood cell count
    c. Negative wound culture
    d. Pale, cool, indurated lesión

22. An adult who was involved in a sports injury has a fractured right radius. His right arm has been casted. While performing assessment of this client, which of the following findings should prompt the nurse to inform the physician immediately?
    a. Pain on the right forearm
    b. Swollen fingers of the right hand

c.   Warm dry fingers on both hands
d.   Diminished capillary refill on the affected arm

23. A 55-year old male client has suffered from low back pain and sciatica for almost three years. He is admitted to the hospital for further evaluation and treatment of his condition. The nurse understands that the primary reason why assessment of the level of pain is important is that
a.   This is important for identifying people with sciatica
b.   This will serve as a baseline data for a later evaluation
c.   Clients with low back pain that radiates to an extremity are not candidates for surgery
d.   Surgery is not indicated for people in pain for less than 2 years

24. Which statement is most accurate in describing a nurse's assessment of a client with rheumatoid arthritis?
a.   Pain is best assessed by observing the client's facial expression during her interview as well as the limitation of mobility caused by the pain
b.   Vital signs are more accurate indications of the client's level and character of pain
c.   Assessment should be done on the musculoskeletal, cardiopulmonary and renal systems
d.   Physical findings are more reliable than history data

25. Which of the following assessments is critical to be performed by the nurse whose client has sustained fracture on the tibia and fibula?
a.   Palpating for skin temperature proximal to the site
b.   Observing for the degree of deformity
c.   Palpation of the dorsalis pedis pulse
d.   Cutting away clothing on the affected leg

26. The nurse is assessing a female client with midline back pain. Which of the following disorder will the nurse NOT consider as the cause of her pain?
a.   disc herniation
b.   vertebral collapse
c.   spinal cord metastases
d.   trochanteric bursitis

27. A nurse is to perform assessment on the ROM abilities of a client's elbow. The nurse prepares which instrument?
a.   Tuning fork
b.   Goniometer
c.   Reflex hammer
d.   Posture analyzer

28. A nurse is assessing a client for joint pain. The nurse notes that only one elbow joint is affected. Which of the following disorder is the LEAST probable cause of the client's joint pain?

a. Trauma
b. Septic arthritis
c. Gout
d. Rheumatoid arthritis

29. Which of the following assessment finding is true of rheumatoid arthritis?
    a. Nodes on the distal interphalangeal joint
    b. Nodes on the proximal interphalangeal joint
    c. Subcutaneous nodes
    d. Gritty node on the proximal interphalangeal joint of the index finger of the left hand

30. A nurse is assessing the range of motion of a client's wrist. The nurse asks the client to stretch the fingers from a clenched fist. Which wrist movement is the nurse assessing?
    a. Flexion
    b. Extension
    c. Adduction
    d. Abduction

31. A nurse is establishing care for a client suspected of having carpal tunnel syndrome. Which of the following history data is most critical in her having the condition?
    a. Occupation as a court transcriptionist for >10 years
    b. Repeated exposure to cold temperatures
    c. Infection with syphilis 4 years ago
    d. Repeated antibiotic use

32. A client suspected of having carpal tunnel syndrome tested positive of the Phalen's sign. What is the correct interpretation of the nurse's findings?
    a. Aching and numbness in the course of the median nerve when the area of the nerve is tapped lightly
    b. Weakness on thumb abduction
    c. Throbbing pain on thumb adduction
    d. Numbness and tingling in the median nerve distribution within 60 seconds of wrist flexion

33. Which of the following findings is consistent with scoliosis?
    a. Port-wine stains on the back
    b. Hairy patches
    c. Pelvic tilt
    d. Café-au-lait spots

34. The nurse is assessing a group of clients. Who among these clients is at most risk for having osteoporosis?
    a. A 40 year old female encoder with a BMI (body mass index) of 16

b. A 33 year old male laborer with low back pain
c. A 16 year old obese male student
d. A 25 year old marathoner complaining of calf tenderness

35. A nurse is conducting health teachings to a group of elderly women on the subject of osteoporosis. Which of the following describes a situation wherein a client most likely has low levels of 25-hydroxyvitamin D?
a. Eating meat and fish
b. Housebound in a country with little sunlight
c. Taking health supplements
d. Drinking milk

36. Which of the following client's activities/history data suggest possible cause of his sciatica?
a. Loading of sacks of potatoes on a truck using a forklift a week ago
b. Falling on his back during a soccer game last fall
c. Jogging for 2 miles everyday
d. Squatting while watching TV

37. A client was involved in a vehicular accident and reports bumping his head. A day after admission, he complains about pain and stiffness in the neck. He also has occipital headache, dizziness, malaise and fatigue. Which of the following condition is the patient most likely suffering from?
a. Herniated lumbar disc
b. Sciatica
c. Whiplash
d. Cervical nerve root compression

38. The nurse is assessing a client with neck pain. Which of the following is consistent with cervical myelopathy from cervical cord compression?
a. Torticollis
b. Hyperreflexia
c. weakness in the triceps
d. Localized paracervical tenderness

39. A client who is a star basketball player for over 10 years comes to the clinic for evaluation of his joint pains. Which of the following condition is caused by "wear and tear"?
a. Rheumatoid arthritis
b. Gouty arthritis
c. Systemic lupus erythematosus
d. Osteoarthritis

40. A patient is complaining of joint pains. The nurse wants to determine if there is a migratory pattern of joint pain. Which of the following questions would help assess if the patient's joint pains are

migratory?
a. "Is the pain any worse at a particular time of day?"
b. "Does the pain come and go in different joints?"
c. "Is the pain sharp, dull, achy, or shooting?"
d. "Does anything relieve the pain or make it worse?"

41. A patient tells the nurse that the joints of both their knees and hips are painful especially upon waking up in the morning. The nurse considers many conditions for the patient's complaint, including:
a. Septic arthritis
b. Trauma
c. Gout
d. Rheumatoid arthritis

42. A nurse is assessing the joints of a patient who told the nurse that they tripped while running down the stairs. The nurse is checking for signs of inflammation. Which of the following are signs of inflammation? Select all that apply.
a. Palpable swelling
b. Presence of a mass
c. Coolness
d. Erythema
e. Presence of a lesion

43. A nurse is assessing the calf muscles of a marathoner who came in for their annual physical checkup. The calf muscles are firm and nontender, and appear bigger than average. Which of the following change in muscle structure did the patient exhibit?
a. Dystrophy
b. Atrophy
c. Hypertrophy
d. Pseudohypertrophy

44. A patient with Parkinson's disease exhibits resistance throughout the range of joint movement, especially in flexion and extension. Which of the following correctly describes the patient's muscle tone?
a. Flaccid
b. Spastic
c. Rigid
d. Atonic

45. A nurse is assessing a patient who sustained a T3 spinal injury. The patient could not move or feel any sensation in all four extremities. Which of the following correctly describes the patient's symptom?

a. Hemiparesis
b. Hemiplegia
c. Quadriplegia
d. Paraplegia

46. A nurse assessing the patient's musculoskeletal system gives the patient's muscle strength a grade of 5. Which of the following is about the patient's muscle strength is true?
    a. A barely detectable trace of contraction
    b. Active movement of the body part with gravity eliminated
    c. Active movement against gravity
    d. Active movement against full resistance without evident fatigue

47. The nurse wants to assess the patient's shoulder movement and see if the patient has any difficulty with hyperextension. Which of the following instructions would assess the patient's shoulder hyperextension?
    a. "Raise your arms in front of you and above your head."
    b. "Raise your arms behind you."
    c. "Raise your arms out to the side."
    d. "Lower your arms to your side and bring them across your body."

48. A nurse is assessing the shoulder movements of one patient and asks the patient to place their hand behind their back and attempt to touch their shoulder blades. Which of the following shoulder movements is the nurse asking the patient to perform?
    a. Adduction
    b. Flexion
    c. External rotation
    d. Internal rotation

49. A patient who was involved in a vehicular accident sustained injuries to the shoulders. The nurse decided to test for the 'drop arm' sign to consider possible rotator cuff tear. Which of the following actions correctly elicits the 'drop arm' sign?
    a. Ask the patient to fully abduct the arm to shoulder level and slowly lower their arm
    b. Ask the patient to adduct the arm to the side
    c. Ask the patient to slightly abduct their arm to the side with their palms facing front
    d. Ask the patient to resist as their flexed forearms are pressed outward

50. A nurse is performing the painful arc test on a patient who is complaining of shoulder pain. Which of the following result is positive of subacromial impingement?
    a. Shoulder pain from 60° - 120°
    b. Shoulder pain from 100° - 180°
    c. Shoulder pain at 30°
    d. Shoulder pain at 180°

51. A nurse examining the hands of a patient with osteoarthritis notes that the patient has hard dorsolateral nodes at both the distal and proximal interphalangeal joints. Which of the following refers to the nodes found in the proximal interphalangeal joints?
    a. Haberden's nodes
    b. Bouchard's nodes
    c. Swan neck deformity
    d. Ulnar deviation

52. A patient complains to the nurse that the severe pain in their wrist and forearm could not even make them do simple things such as twisting the lids off jars. Which of the following data in the patient's history strongly suggest carpal tunnel syndrome?
    a. Cultural background: Asian
    b. Childhood diseases: juvenile rheumatoid arthritis
    c. Family history: osteoarthritis
    d. Present occupation: court typist

53. A nurse assesses for possible median nerve compression by asking the patient to press the backs of both their hands together to form right angles with the forearm. The patient felt numbness and tingling in the wrists and forearm after 10 seconds. Which of the following signs did the nurse test?
    a. Tinel sign
    b. Empty can sign
    c. Phalen sign
    d. Obturator sign

54. A nurse is assessing a pregnant patient on her 8th month of gestation. During the examination of the patient's back, the nurse notes concavity of the lumbar spine. Which of the following correctly describes the patient's spinal curvature?
    a. Lordosis
    b. Kyphosis
    c. Scoliosis
    d. Thoracic convexity

55. A nurse is assessing a patient with scoliosis and wants to see if the patient has an unequal height of the iliac crests. Which of the following will the nurse observe in a patient with uneven iliac crests?
    a. Both shoulders appear raised
    b. One arm appears shorter
    c. One shoulder is lower than the other
    d. One leg appears shorter

56. A patient tells the nurse that they feel shooting pain from the lower back, down to their hips, and along the back of the thighs, knees and lower leg. The patient claims that the day before, he helped his neighbor move out by carrying big boxes for them. Which of the following conditions would the nurse consider to be the source of the patient's pain?
    a. Cogwheel rigidity
    b. Osteoarthritis
    c. Rheumatoid arthritis
    d. Herniated lumbosacral discs

57. A nurse is testing the patient's neck movement, specifically the lateral flexion of the neck. Which of the following instructions to the patient would test for the lateral flexion of the neck?
    a. "Look up the ceiling."
    b. "Look over your right shoulder, and then your left."
    c. "Bend your neck toward your shoulder."
    d. "Bring your chin to your chest."

58. A nurse is observing a toddler with uncorrected congenital hip dislocation walk. As the toddler walks, the pelvis drops on the unaffected side. Which of the following correctly describes the patient's gait?
    a. Spastic gait
    b. Waddling gait
    c. Scissoring gait
    d. Lurching gait

59. A nurse is to perform passive range of motion exercises on several patients. With which of the following patients will the nurse will need to verify the limitations to the range of motion exercises for the hips?
    a. A patient post-pneumonia confined to bed for three days
    b. A patient recovering from an abdominal surgery
    c. An older patient who is obtunded
    d. An adult who is post-hip replacement surgery

60. A nurse is assessing a patient whose primary complaint is joint pain that is worse at night. The pain is deep and achy and is felt in the hands and knees. Upon careful examination of the knee, the nurse palpates bony ridges along the joint margins. Crepitus is noted. Which of the following conditions should the nurse consider based on the patient's manifestations?
    a. Osteoarthritis
    b. Gout
    c. Muscular dystrophy
    d. Patellofemoral syndrome

61. The nurse is testing the patient's ankle and foot movements and is asking the patient to bend their heel outward. Which movement of the foot and ankle is the nurse assessing?
    a. Ankle flexion
    b. Ankle extension
    c. Inversion
    d. Eversion

62. A nurse is conducting a health teaching regarding the recommended physical activity to keep oneself healthy. Which of the following recommendations is correct?
    a. At least 2.5 hours a week of vigorous intensity, aerobic physical activity
    b. At least 1.25 hours a week of moderate-intensity, aerobic physical activity
    c. At least 2.5 hours a week of moderate-intensity, aerobic physical activity
    d. Moderate- or high-intensity muscle strengthening activity that involves all muscle groups at least for a day in a week

63. A nurse receives the laboratory result of a patient who had undergone bone density test. Which result or bone density T score will indicate that a patient has osteoporosis?
    a. -0.1 to -0.5
    b. -0.5 to -1.0
    c. -2.5 to -1.0
    d. Less than -2.5

64. A patient is being assessed by the nurse for mechanical neck pain with aching paracervical pain and stiffness. The patient also complains of occipital headaches and vertigo. The nurse is considering whiplash as the cause of the patient's symptoms. Which of the following is the primary cause of whiplash?
    a. Forced hyperflexion-hyperextension injury to the neck
    b. Herniated cervical intervertebral disc
    c. Cervical spinal nerve dysfunction
    d. Degenerative changes of the cervical spine

ANSWERS

1. B
    Inversion is turning the feet inwards on the ankle. Eversion is turning the feet outward.

2. A, C
    Infants and women on their third trimester in pregnancy are normally lordotic. The lordosis is temporary.

3. B
    Joint pains brought about by osteoarthritis worsen later in the day or after carrying heavy things during the day. This is because the weight of the client causes the worn out joints to rub together. The more that the client ambulates, the worse the pain is.

4. A
    Rheumatic fever, which is manifested by fever and joint pains, is a sequalae of a strep throat infection.

5. C
    Passive joint movements are motions that are involuntary and that which are facilitated by the nurse or a machine. Options A and B are active movements while Option D is isometric muscle movement.

6. D
    Radial deviation should reach 20 degrees. Movements less than this means there is limited movement of the joint.

7. C
    The Phalen test is performed to check for carpal tunnel syndrome. The nurse asks the client to flex the elbows, and lift the arms 90 degrees. Then she instructs the client to have the backs of the hand touch each other in front at the level of the upper chest, and to maintain that position for a minute. When numbness, tingling or pain is noted while in this position, the client has carpal tunnel syndrome.

8. B
    The Tinel sign is elicited by percussing the median nerve by the wrist. With carpal tunnel syndrome, there is tingling or burning pain along the distribution of the nerve.

9. D
    Bouchard and Haberden nodes are bony lumps on the interphalengeal joints of the hands. They are manifestations of osteoarthritis.

10. C

The Thomas sign is the deformity of the lumbar spine that becomes evident when the hips are flexed.

11. B

Get Up and Go test identifies elderlies who are at risk for falls. It measures time it takes for a client to complete a task, such as rising from a chair and walking 10 feet.

12. A, C, D

To prevent osteoporosis, the clients should be advised to increase calcium and Vitamin D intake, perform exercises especially weight bearing exercises and avoiding smoking and drinking.

13. A

The signs and symptoms manifested by the client is rheumatoid arthritis wherein synovial tissues are inflamed and painful. Rheumatoid arthritis is an inflammatory disease.

14. B

Ankylosing spondylitis is the swelling and fusion of sacroiliac joints of the spine. It is a form of rheumatoid arthritis and is chronic and progressive. There is a spasm of the paraspinal muscles.

15. B

Osteoporosis is caused by bone resorption more than absorption that leads to low bone mineral density. It is more prevalent among White females, those thin and frail in built. It is also brought about by early menopause, lack of weight bearing exercise and low estrogen levels in women.

16. B

The manifestations of the client indicate torn rotator cuff. It is caused by forceful adduction while the arm is in abduction.

17. C

Frozen shoulder or adhesive capsulitis is a progressive limitation of shoulder movement caused by prolonged immobility. The client will have limitations in abduction, external rotation of the shoulder so that the client will have difficulty reaching for things above her.

18. C

Gouty arthritis is the result of too much uric acid in the blood. The big toe is usually affected. Elbows and knees sometimes manifest too. The toe is extremely swollen, red, and painful to touch.

19. A, C

Swan's neck deformity is the hyperextension of the proximal interphalengeal joints, and Boutonniere deformity is the flexion of the distal interphalengeal joints. They are both evident in rheumatoid arthritis.

20. D

   In rheumatoid arthritis, the small joints of the hands, feet, wrists and ankles are often involved. All other options suggest osteoarthritis.

21. A

   Infections that involve skin and bones would produce warm, erythematous and tender skin on the infected area. The wound culture turns positive to identify the causative microorganism. White blood cell count also increases.

22. D

   Diminished capillary refill suggests perfusion problems. This should be reported to the physician. The cast may need to be readjusted.

23. B

   The importance of an accurate history cannot be overemphasized in assessing the character and location of the pain. A baseline data of assessment findings should be well established to help in evaluating if the client's condition has improved after treatment.

24. C

   Rheumatoid arthritis is an autoimmune disease with multi-system involvement. Other than the musculoskeletal systems, cardiopulmonary and renal systems should also be assessed because of extra-articular manifestations and nephrotoxicity of medications for rheumatoid arthritis.

25. C

   Neurovascular compromise can become apparent with fracture. Distal pulses should be assessed to ensure that there is adequate perfusion in the area. The dorsalis pedis pulses of both feet should be assessed for comparison.

26. D

   Musculoligamentous injury, disc herniation, collapse of the spine, spinal cord metastases, or even epidural abscess can cause midline back pain. On the other hand, pain off the midline, suggests sacroiliitis, trochanteric bursitis, sciatica, or hip arthritis.

27. B

   A goniometer is a device used to measure the range of motion around a joint in the body.

28. D

   Acute involvement of only one joint suggests trauma, septic arthritis or gout. Rheumatoid arthritis usually involves several joints symmetrically.

29. C

Subcutaneous nodules are noted in rheumatoid arthritis. Nodules on the interphalangeal (IP) joints of the hands called Heberden (distal IP) and Bouchard (proximal IP) are observed in osteoarthritis. Gritty nodules in a joint are indicative of uric acid crystals that are apparent in gout.

30. B

Extension is a movement that increases the angle between two body parts. Stretching the fingers from a clenched fist assesses extension.

31. A

Carpal tunnel syndrome is usually brought about by repetitive wrist motion (e.g. typing). It can also be triggered by pregnancy, rheumatoid arthritis, diabetes and hypothyroidism.

32. D

The nurse elicits the Phalen's sign by asking the client to hold the wrist in flexion for 60 seconds or by asking the patient to press the backs of both hands together to form right angles. Numbness and tingling in the median nerve distribution within 60 seconds is a positive test.

33. C

Scoliosis is the abnormal curvature of the spine. Unequal heights of the iliac crests, or pelvic tilt, suggest unequal lengths of the legs and disappear when a block is placed under the short leg and foot. Scoliosis, and hip abduction / adduction cause a pelvic tilt.

34. A

Advancing age and being underweight are risk factors for having osteoporosis. Other risk factors for osteoporosis are: Postmenopausal status in white and Asian women, family history of fracture in a first-degree relative, history of fracture, excessive alcohol intake, delayed menarche or early menopause, smoking, low vitamin D levels, chronic use of corticosteroids, inflammatory disorders of the musculoskeletal, pulmonary, or gastrointestinal systems, including gluten senstivity, chronic renal disease, organ transplantation, hypogonadism, anorexia nervosa, and sedentary lifestyle or extended bed rest.

35. B

Exposing bare skin to sunlight is one of the best ways to acquiring vitamin D. Vitamin D is needed by the body to absorb calcium, a mineral that is deficient in osteoporosis. Low sun exposure predisposes to Vitamin D deficiency.

36. B

Sciatic pain is very sensitive and specific for disc herniation, particularly from herniated intervertebral disc with compression or traction of nerve root(s). Trauma to the lower spine and carrying heavy loads are causes of disc herniation.

37. C

Whiplash is a mechanical neck pain with aching paracervical pain and stiffness, often beginning the day after a hyperextension-hyperflexion type of head injury. The client reports occipital headache, dizziness, malaise and fatigue.

38. B

Patients with cervical myelopathy exhibits hyperreflexia (e.g. clonus at the wrist, knee, or ankle). They also have gait disturbances the Babinski reflex.

39. D

Osteoarthritis is caused by degeneration and progressive loss of cartilage within the joints, damage to underlying bone, and osseous formations at the margins of the cartilage. It is sometimes referred to as a consequence of "wear and tear" and of overuse of weight-bearing joints.

40. B

Migratory joint pain refers to pain that spreads or transfers from one joint to another. It is a usual finding in people with rheumatic fever.

41. D

The joint pain in rheumatoid arthritis is usually symmetrical and involves more than one joint. The joint pain in septic arthritis, trauma, and gout are typically unilateral or felt only on one side.

42. A, D

Signs of joint inflammation include palpable swelling, warmth, tenderness, and erythema. The swelling may involve the synovial membrane, bursae, tendons, and tendon sheath. It may also be caused by effusion within the joint space.

43. C

Hypertrophy of muscles is usually evident in athletes who constantly condition their muscles. The muscles grow and increase in size so that the muscles look bulky. The increase in bulk is accompanied by an increase in strength.

44. C

Muscle rigidity is the presence of resistance to joint flexion and extension or any range of motion. Muscle rigidity is evident in conditions such as Parkinson's disease and it is a manifestation of extrapyramidal tract lesion or impairment.

45. C

If paralysis is evident in all four extremities, it is known as quadriplegia. If it is seen on one side of the body, it is hemiplegia. Paralysis of both legs is known as paraplegia. Hemiparesis is the weakness on one side of the body.

46. D

A grade of 5 in the scale for grading muscle strength means that the patient exhibits an active movement of the muscle against full resistance without evident fatigue. This suggests normal muscle strength.

47. B

To test for the patient's shoulder hyperextension, the nurse instructs the patient to raise their arms behind them. Flexion of the shoulders can be demonstrated by flexing of the arms in front and above the head. Abduction is raising the arms out to the side and overhead, and adduction is bringing the arms back to the side and down in front.

48. D

To assess for the internal rotation movement of the shoulder, the nurse instructs the patient to place one hand behind their back and try to touch their shoulder blades. In this movement, the subscapularis, anterior deltoid, pectoralis major, teres major, and latissimus dorsi muscles are contracting.

49. A

To perform the 'drop arm' sign, the nurse asks the patient to fully abduct the arm to shoulder so that it is forming 90° with the body. The nurse then asks the patient to lower their arm slowly. If a patient could not hold the arm when it is fully abducted at 90°, then the nurse considers rotator cuff tear or bicipital tendenitis.

50. A

The painful arc test is performed by having the patient fully abduct their arms starting from their side up to 180° or until their arm is almost touching their ear. When pain is present when the arms are abducted at 60° - 120°, it is a positive sign for subacromial impingement.

51. B

A patient with osteoarthritis will possibly also have hard dorsolateral nodes on the proximal interphalangeal joints, called Bouchard nodes, and on the distal interphalangeal joints, called Heberden nodes.

52. D

Carpal tunnel syndrome is caused by the compression of the median nerve due to repetitive wrist motion. Examples of these repetitive wrist movements are typing, stamping, and pressing with the fingers. The patient feels pain in the wrist and the forearm.

53. C

The Phalen sign is a test for median nerve compression. The nurse asks the patient to flex their wrists and hold it in that position for one full minute. Alternatively, the patient may press the backs of both hands together to form right angles with the forearms. The test is positive if the patient feels numbness and tingling along the median nerve distribution within 60 seconds of the test.

54. A

Lordosis is the concavity of the lumbar spine. Women who are in their third trimester would have a lordotic posture to maintain their balance as the fetus grows in utero.

55. D

Lumbar scoliosis is the lateral curvature of the lower back. A patient with lumbar scoliosis will have uneven iliac crest height. The hips are uneven, with one side appearing higher, and one leg shorter.

56. D

Intervertebral disc herniation from L5-S1 or L4-L5 cause swelling of the spinous processes, the intervertebral joints, paravertebral muscles, the sacrosciatic notch and the sciatic nerve. The pain felt from the lower back until the back of the lower leg is called sciatica, which is caused by the compression of the sciatic nerve.

57. C

To check for the lateral flexion of the neck, the nurse asks the patient to bend their neck toward one shoulder or to bring their ear to their shoulder.

58. B

Patients with congenital hip dislocation will have a waddling gait because one hip is lower than the other. Waddling gait is also evident in muscular dystrophy and spinal muscle atrophy diseases.

59. D

Patients who had just undergone hip replacement surgeries will have their hip range of motions limited to prevent dislocation of the prosthesis. In the patient who had posterior approach hip replacement, for example, no hip flexion beyond 90°, internal rotation or adduction beyond neutral is allowed.

60. A

The musculoskeletal signs and symptoms of osteoarthritis are numerous. In osteoarthritis, the joint pains are asymmetrical, and they are felt in the hands, hips, and knees. The pain is described as deep and achy. Since osteoarthritis is a result of a 'wear and tear' process, the pain is worst at night after prolonged joint use. Bony ridges and crepitus felt during palpation are also common findings.

61. D

Asking the patient to bend their heel outward so that the sole is turned outward is a test for eversion.

62. C

The current recommendation for physical activity for health maintenance is at least 2.5 hours a week of moderate-intensity, or 1 hour and 15 minutes of vigorous intensity a week of aerobic physical activity. Alternatively, moderate- or high-intensity muscle strengthening activity that involves all muscle groups for at least for two days in a week can also be performed.

63. D

Osteoporosis is a condition wherein the bones become porous, weak and fragile due to demineralization. A bone density T score of less than -2.5 indicates osteoporosis. A score of -2.5 to -1.0 indicates osteopenia, a less severe bone density loss than osteoporosis.

64. A

Whiplash is the sprain or strain of muscles and ligaments of the neck due to forced and sudden hyperflexion and hyperextension of the neck. Whiplash can be caused by rear-end collisions. The mechanical neck pain in whiplash is aching and paracervical with stiffness.

The Nervous System

Questions

1. A client sustained trauma to the head. During recovery, he started having difficulty speaking. He finds that he can understand written and spoken language but cannot make himself speak. He mumbles incomprehensible words. In which area of the brain did the client most likely sustained injury?
    a. Occipital lobe
    b. Parietal lobe
    c. Wenicke's area
    d. Broca's area

2. The nurse is caring for a client who underwent brain surgery. Soon after, he has been exhibiting signs and symptoms of hypothalamic dysfunction. Which of the following is a manifestation of damage to the hypothalamus?
    a. Paralysis of the lower extremities
    b. Expressive aphasia
    c. Altered thermoregulation
    d. Equilibrium

3. A nurse is preparing different samples of food with varying tastes. She then asked the client to taste each sample. She later instructed the client to frown, smile, close the eyes, and move the lips and mouth. She also checked saliva and tear production. Which cranial nerve is the nurse assessing?
    a. V
    b. VI
    c. VII
    d. VIII

4. The nurse is preparing to be assigned in a nursing home and is reviewing her concepts of age-related changes in the nervous system. Which of the following is not considered an age-related change in the nervous system?
    a. Waxing and waning of respiration
    b. Decreased muscle strength
    c. Slow reaction time
    d. Decreased pupillary reflexes

5. A nurse is caring for a client with seizure. She wants to know if the client is experiencing an aura prior to an episode. Which of the following is the most appropriate to ask the client to assess for aura?
    a. "Do you feel numbness anywhere when you are having a seizure?"
    b. "Do you have any warning signs before experiencing a seizure?"
    c. "Do you feel any lightheadedness before having a seizure?"
    d. "Are you having palpitations prior to having a seizure?"

6. A client with multiple sclerosis has dysmetria. In which of the following activities will the client have difficulty performing?
   a. Climbing up and down the stairs
   b. Remembering
   c. Hearing
   d. Equilibrium

7. The nurse is testing the olfactory nerve of a client. Which of the following activity will the client most likely perform?
   a. Read
   b. Sniff
   c. Walk
   d. Talk

8. The nurse asked a client to turn his face against resistance from the hand of the nurse on his face. Which cranial nerve is the nurse assessing?
   a. Vagus
   b. Acoustic
   c. Glossopharyngeal
   d. Spinal accessory

9. A nurse is observing a client with cerebellar disease pouring water from a bottle. It has taken him 5 minutes to take the bottle and open it, dropping it twice in the attempt. He spilled half the contents of the bottle on the table. The entire process of pouring his water and drinking it took 10 minutes. Which of the following accurately describes the client's manifestation?
   a. Tardive dyskinesia
   b. Resting tremor
   c. Dysdiadochokinesia
   d. Dysmetria

10. A nurse has asked a client to perform the Romberg test. The nurse found the client 'positive'. Which of the following is a correct interpretation of the nurse's finding?
    a. The client lost his balance, and fell from a standing position
    b. The client lost his balance, and fell from a sitting position
    c. The client's arm drifted down
    d. The client slightly swayed from a standing position

11. A nurse is testing the client's pain sensation. As the nurse performs the pinprick test, the client retracted the arm pricked and yelled "Ouch! That really hurt!" based on the client's reaction, which of the following should the nurse include in her documentation?
    a. Hypoalgesia
    b. Analgesia

c. Hyperalgesia
d. Amnesia

12. The nurse asks a client who recently had a stroke to close his eyes and then touch several objects, namely a coin, a key, a smartphone, a pen, and a book. The client was unable to identify the objects. But when asked to identify the same items with his eyes open, he had no difficulties doing so. Which of the following is the client most likely exhibiting?
    a. agnosia
    b. stereognosis
    c. aphasia
    d. astereognosis

13. A nurse asked a client to sit comfortably in a chair and to close his eyes. The nurse passively moves the client's forefingers and points the fingers in several directions. The nurse asks the client to identify the directions to which his finger is pointing. Which parameter did the nurse test?
    a. stereognosis
    b. Position (kinesthesia)
    c. vibration
    d. Tactile discrimination

14. A nurse is concerned that a 4-mopnth old infant is developing meningitis. She is running a fever and assumes a position wherein the head and the spine are arched. She encounters resistance as she attempts to flex the neck of the baby. Which of the following describes the client's positioning?
    a. Frog position
    b. Opisthotonos
    c. Decorticate positioning
    d. Decerebrate positioning

15. The nurse is assessing a 4-month old infant. She holds the infant in the air with the infant resting prone on the nurse's arm and hand. Which reflex is the nurse testing?
    a. Moro
    b. Landau
    c. Babinski
    d. Tonic neck

16. The nurse is aware that the aging adult undergoes several changes to the nervous system. Which of the following is NOT an age-related change?
    a. Loss of vibration at the heel
    b. Difficulty performing alternating movements
    c. There is slight scissoring gait
    d. Gait is slow and more deliberate

17. A nurse is interviewing an elderly client. She noticed that in the course of the interview, the client suddenly seemed confused. The nurse also noticed that the eyelids, and one side of the face are not congruent with the other side that reacts normally. The client is also not using one hand for gestures. Which of the following should the nurse perform next?
    a. Immediately inform the physician
    b. Document findings promptly
    c. Provide rest periods
    d. Perform further assessments

18. People with Alzheimer's disease experience several neurologic dysfunctions. Which of the following is an example of abstract failing?
    a. Forgetting where things are placed
    b. Forgetting purpose of why they entered a room
    c. Being given a number code for a safe and forgetting what those numbers are for
    d. Putting on summer clothes during winter

19. A nurse is interviewing a client. As the interview progresses, the nurse notices that the client is repeatedly winking his eyes, and is simultaneously moving his head swiftly to the side. Which of the following correctly describes the client's manifestations?
    a. Tic
    b. Clonus
    c. Athetosis
    d. Chorea

20. A client with multiple sclerosis complains that he is having difficulty making a cup of coffee. He keeps dropping his mugs and spilling water and sugar because of hand tremors. Which of the following accurately describes the client's condition?
    a. Resting tremor
    b. Intention tremor
    c. Athetosis
    d. Chorea

21. A client was admitted after a vehicular accident. The doctor finds him in a comatose state. Which Glasgow coma scale is indicative of coma?
    a. 0
    b. 2
    c. 6
    d. 10

22. A nurse is examining an unconscious client for painful stimuli. The client responded with decorticate rigidity. Which statement best describes this posturing?
    a. Flexion of the upper and lower limbs into a fetal-like position
    b. Plantar flexion with rigid extension of upper and lower limbs
    c. Flaccidity of extremities with neck hyperextension
    d. Flexion of the upper extremities, extension of the lower extremities and plantar flexion

23. The nurse is assessing the optic nerve of a client. Which of the following procedures tests the CN II?
    a. Inspecting pupil's reaction to light
    b. Observing for extraocular movements
    c. Using a Snellen chart
    d. Testing the corneal reflex

24. A nurse is scoring a patient's level of consciousness using the Glasgow coma scale. She obtains the following results: best eye opening 3, best motor response 6, best verbal response 4. Which of the following is the best interpretation of her findings?
    a. Opens eye to speech, obeys verbal commands, and is confused
    b. Opens eye to pain, decorticates to pain and does not speak
    c. Opens eye to pain, no motor response and the speech is inappropriate
    d. There is spontaneous eye opening, obeys verbal commands and is oriented

25. A client who was in a car accident is rushed to the emergency department. The nurse is assessing hypothalamic functions. Which of the following are parameters for assessing hypothalamic functions?
    a. Temperature and urine output
    b. Blood pressure and intracranial pressure
    c. Respiratory rate and pupillary responses
    d. Verbal response and eye opening

26. The nurse is assessing a client who, when asked to extend his legs, reports pain. His temperature reads 103 F. Upon examination, the nurse attempts to flex the neck. In response, the client also flexes the hip and knee. Based on these findings, the nurse suspects which condition?
    a. Meningitis
    b. Brain tumor
    c. Multiple sclerosis
    d. Epilepsy

27. A nurse is assessing the cranial nerves of a male client. In assessing CN VI, the nurse asks the client to perform which movement?
    a. Chewing motion
    b. Looking left and right

c. Blinking the eyes

d. Smelling a wisp of cotton

28. A 54-year old female client reports frequent bouts of fatigue that worsens when she moves and improves when she rests. Which of the following conditions is the most probable cause of her fatigue?

a. Multiple sclerosis

b. Parkinson's disease

c. Transient ischemic attack

d. Myasthenia gravis

29. During a routine assessment, the nurse asks the client to stand upright with the eyes closed for about half a minute while the arms are outstretched and the palms facing upward. The nurse is testing the client for

a. Romberg sign

b. Pronator drift

c. Intentional tremor

d. Resting tremor

30. A nurse asks a client to close his eyes and identify a fairly common object by feeling it. The client fails to identify the object. The nurse documents this as

a. Anosmia

b. Ageusia

c. Ataxia

d. Astereognosis

31. A nurse in the outpatient department is examining a client's deep tendon reflexes. When the nurse strikes the patellar tendon, the nurse was able to elicit very minimal response. What is the most appropriate grade to assign to the client's deep tendon reflexes?

a. 4+

b. 3+

c. 2+

d. 1+

32. A client has been brought to the hospital after being arrested for driving under the influence of alcohol. His blood test shows high levels of alcohol in his system. The nurse is assessing the planter reflex and observes that as she draws an imaginary line from the heel moving up toward the small toe to the ball of the foot, the big toe dorsiflexes and the other toes fan out. The nurse document this finding as

a. Clonus

b. Babinski

c.   Chorea
d.   Downward contraction

33. A nurse is assigned to care for clients in the intensive care unit. During her rounds, she was unable to rouse a client using a shaking motion. The nurse then tries to roll a pencil across a nail bed. Still there was no response. What is the client's level of consciousness based on the nurse's findings?
a.   Lethargic
b.   Stuporous
c.   Obtunded
d.   Comatose

34. A client met an accident while working at a local factory. Upon admission, the nurse finds that the client only opens his eyes when talked to. When asked about the accident, he couldn't give a straight forward answer and seemed not to remember the accident. He lies in a fetal position and protects his injured side. What is the most accurate Glasgow coma score for this patient?
a.   7
b.   10
c.   12
d.   15

35. A nurse is teaching a group of hypertensive clients about the critical warning signs of stroke. Which of the following client responses indicate a need for further teaching?
a.   "I will report any sudden headaches that I feel"
b.   "I will tell my wife immediately if I have any trouble seeing with one or both eyes."
c.   "I will take a rest when I feel suddenly weak."
d.   "I will call the clinic if I feel numbness in my arm."

36. A 13-year old female student reports to the nurse that she often feels dizzy. When assessed further, the client states that it happens when she suddenly stands up from a sitting or squatting position. She also states that she does not lose consciousness. Based on the client's reports, the nurse suspects that the girl has
a.   Vasovagal Syncope
b.   Postural (orthostatic) Hypotension
c.   Drop attacks
d.   Cough syncope

37. A mother confides to a nurse that his 20-year old son has 'strange' activities that the client cannot remember happening. Upon further questioning, the mother states that for about a minute or so, the client unbuttons his shirt without any regard to time and place. She notices that those 'moments' happen after the client sees glaring lights. The nurse considers seizure to be a probable explanation. Which type of seizure is the nurse referring to?
a.   Simple partial

b. Complex partial
c. Grand mal
d. Absence

38. A client has been recently diagnosed with grand mal seizures. Which of the following items on the client's bed side table should be questioned?
   a. Pen light
   b. Tongue depressor
   c. Elbow pads
   d. Extra pillows

39. A nurse is assessing a group of clients with tremors. Which of the following clients reports worsening of intentional tremors?
   a. "Yesterday I dropped my mug twice. Today I dropped it thrice."
   b. "My legs seem more rigid when I walk"
   c. "My pill-rolling movements seem longer when I am at rest."
   d. "I can't control my jerky trunk twisting."

40. A nurse from an earlier shift endorses a client with athetoid movements. Which of the following best describes athetosis?
   a. brief, rapid, jerky, irregular, and unpredictable; occurs at rest or interrupt normal coordinated movements
   b. brief, repetitive, stereotyped, coordinated movements occurring at irregular intervals
   c. Grotesque, twisted postures of the neck or trunk
   d. Slow, twisting and writhing movements; common in cerebral palsy

41. The nurse wants to assess the lateral deviation of the patient's eye. Which cranial nerve test should the nurse perform?
   a. Cranial nerve I
   b. Cranial nerve IV
   c. Cranial nerve VI
   d. Cranial nerve VII

42. The nurse is using the OLD CART mnemonic to assess for the patient's weakness. According to the patient, the weakness started in the legs two days ago, and it is has spread up the knees and thighs as well. The patient's history reveals that the patient had a viral infection the week before. Which of the following should the nurse consider as the cause of the patient's symptom?
   a. Guillain-Barre syndrome
   b. Transient ischemic attack
   c. Myasthenia gravis
   d. Stroke

43. A patient tells the nurse that they feel weak. Which of the following questions will help assess for proximal weakness?
    a. "Do you have difficulty getting out of a chair?"
    b. "Do you experience difficulty opening jar lids?"
    c. "Do you drop the things that you are holding?
    d. "Are you constantly tripping?"

44. A female patient was rushed to the clinic by relatives who later said that the patient fainted after receiving news of her husband's death. After further assessment, the nurse strongly considers that the patient experienced vasovagal syncope. Which of the following factors supports the nurse's analysis?
    a. Sudden onset of loss of consciousness
    b. Onset of seizures while without consciousness
    c. Prodromal symptoms of nausea, diaphoresis, and pallor prior to the loss of consciousness
    d. Sudden change of position from standing to a sitting position

45. A patient was rushed to the emergency room after experiencing an acute symptomatic seizure. Which of the following in the patient's history strongly suggest the cause of the patient's seizures?
    a. Viral gastroenteritis two months ago
    b. Chronic alcoholism
    c. Congenital heart disease
    d. Waddling gait

46. A patient has been recently diagnosed with Parkinson disease. The nurse makes a follow-up assessment. Which of the following characteristics of the patient's tremor will the nurse most likely observe in the patient? Select all that apply.
    a. Unilateral
    b. Low frequency
    c. High frequency
    d. Appears when at rest
    e. Coarse

47. The nurse is testing the patient's pupillary reaction to light. The patient's anisocoria worsens in the light. Which of the following is the correct interpretation of the nurse's finding?
    a. The large pupil has an abnormal pupillary constriction
    b. The small pupil has an abnormal pupillary dilation
    c. The patient is legally blind
    d. The patient is blind in one eye

48. The nurse is asking the patient to raise their brows, frown, tightly close the eyes, smile with the teeth showing and not, and to puff out the cheeks. Which cranial nerve is the nurse assessing?
    a. Trigeminal nerve

b. Vagus nerve
c. Facial nerve
d. Spinal accessory

49. Which of the following can the nurse instruct the patient to do to assess for coordination?
    a. Bend over
    b. Walk
    c. Blink
    d. Clench both fists

50. A patient recently diagnosed with multiple sclerosis exhibits intentional tremors. Which of the following most probably triggered the patient's tremors?
    a. Reaching inside the refrigerator to get milk
    b. Resting in a chair
    c. Dangling the feet by the side of the bed
    d. Leaning forward on an overbed table

51. The nurse is performing the Romberg test on a patient. Which of the following steps is INCORRECT?
    a. Ask the patient to stand with the feet together
    b. Close both eyes for 30-60 seconds without support
    c. The nurse stands behind the patient and supports the patient's back with their extended arms
    d. Observe if the patient can maintain balance and posture

52. A nurse is assessing a patient with diabetes for sensory deficits. The nurse notes that the patient could not feel any pain, heat, or tactile sensation in both their feet. The patient has which kind of sensory deficit?
    a. Symmetrical proximal sensory loss.
    b. Unilateral distal sensory loss
    c. Hemisensory loss
    d. Symmetrical distal sensory loss

53. A nurse instructs the patient to close their eyes and then asks the patient to identify the object placed on their hands. Out of 5 different objects, the patient was not able to identify any. Which of the following accurately describes the patient's manifestation?
    a. Hyperaesthesia
    b. Astereognosis
    c. Analgesia
    d. Graphesthesia

54. A nurse tests a patient's deep tendon reflexes and gives it a grade of 4+. Which of the following associated manifestation will the nurse most likely observe in the patient who has 4+ deep

tendon reflexes?
a. Diplopia
b. Flaccidity
c. Resting tremor
d. Spasticity

55. The nurse is to test the presence of ankle clonus on a patient with a CNS disorder. The nurse supports the patient's knees and maintains it in a slightly flexed position. In quick succession, the nurse dorsiflexes and plantarflexes the foot and then keeps it dorsiflexed. Which of the following when observed in the patient indicates that the patient has ankle clonus?
a. The ankle becomes rigid
b. The ankle recoils and remains plantar-flexed
c. The ankle remains dorsiflexed
d. The ankle dorsiflexes and plantar flexes rhythmically several times

56. A nurse is caring for a comatose patient who sustained an injury to the head in a vehicular accident. Which of the following nursing actions indicates that the nurse needs further teaching in the care of comatose patients?
a. The nurse takes the blood pressure measurement on the arm without an IV line
b. The nurse flexes the neck of the patient to put a pillow under the patient's head
c. The nurse tests the patient's pupillary reactions to light
d. The nurse tests the patient's deep tendon reflexes

57. A nurse is doing a neurologic assessment using a Glasgow Coma Scale. The patient opens their eyes to some painful stimuli and exhibits an extension motor response. They can also be heard groaning a few times. Which of the following is the patient's Glasgow Coma Score?
a. 3
b. 6
c. 9
d. 12

58. A patient presents to the emergency room with a high-grade fever. As the nurse performs further assessments, the patient shows signs of meningeal irritation. The nurse attempts to flex the patient's neck. In response, the patient's hips and knees also flex. Which of the following sign did the patient exhibit?
a. Nuchal rigidity
b. Brudzinski sign
c. Kernig sign
d. Battle sign

59. A patient had a transient ischemic attack (TIA) a few hours back. Which of the following is the current recommendation to determine the possibility of stroke in patients who had TIA?
    a. Neurodiagnostic imaging within 24 hours of a TIA
    b. Nothing by mouth for 24 hours
    c. Low-dose acetaminophen within 24 hours
    d. No blood tests within 24 hours

60. A nurse is assessing a 55-year old female patient's risk for stroke. Which of the following, if noted in the patient's history indicates a risk for stroke?
    a. Gestational diabetes
    b. Childhood asthma
    c. Use of aspirin
    d. Sedentary lifestyle

61. A nurse is caring for several patients in the ward. The nurse observes that in one older patient, their smile has suddenly become uneven, and one side of the face is drooping. The patient also tells the nurse that they could not feel their arms on one side only at that moment. Which of the following is the best action to do next?
    a. Wait for 30 minutes and reassess the patient
    b. Administer a dose of aspirin
    c. Inform the physician immediately
    d. Document findings

62. A nurse is conducting a neurological assessment in a patient. The nurse observes that there is more fatigability than weakness in the patient's extremities, specifically when the skeletal muscles are used. The patient's deep tendon reflexes are normal. They also observe that it is hard to recover from the fatigue. Which of the following describes the patient's condition?
    a. Polio
    b. Myasthenia Gravis
    c. Herniated cervical disc
    d. Muscular dystrophy

63. An older patient exhibits weakness on one side of the face and the body. The patient also exhibited aphasia and was later given a diagnosis of stroke. Based on the patient's manifestations, which vascular territory in the brain was affected by stroke?
    a. Subcortical circulation
    b. Posterior circulation -posterior cerebral artery
    c. Posterior circulation -brainstem
    d. Anterior circulation -middle cerebral artery

64. A patient with Parkinson disease has difficulty speaking because of the loss of muscular control that produces speech. The patient can still produce sounds nasally, and they speak with a slur.

The patient has no difficulty comprehending language. Which of the following refers the patient's manifestation?

a. Dysarthria
b. Aphonia
c. Broca aphasia
d. Wernicke aphasia

65. A nurse is observing a patient walk. As the patient steps to move forward, the patient lifts the foot high and slaps them on the floor, like seemingly walking up the stairs. Which type of gait does the patient have?

a. Cerebellar ataxia
b. Scissoring gate
c. Steppage gait
d. Waddling gait

ANSWERS

1. D
    Damage to the dominant part of the Broca's area will result to expressive aphasia. A client with expressive aphasia will have difficulty producing speech and would only make garbled sounds. However, the client can understand spoken and written language.

2. C
    The hypothalamus regulates temperature, appetite, libido, heart rate and BP. It is also the sleep center of the brain. It regulates anterior and posterior pituitary hormones and is responsible for stress responses and for coordination of autonomic functions

3. C
    The facial nerve or CN VII is responsible for the sensory function of taste in the anterior two-thirds of the tongue. It is also responsible for motor movements of the facial muscles, eyes, lips and mouth, as well as for saliva and tears production.

4. A
    Waxing and waning of respiration is called Cheyne-Stokes respiration, and is apparent in neurologic disorders and decompensated heart failure. It is not a normal age-related change. All other options are expected changes in the elderly.

5. B
    An aura is a sensory experience before a seizure. It can be something that is seen, heard or smelled. It can also be a motor activity.

6. A
    Dysmetria is over- or undershooting with the intended position of the arm, leg and eye because of loss of control of speed and distance. A client with dysmetria will have difficulty climbing stairs.

7. B
    The olfactory nerve is responsible for the sense of smell. The patient will be sniffing different kind of scents.

8. D
    The spinal accessory nerve or CN XI assesses for motor function of the trapezius and sternocleidomastoid muscles. Asking the client to turn his face against resistance from the hand of the nurse on his face assesses this nerve.

9. C
    A client with Dysdiadochokinesia will have slow uncoordinated movements. He will be clumsy and sloppy. It is a manifestation of cerebellar dysfunction.

10. A

The Romberg test is performed by asking the client to stand erect with arms on the side, and feet together. The client then has to close his eyes and maintain his position for 20 seconds. A normal person will sway slightly but will not lose his balance and fall. If a person loses his balance, he tests 'positive'.

11. C

The client exhibited increased pain sensation, or hyperalgesia. Hypoalgesia is decreased pain sensation. Analgesia is absence of pain. Amnesia is loss of memory.

12. D

Astereognosis is the inability to recognize objects by touching without visual clues. Stereognosis is the ability to recognize objects by touching without visual clues. Agnosia is inability to interpret sensory stimuli or inability to recognize familiar objects.

13. B

To test for position or kinesthesia, the nurse asks the client to close his eyes, and then she passively moves the client's toes or fingers to point in a certain direction. She then asks the client to identify to which direction his finger or toe is pointing.

14. B

Opisthotonus happens when there is meningeal irritation or damage to the brainstem. The client assumes a hyperextended position, of the neck and spine and the neck is stiff and resistant to flexion. The extremities are also extended.

15. B

The Laundau reflex can be assessed from 3 months of age and onwards until about 18 months. The nurse holds the baby prone in the air. The baby will normally arch the back, slightly flex the knees and lift the head.

16. C

Scissoring gait is characteristic of Parkinson's disease and is pathologic.

17. A

The client is exhibiting signs and symptoms of stroke, and the physician should be informed immediately. The call for help should not be delayed because this is a life-threatening situation and will have serious consequences if left untreated.

18. C

Abstract failing is having difficulty performing abstract thinking. An example of this is forgetting what numbers are for.

19. A

Tics are involuntary and repetitive movement of a muscle group usually of the muscles of the face and upper body. The muscles appear to be twitching. Examples of tics are repetitive winking, grimacing and head movements.

20. B

Intention tremors are triggered by purposeful movements, such as making coffee. The client will have difficulty finishing purposeful tasks because of tremors. This is associated with multiple sclerosis and cerebellar disease.

21. C

A score of 7 or less defines coma. The lowest score is 3 indicating deep coma. 15 is the perfect score.

22. D

Decortitate rigidity or posturing is the abnormal flexion of the arms with extension of the legs and plantar flexion.

23. C

CN II or the optic nerve is responsible for vision. The Snellen chart will help assess visual acuity.

24. A

Using the Glasgow Coma scale, opening eyes to speech garners 3 points, obeying verbal commands 6 points, and 4 points is for confused verbal response.

25. A

Increased intracranial pressure causes dysfunction of the hypothalamus. Since the hypothalamus regulates body temperature and osmolality of body fluids, the nurse assesses temperature and urinary output of the client.

26. A

Fever, brudzinkski and kernig signs are manifestations of meningeal irritation which are all apparent in meningitis.

27. B

Cranial nerve VI is the abducens nerve. It is responsible for the lateral movement of the eye. To assess its function, the nurse asks the client to look left and right while the head is steady.

28. D

Myasthenia gravis is a rare chronic autoimmune disease characterized by muscular weakness without atrophy. It is caused by a decrease of acetylcholine at neuromuscular junctions. As the body depletes acetylcholine with movement, the body feels weaker. Resting allows the acetylcholine to be preserved and the patient feels an improvement of the fatigue.

29. B

Pronator drift is the pronation of one forearm when the client is asked to stand with the eyes closed for 20-30 seconds while the arms are outstretched and the palms facing upward. It can signify corticospinal lesions. The arm can also drift downward with flexion of fingers and elbow.

30. D

Astereognosis refers to the inability to recognize objects placed in the hand when the eyes are closed.

31. D

Scale for Grading Reflexes

4+ Very brisk, hyperactive, with clonus (rhythmic oscillations between flexion and extension)

3+ Brisker than average; possibly but not necessarily indicative of disease

2+ Average; normal

1+ Somewhat diminished; low normal

0 No response

Hypoactive or absent reflexes (hyporeflexia) are apparent in diseases of spinal nerve roots, spinal nerves, plexuses, or peripheral nerves.

32. B

Dorsiflexion of the big toe and "fanning" of other toes is a positive Babinski response that is usually caused by a lesion in the corticospinal tract. Babinski reflex is also observed in unconscious states from drug or alcohol intoxication or the postictal period following a seizure. It is normal in a newborn.

33. D

A comatose patient remains unarousable with eyes closed. There is no evident response to external stimulus even to repeated painful stimuli.

34. C

The nurse assigns 3 points for eye opening to verbal stimuli, 4 points for confused verbal response and 5 points for localizing pain in the assessment of motor response.

35. C

The nurse advises the patients to seek immediate care for any of the following critical warning signs of stroke: sudden numbness or weakness in any part of the body especially of the face and extremities, trouble speaking or comprehending, sudden incoordination of movement, sudden change in vision, or a severe headache.

36. B

Postural (orthostatic) hypotension is often caused by inadequate vasoconstriction mechanism in both arterioles and veins. This results to venous pooling, decreased cardiac output, and low blood pressure.

37. B

Complex partial seizure may start with an aura and will include automatisms. Automatisms are automatic motor behaviors such as chewing, smacking the lips, walking about, and unbuttoning clothes. Sometimes these automatisms can be as complicated and skilled as driving a car or crossing the streets. The client is unaware of the incident and has no memories of the episodes.

38. B

Grand mal seizures are characterized by tonic extensor rigidity followed by clonic muscular contractions. The jaw is clenched and breathing stops. Tongue depressors and oral thermometers are not used on these clients because of the possibility of injuring the mouth when the jaw is clenched during tonic-clonic episodes.

39. A

Intentional tremors are evident when the client starts a purposeful movement such as holding a cup. The tremor worsens as the objective of the movement is reached. Causes of this tremor include disorders of cerebellar pathways, as in multiple sclerosis.

40. D

Athetosis is characterized by slow, involuntary, convoluted, writhing movements of the fingers, hands, toes, and feet and is commonly seen in cerebral palsy patients.

41. C

The Cranial Nerve VI is the Abducens nerve, which is responsible for the lateral deviation of the eyes. To test the function of the Abducens nerve, the nurse asks the patient to look from side to side without moving their heads.

42. A

Weakness that starts in the lower extremities and spreads upward suggests Guillain-Barre syndrome. Patients with Guillain-Barre syndrome will report that the weakness began as numbness or tingling. The signs and symptoms manifest after a viral infection. This condition becomes life-threatening when the weakness reaches the chest muscles and consequently affects breathing.

43. A

Proximal weakness is felt in the shoulder or hips. To assess for proximal weakness, the nurse must ask the patient if they have difficulty reaching for things above them of if they have difficulty sitting down to and getting up from a chair.

44. C

Patients who experience vasovagal syncope exhibit prodromal symptoms such as nausea, diaphoresis, and pallor prior to the loss of consciousness. The trigger for vasovagal syncope is usually a negative emotion such as those produced by fearful or unpleasant events.

45. B
Common causes of acute symptomatic seizures include epilepsy, brain trauma, meningeal irritation, substance abuse, withdrawal from drugs and alcohol as well as metabolic and electrolyte imbalances.

46. A, B, D
The tremors in Parkinson disease are unilateral and of low frequency (pill-rolling motion). The fine tremors appear when the patient is at rest.

47. A
When the nurse performs a pupillary reactions to light test and notes that the large pupil reacts poorly to light or the anisocoria is worse when the light is flashed, it means that the large pupil has an abnormal pupillary constriction.

48. C
To test the Cranial Nerve VII or the facial nerve, the nurse asks the patient to perform a series of facial movements. The nurse consecutively asks the patient to raise both eyebrows, frown, tightly shut the eyes, to smile with without the teeth showing, and to puff out both cheeks. In Bell palsy, the upper and lower face on one side is affected.

49. B
To assess for coordination, the nurse may ask the patient to make alternating movements rapidly, perform point-to-point movements, walk, or stand in a particular way.

50. A
Intention tremors happen during voluntary purposeful movement, especially toward the end of the deliberate movement. It is evident in patients with multiple sclerosis or those with cerebellar disease.

51. C
To correctly perform the Romberg test, the nurse asks the patient to stand with the feet together and then to close their eyes for 30-60 seconds without support. The nurse should stand beside the patient ready to support the patient in case of loss of balance but should not be touching the patient. At this time, the nurse observes the patient for upright posture and balance. Minimal swaying is normal.

52. D
Patients with uncontrolled diabetes experience peripheral neuropathy, which manifests as loss of sensation of pain, temperature or touch in distal parts such as the feet.

53. B

Astereognosis is the inability to recognize objects that are placed on the hands when the eyes are closed. Hyperesthesia is increased sensitivity. Analgesia is the absence of pain sensation. Graphesthesia is the inability to recognize numbers that are drawn on the palms of the hand while the eyes are closed.

54. D

Grade 4+ deep tendon reflexes indicate hyperreflexia. Hyperreflexia is evident in patients who have lesions along the descending corticospinal tract of the CNS. Associated symptoms are upper motor neuron impairments such as weakness, spasticity, and a positive Babinski sign.

55. D

A clonus is a repetitive rhythmic muscular contraction. Ankle clonus is the repetitive and rhythmic dorsiflexion and plantarflexion of the foot.

56. B

When examining a comatose patient, there are cardinal rules to follow to maintain patient safety. One is to never dilate the patient's pupils because pupillary dilation is a very significant clue as to the severity and cause of coma. Another rule is to never flex the patient's neck unless cervical fracture has been ruled out because doing so could cause cord compression in a fractured neck.

57. B

Using the Glasgow Coma Scale, the results are: the patient's eye opened to a painful stimulus, there was an extension motor response, and they made an incomprehensible verbal response (groaning). Each parameter receives a score of 2 for a total score of 6. A Glasgow coma score of 3-8 is considered coma.

58. B

When the nurse flexes the patient's neck, and in response, the patient involuntarily flexes their hips and knees, the patient exhibits the Brudzinski sign. The Brudzinski sign, as well as nuchal rigidity, and the Kernig sign are an indication of meningeal irritation.

59. A

For patients who had a TIA, the current recommendation by the American Heart Association (AHA) and the American Stroke Association (ASA) is to undergo neurodiagnostic imaging within 24 hours of symptom onset. They also recommend a routine noninvasive imaging of the arteries of the head and neck (carotid and intracranial).

60. A

Risk factors for stroke in women include collagen vascular diseases, such as systemic lupus erythematosus, and history of pre-eclampsia, pregnancy-induced hypertension, and gestational diabetes.

61. C

The American Heart Association (AHA) and the American Stroke Association (ASA) released a list of stroke warning signs and symptoms through the mnemonic FAST. F is for face drooping; A is for Arm weakness; S for speech difficulty; and T is time to call the emergency number, 911.

62. B

Myasthenia Gravis is a chronic autoimmune neuromuscular disease involving skeletal muscles. It is characterized by easy and rapid fatigability of the skeletal muscles. It is hard to recover from the fatigue, but deep tendon reflexes are normal.

63. D

An infarction of the anterior circulation of the brain, particularly the middle cerebral artery (MCA), will have different manifestations because the affected area is the largest vascular bed for stroke. Patients with this kind of stroke will exhibit contralateral weakness of the face and extremities, wherein the weakness in the arm is worse than the legs. There will also be sensory loss, visual field impairment, and aphasia. If the left MCA is occluded, unilateral neglect will be evident. On the other hand, if the right MCA is blocked, apraxia will ensue.

64. A

Dysarthria refers to a mechanical problem of the production of speech. Due to various factors, the patient has little or no control of muscles that produce speech so that the client can only produce sounds nasally or speak with a slur. The patient has no difficulty comprehending language. Common causes of dysarthria are Parkinson disease, motor lesions of the CNS and PNS, and cerebellar disease.

65. C

The step page gait is commonly seen in people with foot drop. Patients will lift their feet high as if they are to climb the stairs, and then bring their foot down with a slap because of leg weakness.

The Male Genitourinary System

Questions

1. A nurse assessing a male client uses the Sexual Maturity Rating (SMR) in Boys. She notes that the male genitalia have few straight thin hairs at the base of the penis. There is no enlargement yet of the penis. At what stage is the client in according to the SMR?
   a. 1
   b. 2
   c. 3
   d. 4

2. A culturally competent nurse is assigned to the pediatric ward where majority of the patients are boys. Which of the following cultural group or race is first to show signs of puberty?
   a. African-American
   b. Caucasian
   c. Asian
   d. Hispanic

3. An elderly male client asks the nurse why erection takes longer now that he is older, and why the penis is not as erect as before. Which of the following response is most appropriate to answer?
   a. "You don't have enough blood volume to cause an effective erection."
   b. "Impotence is a first sign of Alzheimer's disease."
   c. "Your body produces less testosterone, a hormone responsible for effective erection."
   d. "It becomes psychological as you age, thinking that you cannot have an effective erection."

4. A mother who just delivered a baby boy asks a nurse if she should have her baby circumcised. In response, the nurse presents advantages and disadvantages of circumcision to help the mother reach a sound decision. Which of the following are advantages of this procedure? Select all that apply.
   a. It helps in the production of sperm
   b. It helps sustain an erection in the adult life.
   c. It reduces the risk of the circumcised male and his partner acquiring sexually transmitted disease
   d. It reduces risk of phimosis, and cancer of the penis
   e. It will reduce the risk of sterility in later life

5. A client with chronic kidney disease asks the nurse what the causes of his conditions are. Which of the following should be included in the nurse's teaching? Select all that apply
   a. Diabetes
   b. Hyperthyroidism
   c. Parkinson's disease
   d. Myasthenia gravis
   e. Hypertension

6. A nurse wants to assess the urinary pattern of a male client. Which of the following is most appropriate to ask the client to assess for urgency?
   a. "How many times a day do you urinate?"
   b. "Do you awake at night wanting to urinate?"
   c. "Do you feel pain or burning sensation when you urinate?"
   d. "Do you feel that you cannot wait to urinate?"

7. A male client complains to the nurse that it takes him at least two minutes standing over the commode to start the flow of his urine. The nurse documents this manifestation as:
   a. Straining
   b. Hesitancy
   c. Dribbling
   d. Dysuria

8. Several elderly male clients are describing their urinary patterns to the nurse. Which of the following reports warrants immediate evaluation?
   a. Yellowish urine color
   b. Involuntary urine flow when sneezing
   c. Dilute tea colored urine
   d. Cannot wait to urinate

9. A 5-year old boy is reported by his mother to still wetting the bed at night. The nurse documents this manifestation as:
   a. Encopresis
   b. Enuresis
   c. Pyrosis
   d. Regression

10. A mother of an 8-year old boy asks a nurse when her child can be given the Gardasil vaccine. Which of the following correctly answers the mother's query?
    a. At 8 years of age
    b. At 9 years of age
    c. At 26 years of age
    d. At 30 years of age

11. A client complaining of nocturia is receiving instructions from the nurse. Which of the following is best for the nurse to include in her teachings to prevent nocturia? Select all that apply
    a. Limit fluid intake after dinner
    b. Limit fluids to 1 liter per day
    c. Administer diuretics in the morning
    d. Limit caffeine intake
    e. Withhold diuretics

12. A nurse is assessing a male client in pain. During examination, the nurse notes that the foreskin of the penis is retracted and swollen, and that the swelling is constricting the glans. Which of the following conditions is the client most likely suffering from?
    a. Phimosis
    b. Paraphimosis
    c. Hypospadias
    d. Epispadias

13. A nurse is drying a newly delivered male baby. She notes that the urethral meatus is at the ventral side of the penis. The nurse documents this condition as:
    a. Hypospadias
    b. Epispadias
    c. Phimosis
    d. Paraphimosis

14. A 45-year old male shows the nurse his inguinal area that is bulging and painful. The client states that the pain intensifies when he lifts heavy equipment. The bulge also seems to worsen. He says that at night when lying down, the bulge becomes smaller. Which of the following conditions is the client most likely manifesting?
    a. Hernia
    b. Epididymitis
    c. Tumor
    d. Orchitis

15. A client has been recently diagnosed with benign prostatic hypertrophy (BPH). Which of the following are manifestations of BPH? Select all that apply
    a. Dribbling
    b. Anal pain
    c. Urgency
    d. Hesitancy
    e. Burning sensation

16. A male client is admitted to the ward with a primary complaint of sudden severe flank pain that 'travels' to the groin area. He also states that he experienced nausea and vomiting as well. Urinalysis reveals microscopic hematuria. The nurse is prompt to develop a care plan for a client with which diagnosis?
    a. Epididymitis
    b. Nephrosis
    c. Nephrolithiasis
    d. Urethritis

17. A male client has been recently diagnosed with urethritis. A few weeks after, he comes back to the clinic because he feels that he could not completely empty his bladder. That morning, there is complete absence of flow of urine. Which of the following condition is a sequelae of urethritis that caused the client's manifestations?
    a. Gonorrhea
    b. Urethral stricture
    c. Hydronephrosis
    d. Genital herpes

18. A client who lives in a hot climate is seeking consultation because he is having discomfort because of the extreme itch he is experiencing in the groin area. According to the client, he puts on several layers of underpants because he is 'just used to it." During examination, the nurse finds a dark red patch at the groin area of the client. Which of the following will the nurse anticipate to administer topically?
    a. Antibiotic
    b. Anti-fungal
    c. Burrow solution
    d. Betadine

19. A nurse is assessing the genitalia of a male client. She notes a single skin-deep ulceration with scant clear drainage. The client does not report pain although the nurse was able to palpate several inflamed lymph nodes in the groin area. Which of the following medications will the nurse anticipate to administer?
    a. Penicillin G
    b. Steroids
    c. Anti-fungal
    d. Keflex

20. A Mediterranean male client is confined to the hospital because after having an upper respiratory tract infection, he now is experiencing pain in different parts of his body. He is particularly concerned with his sustained painful erection. Which of the following conditions causes sustained painful erection?
    a. Phimosis
    b. Sickle cell anemia
    c. Leukemia
    d. Systemic lupus erythematosus

21. A 65-year old client has been diagnosed with inguinal hernia. Which of the following client actions would warrant further intervention?
    a. The client is wearing a truss
    b. The client carries his 2-year old grandchild
    c. The client performs ROM exercises

d. Client performs deep breathing

22. The nurse is performing physical examination of the newborn and notes that the urethral meatus is found in the topside of the penis. What condition is this called?
    a. Phimosis
    b. Paraphimosis
    c. Hypospadias
    d. Epispadias

23. A nurse notes on inspection of the penis that the glans penis and prepuce are red and swollen. The client reports pain when in contact with clothing or when touched. The nurse is sure to provide care for which condition?
    a. Balanitis
    b. Epidydimitis
    c. Balanophostitis
    d. Urethritis

24. A male client who is sexually active with multiple sexual partners reports a copious amount of yellowish discharge. Which of the following conditions is mostly likely responsible for the client's symptoms?
    a. Trichomoniasis
    b. Chlamydia
    c. Gonococcal urethritis
    d. Nongonococcal urethritis

25. The nurse is performing a clinical testicular examination on a 48-year old client. Which of the following is a normal finding that needs only documenting and no further intervention?
    a. Asymmetric testes without any lumps
    b. Scant whitish discharge
    c. Mild pain on urination
    d. Small skin erosion <1cm

26. The nurse is doing her initial assessment of the client and notes that the scrotum is bigger than usual. Upon palpation, the nurse's fingertips made 2mm indentation on the swelling. The skin also appears taut. Which of the following is the most probable cause for this?
    a. Diabetes mellitus
    b. Diabetes insipedus
    c. Congestive heart failure
    d. Malignant hypertension

27. A 37-year old male client is seen in the outpatient department because he suspects that he has STD. He has multiple sexual partners and is having sex with men. Upon assessment of his

genitalia, the nurse notes an uncircumcised penis with a single nodule 1 cm x 1 cm on the side. It is indurated and is nontender. There is no report of any penile discharge or unusual swelling. The nurse reports her finding to the physician because
a. The client is exhibiting signs and symptoms of penile cancer
b. The client probably has condylomata acuminata
c. The client has herpes simplex
d. The client has a benign mass on the penis.

28. A nurse assessing a male client wants to know if her client has scrotal hernia or a hydrocoele. Which of the following is true of scrotal hernia and hydrocoele?
a. Scrotal hernia comes through the external inguinal ring, so the examining fingers cannot get above it within the scrotum
b. Scrotal hernia is a nontender, fluid-filled mass within the tunica vaginalis
c. Scrotal hernia transilluminates.
d. In Scrotal hernia, the examining fingers can get above the mass within the scrotum.

29. The nurse is assessing a client with condylomata acuminata and plans to conduct health teaching on the transmission mode of the causative organism. The nurse knows that teaching has been effective if the client replies which pathogen as responsible for condylomata acuminata?
a. Herpes simplex virus 2
b. Human papillomavirus (HPV)
c. Treponema pallidum
d. Haemophilus ducreyi

30. A 33-year old male client comes to the clinic for a lesion on his genitalia. After tests were performed, he was found positive for syphilis. The client asks the nurse what pathogen is making him sick. Which of the following is a correct nursing response?
a. Herpes simplex virus 2
b. Human papillomavirus (HPV)
c. Treponema pallidum
d. Haemophilus ducreyi

31. A nurse is seeing the client with painful inguinal adenopathy and suppurative buboes in his penis. The client states that the pus filled lesions started out as a small pimple. The nurse knows that to make an effective health teaching for a patient with chancroid, she has to know what the causative microorganism is for chancroid, and that is
a. Haemophilus ducreyi
b. Herpes simplex virus 2
c. Human papillomavirus (HPV)
d. Treponema pallidum

32. A nurse is teaching a group of teenage boys about sexually transmitted diseases (STDs) as part of

their school awareness program. Which of the following statements, if made by a teenager, would indicate the need for further teaching?
a. "Taking the pill protects me from diseases."
b. "If I get an STD I will be more at risk for getting HIV."
c. "I can get a disease through vaginal, oral or anal intercourse."
d. "If I get an infection my partner should be tested and treated as well."

33. The nurse is providing health teaching to a group of workers in the entertainment industry. Which of the following is true about sexually transmitted diseases?
a. STDs can be transmitted during homosexual activities only.
b. STDs can only be transmitted during penetrating intimate acts.
c. Infected person should be treated and all sexual partners should be screened
d. Two or more STIs can coexist in the same client

34. A 9-year old client comes to the clinic accompanied by his mother due to fever and general malaise. The client also complains of swollen painful scrotum. Upon history taking, the nurse notes that the boy has had mumps a week before. Which of the following conditions most likely is the cause of the client's symptoms?
a. Acute bacterial orchitis
b. Acute viral orchitis
c. Hydrocele
d. Testicular torsion

35. A client agrees to perform self-testicular exam. Which of the following is a correct nursing response for client preparation?
a. "You need to hold your urine as you need a full bladder for the examination."
b. "You will lie on your side for the entire examination."
c. "You will need to take a warm shower prior to the examination."
d. "You will need to take a medication prior to the examination."

36. A male client complains to the nurse that every time he urinates, he seems to wait before starting a stream. He also states that he couldn't make a continuous stream of urine. The nurse prepares the client for which exam?
a. Digital rectal exam
b. Abdominal ultrasound
c. MRI
d. CT scan

37. The nurse is conducting a screening for HIV. Who among the following clients should get tested for HIV?
a. A 13-year old soccer player
b. A 34-year old with homosexual sexual relations

c.   A 55-year old lawyer
d.   All of the above

38. The nurse is palpating the scrotum of a client during a routine comprehensive examination. She notes three small about 0.2cm each on the dorsal side of the scrotum. The round nodes appear pimple like and are yellowish. The patient feels no pain when palpating the nodes. Which of the following conditions does the client most probably have?
a.   Herpes simplex
b.   Epidermoid cysts
c.   Genital warts
d.   Chancroid

39. The nurse is doing a health teaching on blood-borne diseases. Which of the following is not included in the nurse's topics?
a.   Hepatitis A
b.   Hepatitis B
c.   HIV
d.   AIDS

40. A client tells the nurse that he suspects that he has hernia. Which of the following techniques will help the nurse assess the client for the possibility of hernia?
a.   Use white overhead lamp to see clearly the abdomen
b.   Have the client lie supine and palpate the lower abdomen
c.   Have the client lie to his side and inspect the abdomen for a bulge
d.   While standing straight, ask the client to bear down just like moving his bowels and inspect and palpate for any bulges

41. Which of the following questions that aim to explore sexual orientation and gender identity is non-therapeutic?
a.   "How is sex for you?"
b.   "Are you male, female, gay or lesbian?"
c.   "Are you comfortable with your partner's sexual practices?"
d.   "How is your current relationship?"

42. An adolescent male patient is rushed to the emergency room after experiencing sudden and intense scrotal pain. The patient says it started after going out of the house to shovel snow. There are accompanying symptoms of nausea and vomiting. Which of the following is best for the nurse to do next?
a.   Inform the physician immediately
b.   Document the findings
c.   Apply an ice pack to the scrotum
d.   Have the patient sit in bed

43. A male patient has just been found to have an inguinal hernia. Which of the following patient response is consistent with this diagnosis?
    a. "The swelling in my groin gets bigger when I carry bags of groceries."
    b. "The pain in my groin is worse at night."
    c. "I have to wait a minute before my urine flows out."
    d. "The pain in my lower abdomen seems to travel to my back."

44. A nurse is to inspect a male patient's genitalia for any abnormalities. Which of the following should the nurse do prior to the procedure?
    a. Position the patient on their side
    b. Apply petroleum jelly to the hands
    c. Inform the patient that a prostate exam is to be done next
    d. Put on gloves

45. A generalist nurse is making a reproductive system assessment on a male patient. Which of the following nursing actions indicates that the nurse needs further teaching?
    a. Performing handwashing before the examination
    b. Instructing the patient to put on a hospital gown
    c. Palpating the patient's scrotum and performing a prostate examination after
    d. Explaining the procedure to the patient before starting the examination

46. A nurse is inspecting the male patient's genitalia who presents with pain and swelling of the prepuce. The nurse notes that the patient is uncircumcised. The patient says that when they retracted the prepuce, it never went back to cover the glans. Which of the following conditions is the patient most likely manifesting?
    a. Balanoposthitis
    b. Phimosis
    c. Paraphimosis
    d. Balanitis

47. Which of the following information about HIV testing is NOT true?
    a. There is an opt-out approach to HIV testing
    b. One-time testing for low-risk individuals is acceptable
    c. All people aged 13-64 years old are recommended to undergo the test
    d. The test is mandatory and cannot be declined

48. A nurse is conducting a health teaching to male adult patient on the correct way of using a condom. Which of the following instructions if given by the nurse to the patient indicates that the nurse needs further teaching?
    a. Use petroleum jelly as a lubricant
    b. For every sexual act, use a new condom
    c. Apply the condom before stating the sexual act

d. If the condom breaks during the sexual act, hold the condom and withdraw immediately

49. A nurse observes that a male patient's scrotum is swollen. Which of the following will point to the cause of swelling as a scrotal hernia and NOT a hydrocele?
a. It transilluminates
b. It is non-tender
c. The examining fingers can palpate above the mass within the scrotum
d. The examining fingers cannot palpate a border above the mass within the scrotum

50. A male patient tells the nurse that he has small painful wounds in his penis. Upon inspection of the penis, the nurse notes small scattered lesions, some vesicular, and some looked like eroded vesicles. After further examination, the nurse also finds that the patient has a fever, headache, arthralgia, and lymphadenopathy. Based on the patient's manifestations, which of the following conditions does the patient most likely have?
a. Condylomata acuminata
b. Genital herpes simplex
c. Primary syphilis
d. Chancroid

51. A male patient is being seen by the nurse complaining of a swollen painful scrotum, especially when touched. Which of the following when noted in the patient's history will suggest to the nurse that the patient has acute orchitis?
a. Recent mumps infection
b. Trauma to the genitalia three months ago
c. Recent abdominal surgery
d. Present employment – laborer

52. A male patient's testicular exam reveals a movable nontender cyst-like mass above the testis. The mass transilluminates. Which of the following most likely caused the patient's signs and symptoms?
a. Acute epididymitis
b. Varicocele
c. Spermatocele or epididymal cyst
d. Hydrocele

53. A nurse is asking a series of questions to older men in a screening session, inquiring if they have trouble starting the flow of urine, if there is any change in the force or size of their urine, or if there is dribbling. Which of the following conditions is the nurse screening the patients for?
a. Urge incontinence
b. Benign prostatic hypertrophy
c. Bladder overdistention
d. Cystitis

54. A patient has poorly controlled diabetes and is urinating in large amounts. The patient describes their urination as "so much more than usual." Which of the following correctly describes the patient's symptom?
    a. Polyuria
    b. Nocturia
    c. Polydipsia
    d. Anuria

ANSWERS

1. B
    In stage 1 of the Sexual Maturity Rating (SMR) in Boys, the male genitalia are similar to preadolescent size without pubic hair present. In stage 2, a few fine straight hairs appear at the base of the genitalia. The scrotum begins to enlarge although the penis remains preadolescent. At stage 3, the hair is sparsely growing over the pubis. They are coarser and curly. There is also enlargement of the penis. At stage 4, the pubic hair thickens, and penile growth in length and diameter is apparent. At stage 5, the pubic hair extends over the medial thighs. Both penis and scrotum reach adult shape and size.

2. A
    According to Tanner Staging, African-American boys are about 1 ½ years earlier to show signs of puberty that boys of other racial background.

3. C
    The elderly produces less testosterone so that erection takes longer is not as effective. Another factor that may cause impotence in the elderly male is multipharmacy with impotence as a side effect.

4. C, D
    Circumcision has more benefits than disadvantages. Some of the advantages are reduced risks of acquiring sexually transmitted disease in both hetero and homosexual relations, and reduced risk of acquiring urinary tract infection, phimosis and penile cancer.

5. A, E
    Diabetes and hypertension are the main causes of developing chronic kidney disease.

6. D
    Urgency is being unable to wait to urinate. Option A describes frequency. Option B describes nocturia and Option C describes dysuria.

7. B
    Hesitancy is described as difficulty starting urination. The client may find himself waiting for his urine to flow out.

8. C
    Tea-colored urine indicates increased bilirubin in the blood brought about by obstruction of the bile duct. It is a sign of pathology especially if accompanied by other signs and symptoms of biliary obstruction. Urgency and stress incontinence, although manifestations of a possible pathology, do not require urgent evaluation as the tea-colored urine.

9. B

    Enuresis is the involuntary flow of urine at night, or bedwetting. Encopresis is involuntary bowel movement.

10. B

    Gardasil vaccine is given to males aged 9-26 years of age to prevent genital warts.

11. A, C, D

    Nocturia is waking at night because of the urge to urinate. It may be prevented by limiting fluid intake after dinner, administering diuretics in the morning and limiting caffeine that also has a diuretic effect.

12. B

    Paraphimosis is the constriction of the glans penis by the retracted foreskin that had swollen because the foreskin failed to return to its natural position.

13. A

    In hypospadias, the urethral meatus is located at the ventral side of the penis. On the other hand, in epispadias, the opening is at the dorsal side.

14. A

    An hernia is the protrusion of the intestines into the inguinal ring. It is manifested by a bulge at the groin area and pain that is worsened by weight-bearing.

15. A, C, D

    Benign prostatic hypertrophy is non-malignant enlargement of the prostrate and is characterized by dribbling, hesitancy and urgency of urination.

16. C

    Nephrolithiasis or renal calculi are kidney stones made of calcium oxalate or uric acid. When they become dislodged to the ureters, the client will experience severe flank pain with radiation to the abdomen or inguinal area, diaphoresis, nausea and vomiting and hematuria.

17. B

    Urethral stricture is constriction of the urethra secondary to urethral damage usually an inflammation. There is gradual weakness of the flow of urine, and with complete stricture, there is absence of flow of urine.

18. B

    Tinea cruris is a fungal infection of the inguinal area. It is commonly referred to as jock itch. It is extremely itchy. The area looks dark red, crescent shaped patch-like lesion in the inguinal area.

19. A

The client is exhibiting signs and symptoms of syphilis, and the lesion on the genitalia is a syphilitic chancre. The drug of choice for syphilis is Penicillin G.

20. B

Priapism is sustained painful erection of the penis. It is a manifestation of sickle cell anemia.

21. B

Hernia pain and swelling are more likely to occur when internal abdominal pressure increases. Carrying a weight increases abdominal pressure.

22. D

An epispadias is a rare type of malformation of the penis in which the urethra opening is found on the dorsal aspect of the penis.

23. C

Balanophostitis is inflammation of the glans and prepuce. Balanitis is inflammation of the glans. Epidydimitis and urethritis are inflammation of the epidydimis and urethra respectively.

24. C

In gonococcal urethritis the client has profuse yellow discharge. On the other hand, there is scanty white or clear discharge in nongonococcal urethritis. Trichomas infection would have greenish discharge and Chlamydia would have white or off-white discharge. Definitive diagnosis requires Gram stain and culture.

25. A

A testis that is bigger than the other without the presence of any lump is normal. The nurse documents the findings.

26. C

Pitting edema can make the scrotal skin taut. This finding is consistent with congestive heart failure or nephrotic syndrome.

27. A

Carcinoma of the penis appears as an indurated nodule or ulcer that is usually nontender. It is almost limited to men who are not circumcised. Sometimes it is not readily seen because it can be covered by the prepuce. The nurse needs to report this finding because further tests are necessary before a diagnosis of penile cancer can be made.

28. A

Scrotal hernia comes through the external inguinal ring, so the examining fingers cannot get above it within the scrotum. Hydrocele is a nontender, fluid-filled mass within the tunica vaginalis.

It transilluminates, and the examining fingers can get above the mass within the scrotum.

29. B

Causative organism for condylomata acuminata is the Human papillomavirus (HPV), usually from subtypes 6 and 11. Carcinogenic subtypes are rare accounting for approximately 5–10% of all anogenital warts.

30. C

Causative organism for syphilis is Treponema pallidum, a spirochete. The incubation period is 9–90 days after exposure.

31. A

The causative organism for chancroid is haemophilus ducreyi, an anaerobic bacillus. Incubation period is 3–7 days after exposure.

32. A

Pills are effective in preventing pregnancy but not against acquiring STD's. The use of latex condoms with a water-based lubricant or not having sexual intercourse at all are the best ways of preventing an infection. An STD can be transmitted through vaginal, oral or anal intercourse. Both partners should be treated.

33. D

Sexually transmitted disease can be transmitted through both heterosexual and homosexual intimate contacts. 2 or more types of STD's can coexist in the same client. The infected client and all sexual partners should be treated for STD's. STD's can be transmitted even without penetration of the penis.

34. B

Orchitis can be viral or bacterial in nature. Orchitis in young male clients is usually a sequala of mumps, a viral infection. The orchitis is therefore viral in nature. Signs of acute orchitis are: inflamed, painful, tender, and swollen testis, fever and chills, reddened scrotum. It is usually unilateral.

35. C

A warm shower is indicated prior to a testicular exam to relax the scrotum. This will make examination easier.

36. A

Digital rectal examination (DRE) provides a relatively crude estimate of prostate size and is an examination indicated for prostate enlargement.

37. D

In 2006 the CDC issued new recommendations advising universal HIV screening for all people 13 to 64 years, regardless of risk factors.

38. B

Epidermoid cysts are common, frequently multiple, and benign. There may be dome-shaped white or yellow papules or nodules formed by occluded follicles filled with keratin debris of desquamated follicular epithelium.

39. A

Hepatitis A is a viral infection that causes liver inflammation. The Hepatitis A virus is transmitted through fecal-oral route.

40. D

To assess for the presence of hernia, ask the client to strain and bear down (perform the Valsalva maneuver) to increase intra-abdominal pressure, making it easier to observe an hernia. If a bulge is present, the patient should be referred to a physician. Absence of a bulge during inspection does not guarantee absence of an hernia, especially in an obese patient.

41. B

To ask about gender identity, the nurse must use a neutral and open-ended question, such as "How would you describe your gender identity?" Responses to gender identity questions include male, female, transsexual, transgender, intersex, among others.

42. A

Sudden scrotal pain in young males, especially if with accompanying symptoms of nausea and vomiting suggest testicular torsion. Testicular torsion happens when the spermatic cord gets twisted and cause an obstruction to the blood supplying the testicles. The patient will need immediate medical attention to correct the torsion and prevent the cellular death of the testicles.

43. A

An inguinal hernia is a swelling in the inguinal area caused by a part of the intestines protruding through the weakened or enlarged opening of the inguinal canal. With increased abdominal pressure, such as when lifting heavy things, bending over or bearing down, the protruding tissue is pushed out some more, thereby increasing the size of the swelling.

44. D

Prior to the examination of the male genitalia, the nurse must put on gloves. It is possible that the patient may have penile discharges and the use of gloves is a must.

45. C

The palpation of the male genitalia as well as prostate exams are not within the scope of practice of a generalist nurse. The generalist nurse, however, may inspect the genitalia during procedures such as urinary catheterization.

46. C

Paraphimosis is a condition wherein the retracted foreskin does not return to cover the glans. The prepuce swells and constricts the penis. This is considered a medical emergency because if the swelling continues, the cellular death of the penis may ensue.

47. D

The HIV testing is recommended to be done on all adolescents and adults who are aged 13-64 years old, including all pregnant women. There is no need for consent for this test. It is the nurse's responsibility to inform the patient that the HIV test will be conducted but the patient may decline if they do not agree to it. This is the opt-out approach to HIV testing. For low-risk individuals, a one-time testing is already reasonable.

48. A

When teaching about the proper use of a condom to a patient, the nurse must give instructions to use only water-based lubricants. Before starting a sexual act, the condom must be applied and replaced with a new one for every act. If the condom accidentally breaks during use, the patient should be instructed to hold the condom and withdraw the penis immediately.

49. D

A scrotal hernia is a mass that is a part of the intestines that protruded through the external inguinal ring. The nurse will not be able to palpate for the border above the hernia. A hydrocele is a fluid-filled mass that can be transilluminated. Since it is fluid, the nurse can still palpate above the mass.

50. B

The lesions of genital herpex simplex are vesicular in nature. The vesicles are scattered or grouped, but found on the glans and shaft of the penis. The vesicles may erode, which cause pain. The patient may have a fever, malaise, headaches, joint pains and lymph node enlargement.

51. A

The most common cause of acute orchitis is a recent mumps infection. In acute orchitis, there is testicular pain, swelling redness, and tenderness. There may also be general symptoms like fever and malaise. Orchitis caused by mumps is common in prepubertal boys.

52. C

A spermatocele or an epididymal cyst presents as a cyst-like mass above the testis, and it is movable and painless. The mass transilluminates. A spermatocele contains sperm, while an epididymal cyst contains only fluids.

53. B

Because benign prostatic hypertrophy (BPH) is common in older men, the nurse has to ask a series of questions in their review of the renal system. The nurse must ask for the presence of signs and symptoms of BPH such as difficulty starting the flow of urine, decreased force or size of urine flow, and dribbling urine.

54. A

Polyuria is the passing of very large amounts of urine, exceeding 3 liters in a 24-hour period. It is a common manifestation of poorly controlled diabetes and is usually the reason why the patient will seek medical help.

The Anus, Rectum, and the Prostrate

Questions

1. A client is complaining of urinary hesitancy and nocturia. When the doctor examined him, he performed a digital rectal examination. The nurse understands that the specific anatomy that the physician is assessing is the client's:
   a. Urethra
   b. Testis
   c. Rectum
   d. Prostate gland

2. A mother of a 1-year old infant asks the nurse why it takes about two years before a baby can be toilet trained. Which is the best response of the nurse?
   a. "The bladder and rectum are not yet big enough to hold waste products of the body."
   b. "The nerves responsible for control of the bladder and rectum have not yet matured."
   c. "She needs to have the conscious effort to control elimination which she will achieve by age two."
   d. "Your baby will not understand instructions until age two."

3. A nurse is conducting blood screening for prostate disease. She looks at several laboratory tests. Which of the following results should the nurse pay particular attention to?
   a. Red blood cells
   b. PSA
   c. CA 125
   d. AFP

4. A nurse is caring for a client with a problematic bowel movement. She wants to assess if the client is experiencing dyschezia. Which of the following question is most appropriate to ask the client to assess for dyschezia?
   a. "Do you your bowels feel so big to move out?"
   b. "You do hesitate when you go to the restroom to relieve yourself of your bowels?
   c. "Do you feel any pain when you move your bowels?"
   d. "Is there bleeding form your anus when you move your bowels?"

5. An adult client presents to the ER with primary complaint of diarrhea, abdominal cramps, nausea and vomiting for more than 24 hours now. The nurse conducts an interview. Which of the following findings is most significant?
   a. Eating cake with the frosting
   b. Eating thoroughly cooked oysters the night before
   c. Drinking from a bottled water
   d. Swimming in the lake

6. A nurse is reviewing the medical records of several clients with blood in the stools. Who of the following patients will report fresh bright red blood in the stools?

   a.   Intestinal ulcer
   b.   Cancer of the cecum
   c.   External hemorrhoids
   d.   Iron supplementation

7.   A client reports fatty frothy stool that floats on water. Which of the following conditions will have such manifestation?
   a.   Irritable bowel syndrome
   b.   Peptic ulcer
   c.   Cholelithiasis
   d.   Pancreatitis

8.   A nurse is conducting health teaching on the prevention of colorectal cancer. One of her main points is to encourage intake of insoluble fiber foods. Which of the following foods should the nurse include in her list of foods that are high in insoluble fiber?
   a.   Wheat germ
   b.   Beans
   c.   Instant oatmeal
   d.   Apples with skin

9.   A nurse performing a digital rectal exam notes a shiny blue sac near the anal opening. The client reports anal pain when passing stools and sometimes sees fresh blood in the tissue he uses to wipe himself with. Which of the following most likely describes the sac?
   a.   Fistula
   b.   Fissure
   c.   Thrombosed hemorrhoid
   d.   Genital herpes

10.   A client reports to the nurse that he feels uncomfortable every after a bowel movement when he feels that "some flesh protrudes" from his anus. He added that he feels like sitting on a small tennis ball. Upon examination of the anal area, the nurse finds a reddish doughnut-looking tissue protruding out of the anal opening. Which of the following conditions most likely is being manifested by the client?
   a.   Hemorrhoids
   b.   Anal fissure
   c.   Anal tumor
   d.   Rectal prolapse

11.   A nurse is performing a digital rectal exam and she palpates a soft movable mass that seem to protrude from the rectal wall. Which of the following is the client's most likely condition?
   a.   Carcinoma
   b.   Polyp

c. External hemorrhoids
d. Genital herpes

12. A male client is complaining of urinary hesitancy, urgency and dribbling. The competent nurse performs the digital rectal examination to palpate for the prostate gland. Upon examination, the client withdraws from pain. The prostate feels swollen and enlarged but not firm. The client reports some dribbling of urine. Which of the following should the nurse anticipate to perform?
a. Administer antibiotics
b. Prepare for surgery
c. Advise client not to ejaculate
d. Anticipate possible priapism

13. A nurse is performing a genital examination of a female client. She inserts her fingers into the vagina and notes a small, firm round doughnut like structure at the anterior wall of the rectum. Which part of the female anatomy did the nurse palpate?
a. Vaginal wall
b. Cervix
c. Uterus
d. Overy

14. A client reports abdominal pain that is gnawing. The physician orders test for occult blood, stat. However, the client stated that he is taking iron supplements. Which of the following should the nurse do?
a. Perform the Guaiac's test
b. Delay the Guaiac's test for the next day because the iron will create a false positive result
c. Perform the fecal immunochemical test
d. Inform the doctor that the test could not be performed

15. A nurse assesses an 80-year old client, and asks him to perform the valsalva maneuver by bearing down. The client reports spilling a scant amount urine and feces. Which of the following is best for the nurse to do next?
a. Help the client change clothing, and document findings
b. Immediately report her findings to the physician
c. Ask the client to perform isotonic exercises
d. Perform digital rectal examination.

16. Colon cancer is one of the leading causes of mortality in the US. The Centers for Disease Control and Prevention recommends screening to be done for Colon cancer, which should start at what age?
a. 40
b. 50
c. 60

d. 65

17. A 55-year old client asks the nurse how screening for colon cancer will be done. The nurse explains that three tests need to be performed. Which of the following are these tests? Select all that apply.
    a. Sigmoidoscopy
    b. Colonoscopy
    c. Explore laparotomy
    d. Digital rectal examination
    e. High sensitivity fecal occult blood testing (FOBT)

18. A nurse is performing an examination of a 20-year old client who is now lying prone on the examination table. Her observation reveals a small tunnel-like opening with visible thick hair just below the coccyx. The client reports no pain or tenderness. Which of the following should appear in the nurse's documentation of the client's condition?
    a. Anorectal fistula
    b. Mongolian opening
    c. Pilonidal sinus
    d. Fissure

19. A client reports severe constipation and passing of large hard stools. When passing stools, the client reports feeling the anal opening being torn "like broken glass is being passed." Which of the following should the nurse advise the client to do? Select all that apply.
    a. Offer stool softeners
    b. Offer laxatives
    c. Assist in having a warm sitz bath
    d. Apply topical analgesics
    e. Administer steroids

20. A 5-year old child is brought by her mother to the clinic. She reports that her child is not having a restful sleep at night because she keeps on scratching her anal area. Upon examination of the anal area, the nurse notes excoriation of the opening and surrounding areas with the skin reddened, raised and thickened. The nurse anticipates which of the following orders? Select all that apply.
    a. Administer anti-fungal
    b. Perform the scotch tape test
    c. Apply talcum powder
    d. Clean the area with 70% isopropyl alcohol
    e. Administer anti-helminthic

21. The nurse is completing an admission assessment of a client with benign prostatic hyperplasia. The nurse understands that she has to obtain more focused assessment on
    a. Breathing patterns
    b. Urinary patterns

c. Internal bleeding
d. Defecation patterns

22. A nurse is doing a health teaching on a client recently diagnosed with benign prostatic hypertrophy. Which of the following client responses means that the client has understood the teaching?
a. "After this visit, I need not worry about my condition again."
b. "I don't know if I can get used to urinating every 2-3 hours"
c. "I will need to wear elastic stockings when going to work."
d. "I need to force fluids a day to prevent urine dribbling."

23. An elderly client diagnosed with prostate enlargement asks the nurse if his sex life would be affected by his condition. Which of the following is an appropriate nursing response?
a. "You will have erectile dysfunction. It is best to talk to your wife about it."
b. "Your urinary patterns will change but your condition should not affect your sex life."
c. "It is inappropriate to ask such question."
d. "I know how you feel. Let's talk about it."

24. A client is seen by the nurse in the outpatient department and conducts teaching on the prevention of anorectal cancer. Which of the following client response means he has understood his instructions?
a. "I need to include more meat in my diet to help me heal faster."
b. "I need to increase my intake of fruits and vegetables."
c. "I have to undergo abdominal x-rays at least once a year."
d. "I will avoid salty foods."

25. An elderly client found to have prostate enlargement tells the nurse that after voiding, he seems to have more drops of urine as he "shakes" his penis. The nurse documents this as
a. Hesitancy
b. Frequency
c. Dribbling
d. Urgency

26. A 77-yar old male client tells the nurse during a routine examination that he seems to wait for his urine to flow for about a minute or so even if he is already standing in front of the urinal and ready to void. What term is used to best describe this condition?
a. Hesitancy
b. Frequency
c. Dribbling
d. Urgency

27. An elderly male client complains to the nurse that he doesn't get enough sleep because he has

to get up several times at night just to void. When doing her documentation, she writes this as
a. Polyuria
b. Hesitancy
c. Nocturia
d. Oliguria

28. A patient recently diagnosed with prostate cancer asks the nurse why he has urine hesitancy, dribbling and bladder fullness. What is the most accurate nursing response?
a. "Your enlarged prostrate that surrounds your passage for urine constricts the passage and obstructs urine flow."
b. "The substance secreted by your enlarged prostate causes you to void less in the morning and more at night."
c. "A stone from your kidneys has dislodged and is causing urine obstruction."
d. "A tumor in your rectum is pressing the tubes for passing urine."

29. A nurse is conducting health teaching on several clients about the risk factors of anorectal cancer. Which of the following is NOT a risk factor for anorectal cancer?
a. Diet high in processed foods
b. Diet high in saturated fat
c. high-fiber diet
d. family history of polyps

30. A client who has been diagnosed with hemorrhoids asks the nurse what causes him to bleed in the rectum. What is the most appropriate nursing response?
a. "You have weakened veins in your rectum that has become dilated. When these veins are traumatized, they get torn and bleed."
b. "Hardened bulky stool lacerates the anal opening and that causes bleeding."
c. "You have muscular growths from your rectum that bleed when in contact with hardened stools."
d. "Your bowels are constantly inflamed and swollen and the inflammation causes bleeding."

31. A nurse is conducting a health teaching on a male client with varicosities in the rectum. Which of the following client activities would the nurse advice against?
a. Driving a car
b. Painting
c. Wearing a belt
d. Reducing calorie intake

32. A client with a tumor of the rectum comes to the clinic for care. Which of the following stool characteristics should the nurse expect the client to report?
a. Scant and mucoid
b. Frequent bloody and watery

   c.   Fatty and malodorous

   d.   Bloody and pencil-like if soft

33. A client comes to the clinic complaining of anal pain because of a fissure. The client asks the nurse what caused his condition. What is the most appropriate nursing reply?
   a.   "A vein in your rectum has become dilated and torn."
   b.   "Hard bulky stools passed from your anus caused the opening to be torn."
   c.   "A tumor in your rectum has grown so large that it has blocked the opening."
   d.   "Your body has made an opening or a sac that has become filled with pus."

34. A male client has been admitted to the unit due to complaints of anal pain. Upon assessment, the nurse palpates an opening in the rectum that drains pus. Which of the following client history is most significant?
   a.   Recent antibiotic therapy
   b.   Recent digital rectal examination
   c.   Anal abscess
   d.   Appendectomy 3 years ago

35. Which of the following stool characteristics is unique to client with anal fistulas?
   a.   Frequent and watery
   b.   With pus and blood
   c.   Profuse bloody
   d.   Mucoid

36. A nurse is to be assigned to the care of a client with external hemorrhoids. What assessment findings of the anal area does the nurse expect to find?
   a.   Bluish bulges near the anal opening
   b.   Torn bleeding anal opening
   c.   Hard lump about an inch from the opening
   d.   Tender anal area with pus-filled discharge

37. A community health nurse is conducting a health seminar on the risks of colorectal cancer. Who of the following seminar attendees has a risk factor for colorectal cancer?
   a.   A 45-year old mother of three who had appendectomy 4 years ago
   b.   A 15-year old soccer player who suffers from chronic constipation
   c.   A 35-year old male with a BMI of 28 working as an executive
   d.   A 56-year old male with a family history of polyps

38. Which of the following is a sign of advanced prostate cancer?
   a.   Hesitancy
   b.   Dribbling
   c.   Urgency

d.   Anuria

39. A nurse is reviewing her concepts of prostate disorders. Which of the following assessment/ laboratory findings is unique to acute prostatitis?
    a.   Dribbling urine
    b.   Semen contains pus
    c.   Erectile dysfunction
    d.   Decreased sex drive

40. A client comes to the clinic because of rectal bleeding. Which of the following findings alerts the nurse to the possibility of rectal cancer?
    a.   Bluish bulges near the anal area
    b.   Torn anal opening
    c.   Significant weight loss and malaise
    d.   Enlarged tender prostate

41. A nurse is screening several male patients for prostate cancer. Which of the following patients have high risks? Select all that apply.
    a.   A 75-year-old African American male
    b.   A 60-year-old Caucasian male with a brother who died of prostate cancer
    c.   A 40-year-old Asian male with diabetes
    d.   A 36-year old Mediterranean male who has a cousin with benign prostatic hypertrophy

ANSWERS

1. D

   The prostate gland is located at the anterior side of the rectum. It surrounds the urethra at the bladder neck. When it hypertrophies such as in benign prostatic hypertrophy, it constricts the urethra, thereby causing urinary hesitancy, urgency and nocturia.

2. B

   Bladder and bowel control cannot be achieved until the age of two because myelinization of nerves that are responsible for control is not complete until two years of age.

3. B

   PSA means prostate specific antigen and it is found both in semen and in the blood. An increased level indicates prostate disease.

4. C

   Dyschezia is pain when moving the bowels. It can be due to hemorrhoids or constipation.

5. D

   Reasons for having diarrhea can be due to autoimmune disorders, and largely due to contaminated food and water, direct contact with symptomatic people and swimming in contaminated water.

6. C

   Bright red blood in the stools indicates fresh bleeding from a part of the GI tract nearest the anal sphincter. External hemorrhoids will have fresh bleeding.

7. D

   The client is exhibiting steatorrhea or passing of frothy fatty foul smelling stool that floats on water. It is the result of malabsorbed fats and it is manifested in sprue, cystic fibrosis, chronic pancreatitis, and Chron disease.

8. D

   Insoluble fibers are cellulose in food that cannot be digested. It adds bulk to the stool and helps stimulate peristalsis. Examples of insoluble fibers are wheat bran whole grains, apples eaten with skin and some type of cereals made of whole grains.

9. C

   A thrombosed hemorrhoid would appear like a shiny blue skin sac which may bleed when defecating.

10. D

Rectal prolapse is the protrusion of the rectal wall out of the anal opening and it would look like a red doughnut-looking tissue at the anus.

11. B

A rectal polyp would feel like a soft movable mass that seem to protrude from the rectal wall during digital rectal examination.

12. A

The signs and symptoms exhibited by the client indicate prostatitis. The nurse anticipates that the physician would prescribe antibiotics for the client. Surgery is not needed.

13. B

The cervix feels like a small firm round mass at the anterior wall of the rectum. It should be free of any lumps and should be closed.

14. C

The fecal immunochemical test is a newer test that could be administered regardless of iron or food intake that can blacken the stools. This method has two types: the liquid based test that utilizes a hemoglobin stabilizing buffer, and the dry-slide cards that are manually analyzed.

15. A

In the elder elderly, there is relaxation of the musculature of the perineum and anal area as well as decreased sphincter control. The nurse should help the client clean himself and then proceed to document her findings.

16. B

The CDC recommends screening for colon cancer starting from the age of 50.

17. A, B, E

It is recommended that American 50 year old and above be screened for colorectal cancer. Screening methods include high sensitivity fecal occult blood testing (FOBT), sigmoidoscopy and colonoscopy.

18. C

A pilonidal sinus or cyst is seen usually below the coccygeal area. It is a dimple like structure with visible tuft of hair protruding from the opening. It is non-tender if no abscess is noted.

19. A, C, D

The client is manifesting signs and symptoms of anal fissure. The nurse advises the client to take stool softeners and have a warm sitz bath. The nurse may apply a topical analgesic after the bath.

20. B, E

The client is exhibiting signs and symptoms of pinworm parasitic infection. To confirm the diagnosis, the nurse will be ordered to conduct health teaching to the mother on how to perform the scotch tape test wherein a small piece of tape will be attached to the anal opening at night and the tape brought to the clinic in the morning to be examined for pinworm eggs. The nurse also anticipates to administer anti-helminthics.

21. B

BPH is enlargement of the prostate resulting to urine flow obstruction. Symptoms include changes in urinary patterns such as hesitancy, dribbling, decreased force of urine stream, incomplete bladder emptying, nocturia and urgency.

22. B

BPH clients need to void every 2-3 hours to avoid urine stasis that can lead to overflow and infections.

23. B

The enlarged prostate obstructs the flow of urine. The male client will continue to produce semen and it will not affect erection.

24. B

A diet low in fiber is a risk or colorectal cancer while increasing bulk in the diet reduces such risk.

25. C

Dribbling urine seen in prostate enlargement is the intermittent passage of small volumes of urine in the middle of voiding or after voiding. This is due to obstruction of urine flow by the enlarged prostate.

26. A

Difficulty starting or maintaining a urine stream is called urinary hesitancy.

27. C

Nocturia is excessive passing of urine at night causing disrupted sleep patterns. It is common among the elderly male, especially those with prostate enlargement.

28. A

In prostate cancer, the abnormal enlargement of the prostate causes constriction of the urethra thereby obstructing urine flow.

29. C

Risk factors for anorectal cancer include: older age, a personal and family history of colorectal cancer or polyps, inflammatory intestinal conditions, low-fiber, high-fat diet, a sedentary lifestyle, diabetes, obesity, smoking, alcohol and consumption of processed foods.

30. A

Hemorrhoids are varicosities of the veins near the rectum. On examination, the hemorrhoids look bluish. When hemorrhoids get traumatized by the passing of hard tools or by increased abdominal pressure, the varicosities bleed. Scant bleeding will be evident as blood streaks on the toilet paper. With profuse bleeding, blood will leak from the anus.

31. C

A client with hemorrhoids should refrain from doing activities that increase abdominal pressure because these actions may cause the dilated veins to rupture and bleed. Wearing a belt, carrying a load and straining during defecation all increase abdominal pressure.

32. D

An irregular firm mass in the rectum that bleeds is a possible indication of anorectal cancer. The stools of the client may appear pencil-like because of the narrowing of the anal canal.

33. B

Anal fissure is caused by the passage of hard bulky stools through the anal opening that consequently causes the anus to tear and bleed.

34. C

An anal fistula is a small channel that develops between the anal canal, and the skin near the anus. An anal fistula is most commonly caused by an anal abscess. Although causes of abscess formation are often unknown, they are associated with AIDS and inflammatory bowel disorders.

35. B

Clients with anal fistulas will have stools that contain pus and blood because they are the sequelae of abscess formation in the rectum.

36. A

External hemorrhoids are located around the anus. They can be felt when they swell and may cause itching, pain, or bleeding with defecation. Upon inspection, the nurse may note bluish bulges near the anal area.

37. D

Client D has 2 of the risk factors of colorectal cancer which are advanced age and family history of polyps.

38. D

Anuria is non-passage of urine. This is evident in advanced prostate cancer when the enlarged cancerous prostate has completely blocked the ureters.

39. B

Prostatitis is inflammation of the prostate. It is usually caused by a bacterial infection. The prostate becomes swollen, enlarged and filled with pus. The ejaculate and urine contain pus.

40. C

Rectal cancer, like any other cancer, can cause significant weight loss and malaise. Other manifestations of this disorder are rectal bleeding and the presence of a tumor that is hard and irregularly shaped.

41. A, B

The primary risk factors for prostate cancer are advanced age, of African-American race, and with a first-degree relative with prostate cancer.

The Female Genitourinary System

Questions
1. A nurse is examining a female client for genitourinary problems. The nurse palpates the uterus. Which of the following findings should necessitate further evaluation?
   a. Pear-shaped
   b. Fixed and not freely movable
   c. Flattened anteroposteriorly
   d. Anteverted

2. A nurse is conducting teaching to a group of pre-adolescent girls. Which of the following changes should the children anticipate to observe as the first signs of puberty? Select all that apply.
   a. Thelarche
   b. Menarche
   c. Pubic hair development
   d. Increase in height
   e. Increase in appetite

3. A nurse performing a physical examination of a female client's genitalia notes that the pubic hair is coarse, dark and curly, and appearing only over a small area. There are no hairs on the medial thigh. According to Tanner staging, which stage is the client at?
   a. Stage 2
   b. Stage 3
   c. Stage 4
   d. Stage 5

4. A nurse is caring for a pregnant client on her second trimester of pregnancy. Upon physical examination, she notes a bluish hue of the vagina. Which of the following findings should appear on the nurse's documentation?
   a. (+) Goodell sign
   b. (+) Chadwick sign
   c. (+) Hegar Sign
   d. Striae gravidarum

5. A pregnant client in her third gestational month tells the nurse that she is concerned she may have urinary tract infection because she feels like urinating many times. Her urinalysis shows normal WBC and no RBCs. Which of the following should be reflected in the nurse's teaching to account for the client's complaint?
   a. The growing uterus compresses the bladder thereby limiting urine storage space
   b. There is skeletal muscle relaxation during pregnancy
   c. It is due to the folic acid supplement prescribed by the physician
   d. It is due to the use of IUD for contraception prior to being pregnant.

6. An elderly woman asks why her vagina appears smaller, thinner and feels itchy. Which of the

following responses is most appropriate to tell the client?

a. "It is expected of aging."

b. "The decrease in estrogen after menopause causes the vagina to shrink, atrophy, thin and itch."

c. "The vaginal pH becomes more acidic causing the changes."

d. "These appear to be manifestations of a disorder. I will have to inform the physician of your complaint."

7. A nurse is performing the genital area of a female client. The clitoris appears swollen, traumatized and is oozing pus. Upon interview, the client claims that she has undergone genital mutilation as girls her age are also obliged to do. To which cultural/ racial group does such practice exist?

a. European

b. Native Alaskan

c. Aborigines

d. Caucasian

8. A client is diagnosed with uterine polyps and exhibiting signs of menorrhagia. Which of the following correctly describes menorrhagia?

a. Heavy menstrual flow

b. Frequent menstrual cycle

c. Long duration of menses

d. Painful menstruation.

9. A 35-year old female client is concerned that she may have cervical cancer and so she sought medical consultation. Which of the following is the recommended screening for her age?

a. Pap test interval of 2 years

b. Pap test interval of 3 years

c. HPV and Pap smear "co-testing" annually

d. HPV and Pap smear "co-testing" every 5 years

10. A female client comes to the clinic because of fever and malaise. She also reports burning sensation when urinating, and urge to urinate every now and then. She passes scant amount of urine when relieving herself in the toilet. Which of the following conditions is the client most likely manifesting?

a. Dysuria

b. Urinary tract infection

c. Pyelonephritis

d. Urethritis

11. A female client reports passing tea-colored urine, and dull pain at the upper right quadrant of the abdomen. The skin of the client appears yellowish. Which laboratory finding is most significant to check at this time?

a. Urinalysis
b. Liver enzymes
c. Complete blood count
d. T3 T4 levels

12. A nurse is screening for possible child abuse in a 5-year old female client. Which of the following is INAPPROPRIATE to ask the child?
    a. "Is your father or uncle touching you in between your legs?"
    b. "Sometimes that happens to children."
    c. "Children should not think they have been bad."
    d. "Children should try to tell 3 big people that they trust."

13. A woman is to undergo pelvic and genital examination. Which of the following measures would help the client go through the exam comfortably? Select all that apply.
    a. Ask her to urinate before the procedure
    b. Assist the client to assume lithotomy position
    c. Keep the head of the bed flat to facilitate the examination
    d. Tell the client she can say "stop" at any time during the examination
    e. Use deep confident strokes when doing internal examination

14. A 13-year old female client who reports vaginal itching is being seen by the nurse. The client claims to not having engaged in sexual relations yet. Which of the following is expected to be observed in this client?
    a. Vaginal introitus appear as a narrow vertical slit
    b. Cheesy white substance at the vaginal opening
    c. Pubic hair is less coarse, curly and darker than that of an adult
    d. Anal opening is midline and slitlike

15. A newly delivered mother is anxious because she feels something massive in her vagina. She has had a prolonged labor during delivery. Upon examination of her genitalia, the nurse sees a shiny tissue protruding from the vaginal opening. Which of the following condition is the client most likely manifesting?
    a. Vaginal polyp
    b. Pelvic organ prolapse
    c. Abruption placentae
    d. Cervical cancer

16. A nurse is to conduct a speculum examination on a 25-year old female client. Which of the following is NOT an appropriate technique?
    a. Clean the speculum first with cool running water prior to use
    b. Use the dominant hand to hold the equipment and the other hand to support skin and tissue
    c. With the middle and forefingers of the other hand, push the vaginal opening down

d.   Insert the speculum obliquely and downward

17. A 30 year-old client comes to the clinic to be screened for cervical cancer. Which of the following findings during the interview alerts the nurse to a significant risk factor?
    a.   Her mother used Diethyl stilbestrol (DES) while she was pregnant with her
    b.   She smokes 3 sticks of cigarette a day
    c.   She had 3 normal deliveries and one cesarean section
    d.   She had a pap smear 5 years ago

18. A woman is complaining of intense pruritus in the genital area. The nurse performs a genital exam and finds curdy white material with no foul odor inside the vagina. Which of the following findings from client interview most likely indicate the cause of her manifestations?
    a.   14 days intake of aminoglycosides this month
    b.   Sexual contact with long-term boyfriend
    c.   Use of topical steroids
    d.   Use of pH-balanced vaginal wash

19. A female client tested positive to whiff test. Upon microscopic exam of vaginal secretions, 'clue cells' were noted. The vaginal pH also indicates increased alkalinity. These tests confirms the diagnosis of which condition?
    a.   Trichomoniasis
    b.   Bacterial vaginosis
    c.   Candidiasis
    d.   Genital herpes

20. A nurse performing a physical exam palpates the uterus of a female client and notes several small nodes that are firm and tender to palpation. Upon interview, the client states that her menses are painful and irregular, usually less than 3 weeks in frequency and there is heavy flow. The ovaries are also enlarged. Which of the following conditions is the client manifesting?
    a.   Carcinoma of the uterus
    b.   Endometriosis
    c.   Myoma
    d.   Miscarriage

21. A nurse is taking the health history of a client. Which of the following information will be critical in assessing her postmenopausal status?
    a.   Asking about significant weight loss in the last couple of months
    b.   Asking about her nightly sleep patterns
    c.   Asking about her religious affiliations
    d.   Asking about her pregnancies and deliveries

22. The nurse is assisting with community service of screening for sexually transmitted diseases.

Which of the following is the nurse's primary role in relation to sexually transmitted diseases?
a. Recognizing symptoms and health teaching
b. Case reporting
c. Diagnosis and treatment
d. Sexual counseling

23. A young woman in her early twenties has been recently diagnosed with gonorrhea. She asks the nurse what would happen if she goes without treatment. What is the most appropriate nursing response?
a. "It can result in disseminated systemic infections."
b. "It can result to early termination of all future pregnancies."
c. "It can cause sterility, birth defects and miscarriage"
d. "Don't worry about it now. The most important thing is that you receive treatment."

24. A nurse is conducting a seminar on sexual practices to young adolescent girls in the clinic. Which of the following client response needs further reinforcement of health teachings?
a. "We are sure to use KY jelly on condoms."
b. "I will shower with my boyfriend."
c. "I will douche after intercourse."
d. "I will urinate after intercourse."

25. A woman comes to the outpatient department complaining of fatigue, weight gain, dysmenorrhea, heartburn and constipation. Which of the symptoms above indicate the possibility of endometriosis?
a. Fatigue and weight gain
b. Dysmenorrhea
c. Heartburn
d. Constipation

26. A 36-yearold woman has been found positive of candida albicans. Which of the following would the nurse expect to find during physical examination?
a. Thin, malodorous yellowish green discharge
b. Yellowish discharge, no foul odor, scant discharge
c. Thick and white, cottage cheese-like texture
d. Off-white with a fishy odor discharge

27. A young pregnant mother who has been recently diagnosed with syphilis asks the nurse why she needs to be treated even when she doesn't have any symptoms at all. What is the best nursing response?
a. "Syphilis can also infect the baby and cause it to die before being birthed if you are not treated."
b. "Syphilis can cause blindness in your baby"
c. "Untreated syphilis can cause severe mental retardation in your child."

d.   "Syphilis will cause multi-organ failure in your baby."

28. A nurse is conducting a seminar on breast self-examination. Which of the following information should be included in her teaching?
    a.   BSE should be conducted before the start of the monthly menses.
    b.   BSE should be conducted 5-7 days from the start of the monthly period
    c.   BSE should be done at least once a year
    d.   BSE is the most accurate method of determining breast cancer.

29. A nurse is conducting breast self-examination to a group of teenage girls. Which of the following should the nurse teach as a finding to be reported immediately to the doctor?
    a.   Breast tenderness 3 days before the start of the monthly menses.
    b.   Several movable tender lumps on both breasts few days before the start of the monthly period.
    c.   A fixed immovable and hard lump on the upper outer quadrant of one breast
    d.   Nipple stiffness when removing undergarments

30. A teenage girl confides to the nurse that there are days in a month that she is more irritable than usual and sometimes she feels like crying for no reason. She also states that sometimes she notices that her breasts and hands become slightly swollen. She also feels some unexplained minor aches in her body. All her symptoms appear a few days before her monthly period. Which of the following is the client most probably having?
    a.   Premenstrual syndrome
    b.   Primary dysmenorrhea
    c.   Secondary dysmenorrhea
    d.   Depression

31. An 18-year old frail girl has been recently diagnosed with primary amenorrhea. The nurse understands that the diagnosis of primary amenorrhea is only established in which of the following conditions?
    a.   Absence of menses at age 14 and no growth noted or no development of secondary sexual characteristics
    b.   Absence of menses by age 18 years with normal development of secondary sexual characteristics.
    c.   No breast development is evident at 13 years
    d.   No menarche at 18 years of age

32. A 46-year old woman is asking the nurse about menopause. Which of the following statements is NOT true?
    a.   Menopause is caused by a period of fluctuation in pituitary secretion of follicle-stimulating hormone (FSH) and luteinizing hormone (LH) and ovarian function
    b.   Menopausal women experience vasomotor symptoms as hot flashes, flushing, and sweating

c. The advantage of menopause is that client reports better sleeping patterns
d. Menopausal women usually reports vaginal dryness

33. A 56-year old woman who ceased to have periods for 5 years now has reported to the nurse that she started bleeding again. Which of the following conditions is NOT a probable cause of post-menopausal bleeding?
a. endometrial cancer
b. hormone replacement therapy
c. uterine and cervical polyps
d. syphilis

34. A female client confides to the nurse that she experiences pain during sexual intercourse specifically during the time of penetration. She feels it deep inside her. Which is the most probable cause for the client's discomfort?
a. inflammation
b. atrophic vaginitis
c. inadequate lubrication
d. pelvic inflammatory disorder

35. The nurse is to conduct a pelvic examination of a female client. Which of the following is NOT indicated for this examination?
a. Instructions to client to avoid intercourse, douching, or use of vaginal suppositories for 24 to 48 hours before examination
b. Nurse asks the client to empty bladder before examination
c. The nurse washes the speculum with cold running water
d. Nurse obtains client consent before examination.

36. A 14-year girl comes to the clinic to have her scheduled examination. After doing the pelvic exam, the nurse notes lacerations in her vagina. The client is withdrawn but is complying with the nurses' instructions. What is the priority nursing action?
a. Inform the nursing supervisor immediately
b. Sit with the client and encourage the client to verbalize feelings
c. Wash her genitalia with warm water
d. Instruct her to void after examination

37. A female client comes to an STD clinic for a consult on her condition. She complains of severe itching of her vulva. Upon examination, the nurse notes a reddened, inflamed excoriated vulva with thick white non-odorous discharge. The nurse understands that the client probably has what infection?
a. Trichomonal vaginitis
b. Candida albicans
c. Bacterial vaginitis

    d. Syphilis

38. A nurse is seeing a client in the STD clinic. She collects a specimen from a female client's vaginal discharge for the whiff test. Which of the following diseases is the whiff test applicable?
    a. Trichomonal vaginitis
    b. Candida albicans
    c. Bacterial vaginosis
    d. Syphilis

39. A nurse conducting a pelvic examination of a female client notes a muscular cylindrical organ protruding from the vaginal opening. The nurse suspects which condition?
    a. Uterine prolapse
    b. Genital warts
    c. Epidermoid cysts
    d. Chancroid

40. The nurse notes several pimple-like nodules on a female client's vulva. The nodes appear yellowish and are nontender. Which of the following is the client most probably having?
    a. Condylomata acuminata
    b. Epidermoid cysts
    c. Syphilitic chancre
    d. Genital herpes

41. Before taking the patient's history regarding sexual orientation and gender identity, which of the following is important for the nurse to do first?
    a. Identify different types of in vitro fertilization
    b. Reflect on their own biases regarding sexual orientation and gender identity
    c. Learn how to be straightforward and strict with questioning
    d. Prepare health teaching materials on the use of contraceptives

42. A female patient is showing signs of weakened pelvic floor muscles. She has recently lost urine and bowel control. Which of the following in the patient's history is significant and the most probable cause of the patient's symptoms?
    a. Sedentary lifestyle
    b. Significant weight loss
    c. Recent HPV immunization
    d. Recent vaginal delivery of macrosomic twins

43. A 50-year-old female patient tells the nurse that her menses have disrupted patterns. At some months the flow is heavy, at some months the flow is scant. There are times when there is no flow at all. The frequency and duration of menses also changed. The patient adds that there are a few times that they feel hot all over even if the room temperature is comfortable. Which of the

following condition is the patient experiencing?
a. Menarche
b. Menopause
c. Perimenopause
d. Pre-menstrual syndrome

44. A patient is having premenstrual syndrome (PMS). Which of the following information about PMS is INCORRECT?
a. The patient may experience angry outbursts, irritability or anxiety
b. There may be bloating and weight gain
c. The patient may complain of generalized aches and pains
d. Signs and symptoms must be present ten days prior to menses for a minimum of two cycles

45. A 15-year-old patient who has anorexia nervosa has stopped menstruating. Which of the following is the correct documentation of the patient's symptom?
a. Primary amenorrhea
b. Secondary amenorrhea
c. Menorrhagia
d. Dysmenorrhea

46. When the nurse asks about the patient's menstruation, the patient narrates that in between their periods, there is some bleeding that lasts for about two days. Which of the following describes the patient's symptom?
a. Polymenorrhea
b. Menorrhagia
c. Metrorrhagia
d. Postcoital bleeding

47. A female patient confides to the nurse that they experience pain during intercourse. Which of the following follow-up question is most appropriate to ask the patient?
a. "When do you feel the pain, at the start of intercourse near the outside, or in the middle of the sexual act when your partner is deep?"
b. "Which is more painful, the pain outside or the pain inside?"
c. "When was your last intercourse?"
d. "What medication do you take for the pain?"

48. A nurse is assisting a patient to undergo a pelvic examination. Which of the following patient responses indicate that the pelvic examination will need to be rescheduled?
a. "I urinated a few minutes ago."
b. "I douched myself to prepare for this exam."
c. "I feel uneasy when exposing myself even to my doctor."
d. "What could the results be?"

49. Which of the following is included in the current recommended cervical screening for women?
    a. Start screening by age 25
    b. Perform cytology exams every year until the age of 65
    c. By age 50, start HPV testing with cytology
    d. After 65 years of age, no need to test if the last three exams performed on schedule are negative

50. A mother is pregnant for the third time and is already in her second trimester. Her first two children were born at term, and both are still living. She had no previous abortions. Which of the following gynecological data of the patient is correct?
    a. G3P3 (F2, P3, A0, L2)
    b. G3P3 (F0, P3, A0, L3)
    c. G3P2 (F2, P0, A0, L2)
    d. G2P3 (F2, P0, A2, L0)

51. A female patient confides to the nurse that they feel intense itch of their vagina. They have a curdy vaginal discharge that looked like "cottage cheese." When asked if they have noticed any foul odor, the patient says none. She also says that it hurt when she has sexual intercourse. Which of the following conditions most likely caused the patient's signs and symptoms?
    a. Trichomonas vaginalis infection
    b. Candida albicans infection
    c. Bacterial vaginosis
    d. Syphilis

52. A patient tested positive for trichomonads after a saline wet mount. Other than pruritus and vaginal redness, the patient will also have a vaginal discharge. Which of the following characteristics of vaginal discharges will the patient exhibit?
    a. White, curd-like, non-odorous
    b. Yellowish green, profuse, frothy, malodorous
    c. Grayish, thin, small amount, fishy smell
    d. Scant, blood-streaked

53. A nurse is to assess the presence of stress incontinence in a patient. Which of the following questions will correctly ask about stress incontinence?
    a. "Do you rush to the toilet to pass urine but do not get there in time?"
    b. "Does coughing, sneezing, or laughing cause you to lose urine?"
    c. "Do you have difficulty passing urine?"
    d. "Does it hurt when you pass urine?"

54. A patient comes to the emergency department with a primary complaint of dull aching pain that "does not seem to go away." The pain is felt below the posterior costal margin near the

costovertebral angle. Further examination reveals that the patient also has fever and chills. Urinalysis shows microscopic hematuria and increased WBC. Which type of pain should the nurse document in the patient's health record?
a. Flank pain
b. Ureteral colic
c. Visceral pain
d. Parietal pain

55. Which of the following will correctly assess for costovertebral tenderness through percussion?
a. Place the finger pads of the pleximeter finger on the costovertebral angle and strike hard with the plexor finger
b. Place the ball of one hand in the costovertebral angle and strike it with the ulnar surface of the fist
c. Place the finger pads of the pleximeter finger below the costal margin and strike hard with the plexor finger
d. Strike the area of the costovertebral angle with the ulnar surface of the fist

ANSWERS

1. B

   A normal uterus would feel pear-shaped, freely movable mass that is tilted forward just superior to the bladder.

2. A, C

   First signs of puberty in girls are breast development (thelarche) and pubic hair development. These are observed first before menarche or first menstruation that usually happens two years after.

3. C

   According to the Tanner staging of pubic hair development, the client is at stage 4.
   Stage 1 Preadolescent. There are no pubic hairs yet.
   Stage 2 Thin slightly pigmented hair straight or wavy hair appear sparsely gown on the labia
   Stage 3 The hair becomes darker, coarser, curlier and spreads to the mons pubis
   Stage 4 Hair is adult in type, coarse, dark, curly and longer but over smaller area; No hairs present on the medial thigh.
   Stage 5 Hair is adult in type, coarse, dark, curly, longer and thicker appearing as an inverted triangle and include areas in the medial thigh

4. B

   Chadwick sign is the bluish discoloration of the vagina and cervix due to increased vascularity in the area.

5. A

   A pregnant client on her first trimester will complain of urinary frequency because the growing uterus exerts a pressure on the bladder, which prevents it from expanding to store larger amounts of urine.

6. B

   Telling the client that the changes are caused by a decreased of estrogen after menopause provides facts. Although they are age-related changes, telling the client that is being insensitive and does not provide any information.

7. C

   The Aborigines, some Christian denominations, Muslims, West and East Asians, people from the Middle East and Africa practice female genital mutilation.

8. A

   Menorrhagia means heavy menstrual flow. A client with menorrhagia will report frequent pad/tampon changes because they are easily soaked.

9. D

New recommendations for cervical cancer screening for women is:

21 years old and below: no pap tests regardless of sexual activity

21-30 years old: pap test every 3 years

30-65 years old: co testing of HPV and Pap smear every five years

10. B

The signs and symptoms manifested by the client: malaise, fever, dysuria indicate urinary tract infection. If the patient experiences flank pain with these manifestations, it indicates possible pyelonephritis.

11. B

Tea-colored urine when accompanied by other signs and symptoms like dull or colicky right upper quadrant pain and jaundice, may indicate liver disease or biliary obstruction. The liver function test is the most significant to check at this point although other tests can also be performed.

12. A

When screening for sexual abuse in children, the nurse should NOT ask directive or suggestive questions. This may inhibit the child to talk or may cause undue embarrassment.

13. A, B, D

Before a pelvic or genital examination using the lithotomy position, it is important to ask the client to empty her bladder first so that she does not have to relieve herself in the middle of the procedure. The nurse should also position the table so that the perineal area is not exposed to people who may enter the door. Drapes must be secured. The client should be asked to put on a hospital gown, and then to remove underpants. She should be assisted to assume a lithotomy position. The nurse uses slow gentle yet firm touch during internal examination. The client is also instructed to say 'stop' if she wishes at any point in the procedure.

14. A

A client who has not engaged in sexual relations will have a vaginal opening that is narrow and with a vertical slit.

15. B

Pelvic organ prolapse happens because of weak musculature of the pelvis. The vaginal wall, cervix or uterus may protrude out of the vagina. The client may report something massive is felt inside the vagina or feels like sitting on a ball. Bleeding and increased vaginal discharge may accompany the protrusion.

16. A

The speculum should be warmed with warm running water to facilitate comfort upon insertion.

17. A

Di-ethylstilbestrol os DES is synthetic estrogen prescribed until 1970's for woman who had miscarriages or premature deliveries. It is found to cause cancer of the reproductive organs of the children whose mother received the estrogen while pregnant with them.

18. A

The intake of antibiotics like aminoglycosides alter normal flora of the body including vaginal flora. It encourages the growth of the fungi candida. Candidiasis is manifested by intense genital pruritus, and cottage-cheese-like discharge without any foul odor.

19. B

A client with bacterial vaginosis will test positive to whiff test. Vaginal pH will show an alkaline environment. Microscopic exam of the vaginal specimen will reveal characteristic "clue cells."

20. B

Endometrioses are myometrial-like growths outside the uterus that also react to hormonal changes like the myometrium of the uterus. The client will experience heavy or irregular menses and dysmenorrhea. The ovaries will be enlarged.

21. B

Postmenopausal women experience vasomotor instability that cause night sweats and interrupted sleep.

22. A

Early recognition of STD's reduces the risk of serious complications as well as helps prevent its spread through health teaching. The critical role of the nurse is to recognize symptoms of STD's in order to teach clients how to comply with medication and treatments, and how to prevent reinfection and spread.

23. C

Untreated gonorrhea can result to birth defects, sterility, and miscarriage. It is the nurse's role to provide health teachings on the importance of complying with treatment and of prevention of reinfection and spread of sexually transmitted disease.

24. C

Douching does not prevent the spread of sexually transmitted diseases and can also cause alteration of the normal flora and protective barriers of the vagina.

25. B

Pelvic pain related to menstruation (dysmenorrhea) is the most common symptom of endometriosis. The pain usually ends when the menses stop.

26. C

Candida albicans is a fungal infection of the vagina. The nurse notes redness and some degree of inflammation of the vulva. Itching is reported by the client. The discharge is white and thick like cottage cheese. It is not odorous.

27. A

Syphilis is associated with stillbirth, premature birth and neonatal death.

28. B

The breasts are softer and less tender and with less hormonal influence about a week from the start of the monthly period.

29. C

Lumps that are felt on one breast that are hard and fixed on the chest wall should be further evaluated for the possibility of breast cancer.

30. A

Premenstrual syndrome (PMS) includes emotional and behavioral symptoms such as depression, angry outbursts, irritability, anxiety, and confusion; also of crying for no reason, sleep disturbance, poor focus, and even social withdrawal. There can also be reports of bloating and weight gain, swelling of the hands and feet, and generalized aches and pains. To be diagnosed with premenstrual syndrome, the onset of signs and symptoms should have started 5 days prior to menses for at least three consecutive cycles and the disappearance of manifestations of PMS 4 days after onset of menses. There should also be reports of interference with daily activities.

31. A

Primary amenorrhea is defined either as absence of menses by age 14 years with the absence of growth or development of secondary sexual characteristics (eg, breast development) or as absence of menses by age 16 years with normal development of secondary sexual characteristics.

32. C

Menopause usually occurs between 48 and 55 years, following a period of fluctuation in pituitary secretion of follicle-stimulating hormone (FSH) and luteinizing hormone (LH) and ovarian function. The client also experiences vasomotor symptoms as hot flashes, flushing, and sweating. Sleep disturbances are also reported. After menopause, there may be vaginal dryness and dyspareunia.

33. D

Postmenopausal bleeding is evident in endometrial cancer, hormone replacement therapy, and uterine and cervical polyps.

34. D

Superficial pain of dyspareunia (pain or discomfort during intercourse) suggests local inflammation, atrophic vaginitis, or inadequate lubrication; deeper pain may be from pelvic disorders or pressure on a normal ovary.

35. C

For a successful pelvic examination, the nurse instructs the client to avoid intercourse, douching, or use of vaginal suppositories for 24 to 48 hours before examination. She asks the client to empty the bladder before examination. The nurse also obtains permission, acts as chaperone and provides explanations for the procedure. The nurse also warms speculum with warm water.

36. A

In suspected cases of sexual abuse, the nurse keeps the client safe and informs the nursing supervisor immediately so that the case may be reported to the authorities. If the abuse is suspected to have happened recently, the nurse is also responsible in preserving evidence for legal purposes by not washing the client's genitalia or by not allowing the client to take a bath.

37. B

Candida albicans is a yeast infection that may be the result of overgrowth of vaginal flora. The client experiences pruritus, vaginal soreness, excoriation, pain on urination (from skin inflammation) and dyspareunia. The vulva is often inflamed and sometimes swollen. Vaginal discharge is white and curdy; may be thin but is typically thick.

38. C

The whiff test is used to help sniff for fishy odor after applying KOH to a vaginal discharge specific to bacterial vaginosis.

39. A

Uterine prolapse occurs when the uterus protrudes into the vagina. The protruding part appears smooth cylindrical and muscular.

40. B

Epidermoid cysts are small, firm, round cystic nodules in the labia that appear yellowish in color. A dark punctum can be noted marking the blocked opening of the gland.

41. B

Before discussing sexual orientation and gender identity information with the patient, it is important to reflect on one's own biases to be able to render proper care. Throughout the interaction with the patient, the nurse must use a neutral and supportive approach to cater to the patient's well-being.

42. D

The weakening of the pelvic floor muscles is commonly caused by advanced age, pelvic surgery or trauma, multiple gestations, vaginal delivery, and medical conditions that affect muscles and nerves to the pelvic area. Signs of weak pelvic muscles include urinary and fecal incontinence, pain, and pelvic organ prolapse.

43. C

Perimenopause is the period before menopause. The patient's menstrual cycle and pattern changes. Some symptoms of menopause may also be felt, such as hot flushes and headaches.

44. D

Premenstrual syndrome (PMS) is a collection of emotional and behavioral symptoms that are experienced within the five days before menstruation. The signs and symptoms should all have disappeared by the 5th day of the start of the monthly flow. The pattern should be evident for three consecutive cycles. Signs and symptoms of PMS include anxiety, depression, anger, irritability, crying spells and sleep disturbances, among others.

45. B

Secondary amenorrhea is the cessation of menses after they have been established in the patient. Anorexia nervosa is one example of a condition that causes secondary amenorrhea.

46. C

Metroragghia is bleeding in between menses. Menorrhagia is excessive bleeding during menstruation. Polymenorrhea is having menstruation cycles that are shorter than 21 days. Postcoital bleeding is bleeding after sexual intercourse.

47. A

Dyspareunia is pain or discomfort during intercourse. When a patient says that they experience dyspareunia, the nurse must explore further by asking where and when they feel the pain. This follow-up data-gathering localizes the symptom so that the nurse would be able to determine possible causes of the patient's symptom. Superficial pain is likely caused by inflammation, atrophic vaginitis, or inadequate lubrication. On the other hand, pain that is felt deeper during the sexual act may be caused by pelvic inflammation and other disorders.

48. B

For pelvic examinations, the nurse must instruct the patient to avoid intercourse, douching, and using tampons and vaginal medications for 24 hours before the scheduled examination. Doing so will change the normal condition of the vagina for obtaining an accurate baseline result.

49. D

The current recommendation for cervical cancer screening is to start screening women at age 21. Cytology should be performed every three years thereafter until the age of 65. By age 30, women may opt to have HPV testing with cytology every five years instead of the 3-year interval, cytology-only exam. After age 65, screening stops if in the last three scheduled cytology-only exam or the last two cytology + HPV testing are negative.

50. C
    G refers to gravida, the number of times the patient got pregnant regardless of outcome. P refers to para or parity, the number of pregnancies wherein the fetus reached a viable age. F refers to full-term or delivered at least at 37th week of gestation. P refers to pre-term births or deliveries after 20 weeks but before 37 weeks. A refers to abortion or births that did not reach the age of viability whether induced or spontaneous, and L refers to live births.

51. B
    Candida albicans is a yeast that causes intense pruritus of the vagina. There is white curdy cheese-like odorless discharge. The vulva is inflamed. The patient will also most likely report dyspareunia.

52. B
    The vaginal discharge of women with trichomonal vaginitis is yellowish green or gray that is profuse, frothy and malodorous. Women with trichomonal vaginitis would also have pruritus, vaginal erythema, dysuria, and dyspareunia.

53. B
    Stress incontinence is urine leakage during an increase in abdominal pressure, such as when coughing, sneezing or laughing.

54. A
    Flank pain is also known as kidney pain, and it is produced by the distention of the renal capsule in acute pyelonephritis. Kidney pain is dull, aching, and steady, and specifically felt near the costovertebral angle. The pain may radiate to the front toward the umbilicus.

55. B
    To assess for costovertebral tenderness, the nurse should place the ball of their non-dominant hand in the costovertebral angle and strikes it with the ulnar surface of their other fist. The force should be strong enough as to cause a perceptible thud. When pain is felt in the costovertebral angle, it suggests pyelonephritis.

Assessing Children

Questions
1. The nurse is taking blood pressure measurements in a 5 month old infant using a pediatric cuff. Upon assessment, she noticed that blood pressure on her thigh is lower than that of her arms. She also appears flushed on her face and pale on her lower extremities. Which of the following should the nurse suspect?
   a. Patent ductus arteriosus
   b. Trigeminal neuralgia
   c. Coarctation of the aorta
   d. Heart failure

2. During the assessment of a 2-day old newborn, the nurse notes bruising and cephalhematoma. The baby also appears jaundiced. The nurse observes the mother breastfeeding her newborn. What is the most probable interpretation of the jaundice?
   a. Pathologic jaundice that necessitates blood transfusion
   b. Hyperbilirubenemia due to the bruising and cephalhematoma
   c. Breast milk jaundice
   d. Hyperbilirubinemia caused by Rh incompatibility

3. A 4-year old child is accompanied by his mother to the emergency room because of high fever and difficulty swallowing. Upon assessment of the mouth and pharynx, the nurse notes that the tongue is strawberry-like, and the tonsils are swollen with yellowish exudates. The uvula is erythematous and there are pinpoint red rashes on the inner cheeks. Which of the following is the priority nursing action?
   a. Institute droplet precaution
   b. Inform the physician
   c. Provide nourishment and hydration
   d. Keep the child in restraints

4. A newborn weighs 1.45kg and has weak and extended extremities. The baby's pinna is flat and do not easily recoil. The soles have deep indentation at the upper third part. The nurse also was able to palpate very little breast tissue. Based on the findings, which is the most probable gestational age of the baby?
   a. Full-term infant 38-42 weeks gestation
   b. Premature infant <24 weeks
   c. Premature at 29-33 weeks gestation
   d. Postterm >42 weeks

5. A full term infant has tachypnea, nasal flaring and intercostal retractions that have been unresolved for 6 hours. IV fluids and oxygen therapy have been instituted. Which of the following assessments indicate that the baby's condition is improving?
   a. The baby has rapid deep respirations with occasional grunting sounds
   b. RR is 45, pulse at 130, no nasal flaring

c.   Weight gain of 150g within 12 hours of birth

d.   SaO2 of 84%

6.   A mother brings her child for his routine immunization. The nurse noticed that the child has short palpebral fissures, thin lips and a flattened and wide philtrum. On further assessment, the head circumference is small for gestational age. Which of the following is most likely the cause of her findings?

a.   Down dyndrome

b.   Fetal alcohol syndrome

c.   Turner's syndrome

d.   Cerebral palsy

7.   A girl was born at 10:15 am. 5 minutes later, the nurse finds her heart rate is at 135 bpm, and that she is crying vigorously and moving all her extremities. Her hands and feet are lightly bluish while the rest of the body is pinkish. Based on the nurse's finding, what is the baby's Apgar score?

a.   10

b.   9

c.   8

d.   7

8.   Which of the following assessment findings in a newborn baby is considered normal?

a.   Passage of green sticky stools within the first 24 hours

b.   Respirations of 75 per minute while at rest

c.   Yellowish skin and sclera after 6 hours of birth

d.   Frank bleeding at the umbilicus

9.   A new mother asks the nurse how much weight loss is expected of the baby after birth. The most accurate reply is

a.   10-15%

b.   5-8%

c.   4%

d.   None

10. The nurse is assessing a 3-hour old newborn while in the nursery. Which of the following findings should the nurse document as abnormal?

a.   Chest circumference 34 cm; Head circumference 32 cm

b.   Two 'soft spots' between cranial bones

c.   Bluish discolorations at the lumbar area

d.   Pinpoint white spots on the baby's nose

11. The nurse collects the following data while assessing a 3-hour old baby. Bluish hands and feet, pinkish body; bluish discolorations on the lumbosacral area, a reddish mark on the face and

pinpoint white spots on the nose. What is the best nursing action for these findings?
a. Document findings as within normal range
b. Institute airborne precaution
c. Refer to a dermatologist
d. Assess nutritional status

12. A nurse is preparing a 3-day old newborn for discharge. As she evaluates the baby, she observes a yellowish tinge on the client's forehead after briefly pressing the skin. The nurse understands that this indicates
a. An infectious liver disorder
b. A normal biologic response
c. An Rh incompatibility problem
d. Related to breastfeeding

13. A 6-year old girl is brought to the clinic by her parents because of fever and painful urination. After careful assessments and laboratory work, she was diagnosed with urinary tract infection. Which of the following parent response indicate a probable cause of her infection?
a. "She likes running around the backyard with our dog."
b. "She enjoys her bubble baths so much."
c. "She is picky with foods and is challenging to feed."
d. "She runs to the bathroom every time she feels she has to pee."

14. A nurse assessing an 8-year old found him positive for the trendelenburg sign. Which of the following is a correct interpretation of this finding?
a. The knees flex when the neck is flexed
b. The pelvis tilts toward the unaffected hip when asked to stand on the leg of the affected side
c. The pelvis tilts toward the affected side when asked to stand on the leg of the affected side
d. There is resistance when the neck is flexed

15. An adolescent has confided in the nurse and requests for confidentiality. Which of the following client responses will prompt the nurse to tell the client that she needs to report their conversation?
a. "I have two boyfriends whom I have sex with at least twice a week."
b. "I masturbate while looking at a mirror."
c. "I plan to use my father's gun on me tonight."
d. "I have an embarrassing vaginal itch and odor."

16. A nurse is assessing a 1-year old infant presenting with honey-colored crusty lesions on the face and the neck. The infant's mother states that the lesions started as a single insect bite-like itch that has become raised and bullous that drains yellowish fluid. It has apparently spread in a span of 1 week. Which skin condition is the baby most likely suffering from?
a. Neurofibromatosis
b. Tinea flava

c. Candida dermatitis
d. Impetigo

17. The nurse is assessing the head and scalp of an adolescent boy and notices a hairless patch on the client's scalp. Further assessment reveals an enlarged lymph node near the nape. What is the most appropriate explanation for this?
    a. Tinea corporis
    b. Tinea capitis
    c. Candida dermatitis
    d. Congenital alopecia

18. A nurse is caring for a school aged boy with Down's syndrome. Which of the following findings is not consistent with this condition?
    a. Simian crease across the palm
    b. Low set ears
    c. Flat and wide philtrum
    d. Flat nasal bridge

19. A 3-year old boy is crying and complaining of pain in his right ear. Otoscopy reveals red, distorted, bulging tympanic membrane in the right ear. Which of the following in the client's history indicate a probable cause for the client's signs and symptoms?
    a. Upper respiratory tract infection 5 days ago
    b. Missed MMR vaccine
    c. Constant chewing of gum
    d. Increased intake of sweets for the last 3 days

20. Which of the following findings in the assessment of the genitalia will prompt the nurse to summon the nursing supervisor immediately?
    a. Healed hymenal transections in the female genitalia of a 4-year old
    b. Undescended testis in a male infant
    c. A blood stained scant discharge on a female newborn's genitalia
    d. Areola that has receded to the general contour of the breast in a 15 year old female

21. A nurse is assessing an 18-month old infant. The nurse is to perform several assessments. Which of the following should the nurse perform last?
    a. Assessment of the symmetry of the eyes
    b. Check for fontanelles
    c. Test for convergence
    d. Otoscopy

22. Children can be assessed by determining if they have reached or performed milestones that are typical for their age. Which principle of child development is this describing?

a. Child development proceeds along a predictable pathway
b. The range of normal development is wide.
c. Various physical, social and environmental factors, as well as diseases, can affect child development and health.
d. The child's developmental level affects how the nurse conducts the history and physical examination.

23. Which of the following questions assesses for safety measures employed by parents for their infant?
    a. "Did you notice any problems with your baby's ability to make sounds?"
    b. "What medications did you take while you were pregnant?"
    c. "In what position does your baby sleep?
    d. "Did your baby have any reaction to the shots?"

24. Which of the following examination procedures done on a 20-month old baby, if performed by the nurse, indicates a need for further teaching?
    a. Allow the mother time to breastfeed her baby when the baby gets cranky during the examination
    b. The nurse does not strictly follow the head-to-toe assessment
    c. The nurse takes the baby to the examination room while the mother waits in the waiting area
    d. The nurse uses a rattle to distract the baby

25. The nurse uses the DENVER II Screening Test to assess a 5-year old male patient. Which of the following parameters will the DENVER II Screening Test NOT assess?
    a. Personal-social
    b. Gross motor
    c. Language
    d. Intelligence

26. The nurse is to measure a 3-month old patient's weight using an infant scale. Which of the following is best for the nurse to do?
    a. Let the mother cuddle the baby while their weights are taken, and then weigh the mother alone and subtract the measurements to get the baby's weight
    b. Let the mother hold the baby while being weighed to prevent anxiety in the baby
    c. Remove all clothes except the diaper and the undershirt
    d. Weigh the baby naked

27. A nurse takes an infant's blood pressure measurements and notes a sustained elevation of blood pressure. Which of the following conditions would possibly cause sustained hypertension in infants?
    a. Coarctation of the aorta
    b. Hypoxia

c. Drug ingestion
d. Heart block

28. Which of the following techniques of counting respiratory rates in infants is correct?
    a. Count for 2 full minutes in a squirming infant
    b. Count a full minute in a quietly sleeping infant
    c. Count for at least 30 seconds in infants with periodic breathing
    d. Count for 2 full minutes in infants with diaphragmatic breathing

29. A nurse observes jaundice in a newborn. Which of the following characteristics of jaundice is NOT normal.
    a. Jaundice that is apparent in the sclerae
    b. Jaundice appearing on the 5th day of birth after breastfeeding
    c. Jaundice that is present on the 4th week of life
    d. Jaundice that is evident in the buccal mucosa of a dark-skinned infant

30. A nurse is assessing the back of an Asian newborn and notes a bluish gray discoloration in the lumbosacral region. Which of the following is the correct documentation entry for the nurse's findings?
    a. Mongolian spots
    b. Stork bite
    c. Spider nevus
    d. Café-au-lait spots

31. A nurse assessing a 9-year old patient finds that the patient is positive for Trendelenburg sign. Which of the following correctly describes the nurse's findings?
    a. The pelvis remains level when weight is shifted from one foot to the other
    b. The pelvis tilts toward the unaffected hip when weight is shifted from one foot to the other
    c. The pelvis tilts toward the affected hip when weight is shifted from one foot to the other
    d. The patient would be outbalanced when they attempt to shift their weight from one foot to the other

32. A 4-year old patient is seen by the nurse standing up by rolling on their abdomen before pushing off with their arms to prop themselves up before standing up. Which of the following refers to the patient's manifestations?
    a. Gower sign
    b. Ataxia
    c. Talipes equinovarus
    d. Turner's syndrome

33. A nurse asks a 5-year old child to stick out their tongue all the way. Which cranial nerve is the nurse assessing?

a. VII
b. IX
c. XII
d. V

34. Which of the following reflects anticipatory guidance for a school-aged child?
    a. The use of a rear-facing car seat
    b. The use of helmets and protective pads when riding a bicycle
    c. The use of floaters when bathing in a tub
    d. The use of condoms when engaging in sexual behavior

35. A nurse wants to assess an adolescent client and ask about their sexual health. Which of the following questions would be most therapeutic and would most likely elicit the cooperation of the patient?
    a. "Other kids your age often have questions about sex and relationships. You can ask me any questions."
    b. "Are you having sex already?"
    c. "It's really ok having a boyfriend. You can count on me to make our conversation confidential. Are you having sex?"
    d. "I am your nurse, and it is important that you are honest with me. Are you sexually active?"

36. A nurse is determining the sexual maturity of an adolescent girl. As the nurse examines the labia, and some growth of pubic hair is noted. The hairs are straight and downy. Using the Tanner staging, what is the stage of sexual maturity of the patient?
    a. Stage 1
    b. Stage 2
    c. Stage 3
    d. Stage 4

37. A nurse is performing the plumb line test. Which of the following disorders is the nurse trying to assess the patient for?
    a. Incoordination
    b. Seizure
    c. Presyncope
    d. Scoliosis

38. A 3-month old patient has reddish appearing rashes in the diaper area. The patient is showing signs of irritation as the perianal area is cleaned. Which of the following factors most probably triggered the patient's manifestations?
    a. Breastfeeding
    b. Intake of cough medications
    c. Dehydration

    d.   Diarrhea

39. As the nurse is examining a 5-year-old patient's scalp, the nurse notes patches of hair loss with some scaling of the bald areas. Which of the following microorganism most probably caused the patient's manifestations?
    a.   Bacteria
    b.   Fungi
    c.   Virus
    d.   Protozoan

40. A nurse is examining a 3-year old male patient. The nurse noticed that the child appears small for his age. The child has a small head with a flat philtrum and thin upper lips. Which of the following would be noted in the mother's prenatal history?
    a.   Heroin abuse
    b.   Alcohol abuse
    c.   Malnutrition
    d.   Gestational diabetes

41. A 2-year old male patient is being assessed by the nurse. The toddler has a flattened nasal bridge, oblique short palpebral fissure, and a palmar crease is prominent transversing the entire palm horizontally. Which of the following most likely suggest the patient's manifestations?
    a.   Down's syndrome
    b.   Tetralogy of Fallot
    c.   Congenital hypothyroidism
    d.   Fetal alcohol syndrome

42. A nurse is assessing a newborn with patent ductus arteriosus. Which of the following findings would the nurse most likely note in the patient?
    a.   Low heart rate and peripheral cyanosis
    b.   Continuous hypertension
    c.   Full bounding pulses, hyperdynamic precordium, atypical murmur
    d.   Intense generalized cyanosis with marked signs of heart failure

43. Which of the following assessment findings suggest a possible sexual abuse in a young child?
    a.   Pain in the lower abdomen in a 3-year-old male
    b.   Marked dilatation of the anus of a 2-year-old male when examined in the knee-chest position
    c.   Prominent mons pubis in a 2-year-old female
    d.   Painful scant urination in a 3-year old female

44. A male newborn was assessed by the nurse and found to have hypospadias. Which of the following will be found in the patient?
    a.   The urethral meatus opens abnormally on the ventral side of the penis

b.   The urethral meatus opens abnormally on the dorsal side of the penis
c.   The testis is felt in the inguinal area
d.   The prepuce cannot be retracted

45. A 5-year-old child is exhibiting fever with violent coughs that feels like it is difficult to stop. After several bouts of hacking coughing, the patient struggles to catch breath producing the 'whoop' sound. Which of the following childhood disorders produce these symptoms?
a.   Rubella
b.   Mumps
c.   Diphtheria
d.   Pertusssis

ANSWERS

1. C

    In children, as well as in adults, systolic blood pressure readings from the thigh are approximately 10 mm Hg higher than those from the upper arm. If they are equal or lower, coarctation of the aorta is suspected.

2. B

    The increased bilirubin levels are caused by the bruising and cephalhematoma secondary to free circulating bilirubin from the reabsorbed blood that had been displaced. Pathologic jaundice is evident in the first 24 hours of life while breast milk jaundice is seen after a week.

3. A

    The signs and symptoms exhibited by the client are characteristic of streptococcal pharyngitis, a highly infectious disease. It is appropriate to institute droplet precaution immediately. Informing the physician and providing nourishment and hydration can follow right after.

4. C

    A birth weight of 1450g is within the normal (within the 10-90th percentile) of a 30-week gestation baby. Arms that do not recoil and the characteristic flat pinna are also apparent at this age.

5. B

    Respiratory rate and heart rate are already at normal range and no nasal flaring is observed. These indicate that the baby has no more respiratory distress and that his condition has improved.

6. B

    Babies born to alcoholic mothers are typically small for gestational age and have microcephaly, mental retardation and developmental delays. They have short palpebral fissures, a wide and flattened philtrum (the vertical groove in the midline of the upper lip), and thin lips.

7. B

    All parameters of the Apgar scoring garner 2 points except for acrocyanosis that is given 1 point. Four perfect scores and a 1 yield 9 as the Apgar score.

8. A

    Meconium is the greenish and sticky stool of the newly born baby. It is normally passed within 24 hours of birth.

9. B

    A weight loss of 5-8% of a newborn's weight within 3-4 days of life is normal. This is due to passage of urine and feces, and also of metabolic and physiologic adjustments to extrauterine feeding.

10. A

The circumference of a newborn's head is typically 2cm greater than that of the chest. This proportion is expected in the next few months. If the head circumference is >2cm larger than the chest, it can indicate hydrocephalus. On the other hand, if the chest circumference is equal or bigger than the head, microcephaly is suspected.

11. A

The findings are normal in a newborn. The bluish hands and feet with a pinkish body is termed acrocyanosis. Bluish discolorations on the lumbosacral region are called Mongolian spots, and the white spots on the nose are milia. The red mark on the face is nevus simplex.

12. B

Jaundice that appears after 24 hours of birth is called physiologic jaundice. It is caused by accelerated destruction of fetal RBC's, immature conjugation of bilirubin, and increased reabsorption of bilirubin from the intestines. These conditions are not pathologic.

13. B

Bubble baths are a risk factor for acquiring urinary tract infection in a child. Bubble baths are therefore not encouraged.

14. B

With a positive Trendelenburg sign, the pelvis tilts toward the unaffected hip during weight bearing on the affected side. Disorders that have this sign are congenital dislocation of the hip (CDH), dysplasia of the hip (DDH) and congenital coxa vara or of muscular dystrophy.

15. C

It is the nurse's role to offer confidentiality to adolescent clients. The nurse will need to explain that the purpose of confidentiality is to improve health care and not to keep secrets. However, confidentiality should not be made unlimited. The nurse should always state explicitly that she will act on information and tell appropriate people if safety will be a concern.

16. D

Bullous impetigo is an infectious bacterial disease caused by streptococci or staphylococci. The infection usually starts on the face as a single raised papule that becomes bullous and drains with pus. Within days, the lesion can spread to involve the neck, chest and arms. When the bullae are ruptured, they dry and crust over giving an appearance of honey-colored crusts.

17. B

Scaling, crusting, and hair loss are seen in the scalp of individuals with tinea capitis. Usually, a painful plaque called kerion and an enlarged occipital lymph node accompany this baldness.

18. C

Flattened and wide philtrum is characteristic of fetal alcohol syndrome. All other findings are evident in Down's syndrome.

19. A

A red, distorted, bulging tympanic membrane that can have a yellowish exudate is a sign of acute otitis media. The client will report pain on the affected ear. The usual cause of otitis media is a recent upper respiratory tract infection.

20. A

Strong indications of sexual abuse should immediately be reported to the nursing supervisor so that the appropriate authorities can be informed. Strong indicators include lacerations, ecchymoses, and newly healed scars of the hymen or the posterior fourchette, no evidence of hymenal tissue, healed hymenal transections, and perianal lacerations extending to the external sphincter.

21. D

When examining infants and young children, it may be necessary to change the sequence of the examination wherein the most distressing or invasive procedures should be done last. This technique is helpful in successfully completing the examination without causing undue stress to the patient.

22. A

The development of children proceeds in a predictable pattern which makes it possible to assess them in terms of milestones that are typical of their age.

23. C

To assess for measures that the parents of an infant are taking for their child's safety, the nurse asks in what position do they put their baby to sleep. This question determines the baby's risk for SIDS or Sudden Infant Death Syndrome, which is associated with letting babies sleep in the prone position.

24. C

When examining young infants, it is preferable that they are seated on their parent's lap to prevent the baby from being anxious due to separation from the parent. Taking the child to the examination room away from the mother will make them distressed. If a thorough examination is needed, have the parent hold the baby in any way.

25. D

The DENVER II Screening Test is a development screening tool for children 0-6 years of age. It uses four parameters to determine developmental delays. The four domains of development that it screens are personal-social, fine motor-adaptive, language, and gross motor. It does not measure intelligence.

26. D

When using an infant scale to take a baby's measurement, weigh them only in dry diapers or naked to obtain accurate measurements.

27. A

Sustained hypertension in infants is possibly caused by stenosis or thrombosis of the renal arteries, congenital renal malformations, or coarctation of the aorta.

28. B

Infants are periodic breathers, meaning they have periods of rapid and slow breathing. They also exhibit diaphragmatic breathing. It is best to count their respirations while they are quietly sleeping for one full minute.

29. C

Jaundice that persists beyond 2-3 weeks of life is pathologic and signal biliary obstruction or liver disease.

30. A

Mongolian spots are bluish gray discoloration in the newborn's buttocks that is sometimes seen in Asian or dark-skinned patients. These spots usually disappear before the baby reaches 4 years of age.

31. B

Patients with hip dysplasia will have their pelvis tilted toward the unaffected hip when asked to shift their weight from one foot to the other.

32. A

Patients with muscular dystrophy will have pelvic girdle weakness so that they cannot stand up normally. To stand up when they are sitting on the floor, they roll over to their abdomen and pushes with their arms before they stand up. This is the Gower's sign.

33. C

The hypoglossal nerve or the Cranial nerve XII assesses for the motor function of the tongue. To assess the movement of the tongue, the nurse asks the patient to stick out their tongue.

34. B

School-aged children usually like riding bicycles and participate in organized sports. They are at high risk for head injuries and fractures so advising them to wear protective gears when they play is a kind of anticipatory guidance for school-aged children.

35. A

Adolescents may sometimes feel embarrassed to ask about sensitive topics such as sexual practices. To be therapeutic, the nurse may tell the patient that other kids have sensitive questions to ask, too and that it is ok to ask them.

36. B

At Stage 2 of the Tanner staging for sexual maturity ratings in girls, there is some sparse growth of pubic hair on the labia. The hairs are long, fine and downy or slightly curved.

37. D

The plumb line test is performed to assess for scoliosis or the abnormal curvature of the spine. A plumb line, a string with a weight attached, is suspended near the cervical spine of the patient in between shoulder blades as the patient stands. The spine of the patient will appear deviated from the midline.

38. D

Diarrhea causes skin irritation especially if the perianal area is not cleaned immediately after soiling. The patient with red skin lesions has contact diaper dermatitis. The irritated skin is painful when the area is cleaned.

39. B

Tinea capitis is a fungal infection of the scalp and is manifested by patches of hair loss where the bald areas will be scaly and crusting.

40. B

Alcohol intake in a pregnant mother will result in a child with fetal alcohol syndrome. The patient will be small for age, with microcephaly and cognitive difficulties. The patient will have short palpebral fissures, wide and flattened philtrum, and thin upper lips.

41. A

A child with trisomy 21 or Down's syndrome will have a small round head, flattened bridge of the nose, low-set ears, and slanted palpebral fissures. A simian crease will also be noted on the palms of the patient, a prominent line transversing the entire palm horizontally.

42. C

Newborns with patent ductus arteriosus will have full bounding pulses. In the premature newborn, the precordium would be hyperdynamic, and an atypical murmur would be noted.

43. B

In the absence of neurologic disorders or if negative of constipation, a marked dilation of the anus in young children, suggests sexual abuse.

44. A

In hypospadias, the urethral meatus is found on the ventral side of the penis. On the other hand, it is found on the dorsal side of the penis in epispadias.

45. D

Pertussis is sometimes referred to as whooping cough. The patient with pertussis would have symptoms of upper respiratory infection, such as fever and coryza. The characteristic cough is violent and continuous that the patient catches their breath after several bouts of coughing.

The Pregnant Woman

Questions

1. A pregnant mother is asking how hormones influence her pregnancy. Which of the following is an accurate information that should be included in the nurse's teachings?
   a. The estrogen supports the implantation of the placenta into the uterine wall
   b. Progesterone maintains the endometrium of the uterus and increases the milk-producing sacs in the breast
   c. Progesterone increases the weight of the uterus
   d. The hCG stimulates the production of ducts of the breast

2. A woman is in her 27th week of gestation. The nurse prepares to care for a client in which trimester of pregnancy?
   a. First
   b. Second
   c. Early third
   d. Late third

3. A woman's obstetrical record says G4 T2 PT1 A1 L2. What is the correct interpretation of this?
   a. Four times pregnant, three times delivered, two term births, one preterm, one miscarriage and two living children
   b. Four times delivered, three pre terms, two term births, one post-delivery trauma, one abortion two living children
   c. Four times pregnant, three times delivered, two term births, one preterm, one abnormal and two living children
   d. Four times pregnant, three times delivered, two term births, one preterm, one abnormal and two live births

4. A woman comes to the clinic because she thinks she is pregnant. Which of the following would confirm pregnancy?
   a. Positive urine pregnancy test
   b. Fetal heart sounds heard through a Doppler
   c. Nausea and vomiting
   d. Cessation of menses

5. A pregnant woman in her first trimester asks the nurse why she feels nauseous all the time. Which of the following are probable reasons for nausea and vomiting during pregnancy? Select all that apply
   a. hyperglycemia
   b. slowed peristalsis
   c. gastric overloading
   d. dehydration
   e. enlarged uterus

6. A primipara on her 19th week of gestation reports feeling a fluttering sensation in her abdomen. How should the nurse document this finding?
    a. Premature labor contractions felt during second trimester
    b. Hyperactive bowel sounds due to increase in appetite
    c. Peristaltic waves felt at upper right quadrant of the abdomen
    d. Quickening at 19th week of gestation

7. A primipara is being seen during her prenatal visit. The nurse noticed that both sides of the breasts, the hips and the abdomen have visible purplish striae that are irregularly elongated. Which of the following correctly describes this finding?
    a. Linea nigra
    b. Hyperpigmentation
    c. Striae gravidarum
    d. Spider nevi

8. A nurse prepares herself to care for clients in the prenatal clinic. Which of the following reflects accurate information on the physiologic changes in pregnancy?
    a. Hypereflexive deep tendon reflexes
    b. Burning sensation during urination
    c. Decreased tone of esophageal sphincter and the stomach
    d. Decreased respiratory effort

9. A client who is on her second trimester of pregnancy is concerned because her gums bleed during brushing. The nurse understands that this condition is because of increasing vascularity in the gums. Which of the following conditions accurately describe the client's manifestation?
    a. Chronic periodontal disease
    b. Epulis of pregnancy
    c. Epistaxis
    d. Bleeding tendencies

10. A client is well in her third trimester of pregnancy. Which of the following should the nurse report to the physician immediately?
    a. Tighter shoes at night but relieved in the morning
    b. Persistent vomiting
    c. Varicose veins
    d. Increased pulse rate than prepregnant HR

11. A client's last menstrual period is September 3, 2015. The current date is June 30, 2016 and the client is showing signs of imminent labor. Which of the following is true regarding the status of the newborn?
    a. Preterm
    b. Term

   c.   Postterm
   d.   Undetermined

12. A nurse is caring for several new mothers who just delivered. Which client would need additional teaching from the nurse?
   a.   A mother sleeps besides her baby while having visitors
   b.   A mother who abused drugs during pregnancy who is seen changing her child's diapers
   c.   An HIV-positive mother who is breastfeeding
   d.   A diabetic mother who props the formula bottle of her newborn while feeding

13. A G3P2 woman asks the nurse if she can have a normal delivery. The client had a previous cesarean birth. Which of the following conditions must apply before a woman can consider vaginal birth after cesarean (VBAC)?
   a.   Classical incision of the uterus during previous cesarean section
   b.   Low transverse incision of the uterus during previous cesarean section
   c.   Normal glucose level
   d.   Normal hemoglobin level

14. A nurse is caring for a client who is a known cocaine addict. The nurse anticipates possible risks and complications of cocaine addiction during pregnancy. Which of the following is NOT a risk/ complication related to cocaine use while pregnant?
   a.   Congenital malformations
   b.   Abruption placentae
   c.   Fetal addiction
   d.   Macrosomia

15. A nurse is caring for a pregnant client who has asked the nurse which foods are safe to consume during pregnancy. Which of the following foods should the nurse discourage to eat at this time?
   a.   Mackerel
   b.   Avocado
   c.   Hard-boiled eggs
   d.   Pasteurized milk

16. A pregnant client's blood pressure has risen as compared to her baseline before being pregnant. Her urinalysis indicate proteinuria. She also reports that her ring is unusually tight these past few days. Upon further examination, the nurse deep tendon reflexes at 3+. Based on the client's signs and symptoms, the nurse should prepare to care for a client with which condition?
   a.   Diabetes
   b.   Abruption placentae
   c.   Placenta previa
   d.   Pre-eclampsia

17. A nurse uses a tape measure to measure fundal height. She finds that the results are more than 4cm than expected for gestation. Which of the following should the nurse consider as possible causes of an abnormally increased fundal height? Select all that apply.
    a. Polyhydramnios
    b. Fetal kidney disease
    c. twin pregnancy
    d. substance abuse
    e. malnutrition

18. A nurse is performing Leopold's maneuver. She palpates the fetal back on the left lateral side of the maternal pelvis. Which of the following refers to the nurse's findings?
    a. Position
    b. Variety
    c. Lie
    d. Attitude

19. A 26-year old pregnant client still at 30 weeks gestation is manifesting signs and symptoms of true labor. Which of the following factors that are true of the client possibly caused the her premature labor?
    a. Heavy cigarette smoking
    b. Large intake of cruciferous vegetables
    c. Non-adherence to supplementation regimen, taking prescribed diet
    d. Age

20. A diabetic mother gave birth to a baby with macrosomia. Which of the following complications is related to delivering a large for gestational age baby?
    a. Candidiasis
    b. Precipitous labor
    c. Placenta previa
    d. Vaginal tissue trauma

21. A 25-year old woman comes to the clinic because she has missed two of her monthly periods. The physician has confirmed her pregnancy. To determine her expected date of delivery, which of the following assessments is necessary?
    a. Date of first menstruation
    b. Date when her last period started
    c. Date when her last period has ended
    d. Age at first menstruation

22. A nurse is providing health teachings to a group of expectant mothers. Which of the following is NOT a danger sign of pregnancy?
    a. Dizziness when lying supine

b. Facial swelling
c. Gush of fluid from the vagina that is not urine
d. Sudden change in vision

23. Which of the following statements is most accurate in describing how maternal hormones affect the body during pregnancy?
    a. Progesterone causes the blood pressure to drop 20mmHg
    b. HPL raises resistance to insulin
    c. HCG causes relaxation of esophageal sphincter causing heartburn
    d. Thyroid hormone decreases causing a decrease in metabolism

24. A pregnant woman on her 26th week of gestation confided to the nurse that she seemed to have urinated without her feeling an urge. When further questioned, she stated that she noticed that after sexual activity. What is the most appropriate nursing action?
    a. Document this as normal
    b. Inform the physician immediately
    c. Let the client lie on her side and assess fetal heart tones
    d. Advise her to use a cotton pad and encourage hygiene measures

25. A 25-year old pregnant woman comes to the clinic to receive missed vaccinations. Which of the following vaccines is contraindicated during pregnancy?
    a. Pneumococcal
    b. Meningococcal
    c. Hepatitis B
    d. MMR

26. A pregnant woman at her 28th week of gestation comes to the clinic and had her blood works done. The results are as follows: blood type AB (-); rubella titer 2 IU/mL IgG antibodies. Which of the following vaccines is most appropriate to be administered at this time?
    a. RhoGAM
    b. MMR
    c. Varicella
    d. Polio

27. A 28-year old obese woman in her first trimester has poor diabetic control. The nurse understands that hyperglycemia in the first trimester will have which result in the fetus?
    a. Hyperinsulinemia
    b. Large for gestational age baby
    c. Fetal malformation
    d. Abnormal presentation during delivery

28. A 33-year old woman comes to the outpatient department because of 2 successive missed

periods. Which of the following is a positive sign of pregnancy?
a. Fetal heart tones
b. Nausea and vomiting
c. Positive pregnancy test
d. Chadwick's sign

29. A noted career woman has just been confirmed pregnant. Based on the ultrasound reports, she is at 7th week gestation. In relation to normal maternal acceptance of pregnancy, the nurse also expects the client to feel
a. Some ambivalence after pregnancy has been confirmed
b. Overjoyed in the changes that are about to happen
c. Indifferent toward the change
d. Uncaring toward self and baby

30. A woman who has been confirmed pregnant and in her first trimester called the clinic to report that she is experiencing some bleeding. Which of the following question is most pertinent to ask the client?
a. "When did you last feel the baby moved?"
b. "Are you having any abdominal cramping?
c. "When was your last menstrual period?"
d. "When did you last take your antihypertensive medication?"

31. A woman complaining of right lower abdominal pain was admitted to the unit for a possible ectopic pregnancy. Which of the following data on the client's history can be responsible for this condition?
a. Age under 20
b. Asthma
c. Previous long-standing chlamydial infection
d. Previous spontaneous abortion

32. After a prenatal class on good habits during pregnancy, the nurse decides to conduct further teaching to which of the following clients?
a. A 23-year old who says a jigger of red wine is good for the heart
b. An 18-year old in her first trimester who says she still enjoys intimate relations with husband
c. A 35-year old who says she walks around the block every morning
d. A 30-year old who says she is still so fond of swimming

33. A nurse is preparing a client for a pelvic ultrasound to assess fetal status. Which of the following is an appropriate advice prior to the procedure?
a. Void prior to the procedure
b. Drink a glass of water and refrain from voiding prior to the procedure
c. Take a warm bath prior to the procedure

d.   Drink something cold prior to the procedure

34. A 23-year old pregnant for the first time is annoyed for being nauseous most of the time. She asks the nurse what causes her symptom. Which of the following responses is most accurate to tell the client?
a.   "Progesterone causes relaxation of the esophageal sphincter causing spillage of stomach content out into the mouth."
b.   "HPL causes abdominal muscles to contract that causes the vomiting."
c.   "HCG is linked to nausea and vomiting in the first trimester."
d.   "Estrogen casing insulin resistance causes you to feel like throwing up."

35. A nurse is conducting a prenatal class on what to expect during delivery. A client asks what fetal presentation is most preferable for a vaginal delivery. Which is the most appropriate nursing response?
a.   Cephalic
b.   Complete Breech
c.   Franck
d.   Footling

36. The nurse performs the Leopold's maneuver and determines that the baby is at LOA position. Where is the best position to place the fetoscope for auscultating heart tones?
a.   Upper right quadrant
b.   Upper left quadrant
c.   Lower left quadrant
d.   Lower right quadrant

37. A nurse from an earlier shift endorses her care of a patient awaiting labor. She stated that the baby has just engaged. What is the present station of the baby?
a.   -1
b.   0
c.   +1
d.   +2

38. A nurse is describing the uterine contractions of a mother in labor. Upon assessment, she notes that the contractions are lasting 90 seconds. What parameter is the nurse referring to?
a.   Frequency
b.   Regularity
c.   Intensity
d.   Duration

39. A nurse is assessing a pregnant mother in her 37th week gestation in the clinic. Which of the following assessment findings should the nurse report immediately?

a. Pinpoint pupils
b. Purple striae over the abdomen and the legs
c. Slight edema of the feet
d. Dizziness when lying supine

40. A pregnant mother who has missed 2 of her prenatal check-ups is admitted to the unit and has been diagnosed with disseminated intravascular coagulation (DIC). She is currently receiving blood transfusion. Which of the following conditions most probably caused her DIC?
    a. Infection with rubella
    b. Missed abortion
    c. Hypertension
    d. Alcohol consumption

ANSWERS

1. B

    Progesterone increases the vascularity of the myometrium that will support pregnancy. It is also responsible for the increase in the milk-producing sacs in the breasts called alveoli. Estrogen stimulates the ducts of the breasts and helps increase the weight of the uterus. hCG stimulates the increase in progesterone and is responsible for implantation of the placenta.

2. B

    The first 12 weeks of gestation refers to the first trimester. From the 13th to the 27th week, the pregnant woman is in her second trimester. From the 28th week up to delivery, it is the third trimester.

3. A

    The acronym G-P-T-PT-A-L stands for Gravida, Para, Term, Preterm, Abortion and Living children. Gravida refers to how many times a woman got pregnant regardless of outcome, and Para refers to number of deliveries regardless of outcome. Abortion refers to either spontaneous or induced abortions.

4. B

    Positive signs of pregnancy confirm pregnancy. Examples are heart sounds heard through a Doppler or through auscultation and evidence of fetal outline seen in ultrasound.

5. B, C, E

    The real cause of nausea during pregnancy is unknown, however, several factors may cause it such as hormonal changes, hypoglycemia, increased gastric content, slow peristaltic movement and the growing uterus.

6. D

    Quickening is the first fetal movement that is felt by the mother. In primiparas, it occurs at the 18th-20th week. It is felt as a fluttering sensation.

7. C

    Striae gravidarum are stretch marks that are off-color and are the result of rapid weight gain more than normal elasticity of the skin can handle.

8. C

    During pregnancy, several physiologic changes are expected. Some of these are decreased tone of the esophageal sphincter and the stomach, increased respiratory effort, sluggish biliary activity, and increased cholesterol, among others.

9. B

    Epulis of pregnancy or gingivitis of pregnancy refers to the bleeding of the gums due to growth of capillaries of the gingigivae.

10. B
Persistent vomiting beyond the first trimester should be reported to the physician because it may indicate hyperememesis gravidarum. Edema of the lower extremities observed at night and which disappears at rest, varicose veins, hemorrhoids and increased HR and RR than baseline are all expected changes in the last trimester.

11. C
According to Naegele's rule, the client's expected date of delivery is June 10, 2016. The delivery was long overdue, and the mother will deliver a post-term baby.

12. C
HIV positive mothers cannot breastfeed because the HIV can be transmitted through breastmilk.

13. B
VBAC is possible only if the previous cesarean section incision is low transverse. A uterus with previous classic incision will have high risk of rupturing during labor.

14. D
Cocaine addiction during pregnancy can result to congenital malformations and abruption. The newborn will also show signs and symptoms of cocaine addiction. A newborn with macrosomia is born to a diabetic mother.

15. A
Some foods are discouraged during pregnancy. Sea fish such as swordfish and mackerel contain high amounts of mercury. Raw eggs, soft cheeses and fresh milk that are not pasteurized can cause salmonellosis. The pregnant woman should also avoid raw or undercooked meats.

16. D
Signs and symptoms of pre-eclampsia are elevated blood pressure, edema, proteinuria. Hyperreflexia may also be noted.

17. A, B, C
Fundal height increases as pregnancy progresses. Fundal measurement should approximately equal the number of weeks of gestation until the 36 th week. A fundal height of more than 4cm than expected for gestation suggests polyhydramnios, fetal kidney disease or multiple pregnancy.

18. B
Variety refers to the location of the fetus's back in relation to the maternal pelvis, at either anterior, posterior or lateral sides.

19. A

The client is manifesting signs and symptoms of preterm labor: factors that lead to preterm labor are cigarette smoking, substance abuse, malnutrition, advanced age of the mother, strenuous activities, and psychological stressors.

20. D

Complications of delivering a macrosomic baby are: incurring vaginal lacerations, dystocia and bladder trauma in the mother, low Apgar scores, and clavicle and brachial plexus damage in the newborn.

21. B

The date when her last period started is considered the last menstrual period (LMP). It will be used in applying Naegele's rule to estimate the date of delivery.

22. A

Dizziness when a pregnant woman in her 2nd and 3rd trimester of pregnancy is a sign of supine hypotensive syndrome. Supine hypotensive syndrome occurs when the central vessels (aorta and inferior vena cava) are compressed by the gravid uterus when the pregnant woman lies on her back. It is characterized by pallor, bradycardia, sweating, nausea, hypotension and dizziness. The symptoms resolve with a change of position to left lateral. All other options are danger signs of pregnancy.

23. B

The human placental lactogen is a major contributor in increasing resistance to insulin utilization. Normally, this allows transport of glucose to the placenta and also prevents blood sugar of the mother to drop drastically. This mechanism is disrupted in gestational diabetes.

24. C

Fluid that gushes from the vagina other than urine is a danger sign during pregnancy. It can mean ruptured amniotic membrane. The initial action of the nurse is to have the mother lie on her side and assess fetal tones. The physician should be informed immediately after.

25. D

The following vaccines are safe during pregnancy: pneumococcal, meningococcal, and hepatitis B. The following vaccines are NOT safe during pregnancy: measles/mumps/rubella, polio, varicella. The weakened virus in attenuated vaccines may still have untoward effects on fetal development.

26. A

Rho (D) immunoglobulin, or RhoGAM, should be given to all Rh-negative women at 28 weeks' gestation and again within 3 days of delivery to prevent sensitization to an Rh-positive infant. MMR, polio and varicella are contraindicated during pregnancy because they contain live attenuated viruses.

27. C

In diabetic pregnant women with poor metabolic control in the first trimester, congenital fetal malformations are likely to happen.

28. A

Positive signs of pregnancy are those that are conclusive for a fetus in utero. Examples are fetal heart tones, fetal movements and fetal outline on palpation.

29. A

During the first trimester of pregnancy, women may feel some ambivalence about being pregnant, especially first time mothers.

30. C

Vaginal bleeding in a pregnant woman will necessitate the nurse to get information on her last menstrual period to approximate how long the client has been pregnant. This is pertinent because management of bleeding is different for each trimester of pregnancy.

31. C

Sexually transmitted disease that progressed to pelvic inflammatory disease can cause ectopic pregnancies secondary to strictures of the fallopian tube.

32. A

Prenatal exposure to alcohol cause fetal malformations and mental retardation in the baby. Any amount should not be encouraged during pregnancy.

33. B

A full bladder will aid in better visualization during a pelvic ultrasound. The nurse advises the client to drink fluids and refrain from voiding just before the procedure.

34. C

Although not clearly understood, human chorionic gonadotropin (HCG) which is abundant in the first trimester is linked to nausea and vomiting in this phase of pregnancy. As HCG levels diminish with the growing placenta, nausea diminishes, too.

35. A

The cephalic presentation is the most favorable position for a vaginal birth because the head that has the biggest circumference is delivered first.

36. C

The LOA (left occiput anterior) position means that the fetal occiput is on the maternal left side and toward the front, and the fetal face is down. Fetal heart tones are best heard at the fetal back.

Therefore the fetoscope should be positioned at the left lower quadrant because that is where the fetal back is located.

37. B

Station is the measurement of how far the fetal presenting part has descended into the pelvis. At 0 station, the presenting part is said to be engaged and is now at level with the ischial spines.

38. D

Duration refers to the length of a contraction. Uterine contractions lasting more than 90 seconds should be reported immediately.

39. A

Pinpoint pupils can indicate opiate addiction and should be reported immediately because of the detrimental effects of the drugs to the unborn child and to the mother herself. It is important to ask when her last take was to determine when withdrawal symptoms are expected.

40. B

Disseminated intravascular coagulation (DIC) is a condition wherein the body creates massive amounts of microthrombi which in turn cause depletion of clotting factors. With clotting factor depleted, the patient with DIC presents with bleeding that is unanticipated and can be massive. DIC can be triggered by abruptio placenta, dead fetus syndrome (missed abortion), amniotic fluid embolism, pre-eclampsia, H-mole and hemorrhagic shock.

The Older Adult

Questions

1. Which of the following is an expected age-related change to the vital signs system that would be observed in a 70-year-old patient?
    a. Heart rate is increased than that of adults
    b. Systolic hypertension with a widened pulse pressure is noted
    c. Core body temperature increases
    d. Respiratory rate increases in depth and rate

2. Which of the following age-related skin changes refers to actinic purpura?
    a. Purple and reddish macules that fade over time
    b. Loose transparent skin
    c. Decreased vascularity of the skin
    d. Large bluish and sometimes greenish discoloration of the skin after trauma

3. Which of the following is an expected age-related change in an older person's eyes and visual acuity?
    a. The eyeball is pushed forward
    b. Fatty deposits increase within the bony orbit
    c. The pupils become larger
    d. Dry eyes

4. Which of the following age-related change is expected in an older patient's pulmonary system?
    a. Increased alveolar elasticity
    b. Increased lung capacity
    c. Increased anteroposterior diameter
    d. Increased lung recoil

5. Which of the following heart sounds is pathologic in older adults?
    a. S1
    b. S2
    c. S3
    d. S4

6. Which of the following age-related change is NOT expected in an older male patient's genitourinary system?
    a. Sexual interest declines
    b. Penis decrease in size
    c. Testicles drop lower in the scrotum
    d. Erections happen because of tactile stimulation more than erotic cues

7. Which of the following age-related change is NOT expected in an older female patient's genitourinary system?

a. Mucopurulent vaginal discharge
b. Pale and dry, atrophic vagina
c. Non-palpable ovaries
d. Pubic hairs become sparse and gray

8. A nurse is assessing an older patient's hearing acuity. Which of the following will the patient with age-related hearing deficit have difficulty hearing?
a. High-pitched sounds
b. Low-pitched sounds
c. Loud noises
d. Music

9. Which of the following will be most likely observed in an older patient with hyperthyroidism?
a. Heat and cold intolerance
b. Weight loss
c. Hyperreflexia
d. Dry skin

10. Which of the following is NOT included in the mnemonic SPICES that comprise geriatric syndromes?
a. Confusion
b. Sleep disorders
c. Incontinence
d. Skin allergies

11. Which of the following is an example of Instrumental Activities of Daily Living?
a. Using the telephone
b. Feeding
c. toileting
d. ambulation

12. Which of the following is a risk factor for adverse drug reactions in hospitalized patients?
a. Age 60-80-years old
b. Presence of heart failure
c. Length of stay: 3 days
d. No history of adverse drug reaction

13. Which of the following is a cause of acute pain in the older patient?
a. Cancer pain
b. Arthritic pain
c. Post-surgical pain
d. Neuropathic pain

14. Which of the following parameters included in the DIAPERS mnemonic would correctly assess for incontinence in the older patient?
    a. Infection -intestinal
    b. Restricted mobility
    c. Post-surgery
    d. Actinic keratosis

15. An older female patient scores 3 on the AUDIT-C assessment tool for Alcohol use. Which of the following is a correct interpretation of her score?
    a. No alcohol use
    b. Negative
    c. Positive
    d. The patient is an occasional drinker

16. An older patient tells the nurse that when they suddenly stand from a reclining position, they feel faint, weak, an unsteady. The patient also reports visual blurring. Which of the following did the patient most likely experience?
    a. Orthostatic hypotension
    b. White coat hypertension
    c. Post-prandial sickness
    d. Diabetic hypertension

17. Which of the following is characteristic of melanoma?
    a. A dark raised lesion with irregular borders
    b. Superficial flattened papules that are scaling
    c. Thickened and yellowed skin
    d. A translucent nodule that spreads, and has a pit and elevated borders

18. An older patient has cataract. Which of the following factors contributed to his having cataract aside from aging?
    a. Allergies
    b. Smoking
    c. Drug abuse
    d. Hypotension

19. Which of the following causes a holosystolic murmur originating from the apex and radiating to the axilla?
    a. Mitral regurgitation
    b. Patent ductus arteriosus
    c. Aortic sclerosis
    d. Heart block

20. A nurse suspects that an older patient has peripheral vascular disease. Which of the following can the nurse perform to support her assessment?
    a. Obtain the Ankle-Brachial Index
    b. Measure the patient's calf circumference
    c. Ask the patient to drink more water
    d. Take the brachial pulse instead of the radial pulse

21. The nurse is using the TRAP mnemonic to assess the patient. Which of the following disorder is the TRAP mnemonic describing?
    a. Myasthenia Gravis
    b. Heart Failure
    c. Parkinson disease
    d. Diabetes

22. A nurse is conducting health teachings on several older adult patients. Which of the following exercise would the nurse recommend to the patients?
    a. 2.5 hours of moderate intensity aerobic activity every week
    b. 2.5 hours of vigorous intensity aerobic activity every week
    c. 1.5 hours of moderate intensity aerobic activity every week
    d. 3.5 hours of vigorous intensity aerobic activity every week

23. A nurse is visiting the home of an older patient. Which of the following if observed by the nurse indicates that the family needs additional teaching on safety?
    a. A big jar in the corner behind the couch
    b. Pots and pans stored on the highest shelf in the kitchen
    c. Throw rugs that are fixed
    d. Grab bars in the bathroom

24. An 80-year old older female patient was admitted because of urinary tract infection. Upon assessment, the patient is not aware that she is in the hospital. She also could not recognize her daughter who is with her. The nurse could not make a comprehensible sense of what she is saying. Which of the following details of the nurse assessment gives a clue that the patient is experiencing delirium and not dementia?
    a. The patient is disoriented
    b. The patient could not recognize her daughter
    c. The diagnosis of urinary tract infection
    d. The patient's speech is incomprehensible

25. A hospice older patient is receiving palliative and end-of-life care. Which of the following is not part of the care plan?
    a. Pain medications

b. Nutrition
c. Hydration
d. Chemotherapy

26. A nurse is preparing to work in a geriatric setting. The nurse understands that to make functional assessments, she has to assess three parameters. Which of the following is NOT included in functional assessments?
a. Activities of daily living
b. Cognition
c. Instrumental activities of daily living
d. Mobility

27. A nurse is to assess an elderly client's activities of daily living (ADL). Which of the following is an example of an ADL?
a. Housekeeping
b. Doing laundry
c. Buying groceries
d. Grooming

28. After the nurse utilized the Katz Index of ADL, the client garnered a score of 1. Which of the following is a correct interpretation of the client's Katz index score?
a. The client is dependent on majority of ADLs
b. The client is independent on majority of ADLs
c. The client is dependent on all of ADLs
d. The client is independent on all of ADLs

29. A nurse wants to assess and measure what a client actually does in the performance of ADLs. At the moment, the only available person to talk to is the client's wife who is living with the client. Which of the following ADL assessment tools is most appropriate for the nurse to use?
a. Katz Index
b. FIM
c. Barthel Index
d. RDS-2

30. The nurse asks a client's participation in the assessment of instrumental activities of daily living (IADL). The nurse mentions all of the following EXCEPT:
a. Managing finances
b. Meal preparation
c. Eating
d. Taking medications

31. The nurse is to use the Lawton IADL scale. Which of the following parameters are included in the

assessment? Select all that apply.
a. Gardening
b. Use of internet
c. Use of telephone
d. Shopping
e. Driving

32. An elderly client has been asked of his functions in five areas of his life namely social, economic, physical and mental health and capacity for self-care. Which of the following tools did the nurse use in assessing the client's IADLs?
a. Lawton IADL instrument
b. Older Americans Resources and Services Multidimensional Functional Assessment Questionnaire-IADL (OARS-IADL)
c. Direct Assessment of Functional Abilities (DAFA)
d. Get up and Go Test

33. The nurse is observing an elderly client sit on a chair, stand up from a sitting position, walk and return to his seat. The nurse is performing which test?
a. OARS-IADL
b. Lawton IADL
c. Katz Index Instrument
d. Get Up and Go test

34. A nurse has asked for the elderly client's age and then proceeded to test his mental state, particularly on orientation, registration, attention and recall. She then proceeded to assess his IADLs. The client is to be discharged after a bypass procedure. Which of the following assessment instruments is the nurse most likely using?
a. HARP
b. MMSE
c. Tinetti
d. OARS-IADL

35. An elderly client becomes disoriented to time, place and person after having been hospitalized for urinary tract infection. Which type of altered cognition is the client experiencing?
a. Dementia
b. Delirium
c. Depression
d. Desolation

36. The nurse knows that depression in the geriatric population is on the rise. The nurse institute measures to prevent depression. Which strategies should she focus on? Select all that apply.
a. Timely administration of antidepressants

b. Provision of rest and recreation
c. Increase period of independence
d. Provide access to televisions and similar media
e. Reduce functional decline

37. A client's wife confides to the nurse that her role as a caregiver is becoming so stressful. She always feels fatigue and burned out. The nurse prioritizes her care to prevent which risk of caregiver burnout?
a. Caregiver resignation
b. Lack of sleep of caregiver
c. Missed meals of client
d. Elder mistreatment

38. An elderly client who requires home care asks which services would be available to him. Which of the following services are included in home care? Select all that apply.
a. Primary care
b. Case management
c. Hospice
d. Legal advice
e. Speech therapy

39. An elderly client wishes to live independently in an apartment. He still wants social interaction like dining with friends, although he still needs assistance with house chores and some personal care. Which facility is best for the client?
a. Assisted living
b. Continuing care retirement community
c. Hospice
d. Home care

40. The nurse encourages exercises in home care facility. Which of the following is an advantage of exercise?
a. Decreases body fat
b. Decreases body temperature
c. Increases risk of fracture
d. Causes peripheral vascular disease

41. An elderly client is aware of the benefits of exercise for his health. He asks about the type and duration of exercise he needs in a week. Which of the following should the nurse recommend to the client?
a. 200 minutes of moderate intensity aerobic exercise
b. 150 minutes of isometric exercise
c. 2 ½ hours of moderate intensity aerobic exercise

d.   75 minutes of moderate intensity aerobic exercise

42. A nurse is assessing the home environment of an elderly client. Which of the following would necessitate calling the attention of the client?
    a.   Throw rugs with a plastic base
    b.   Grab bars by the toilet and shower
    c.   Big jars placed in the corner of the room
    d.   Lights at both ends of the stairs

43. An 85-year old client has just been admitted to the ER. He sustained injuries due to a fall while bathing. The nurse assesses the possible reasons for sustaining a fall. Which of the following client report suggest a reason for his fall?
    a.   Constipation
    b.   Poor hearing
    c.   Syncope
    d.   Astereognosis

44. A 67-year old client with worsening dementia wears glasses when driving. He drives to the grocery store and back. Which of the following factors in the client's status indicates that the client needs to stops driving?
    a.   Age
    b.   Wearing of glasses
    c.   Worsening dementia
    d.   Driving distance

45. An elderly client asks the nurse if he can take vodka to help him sleep. Which of the following is the nurse's best response?
    a.   "You are not allowed to take alcohol anymore."
    b.   "You may take 1 standard drink only, but you have to take it in the afternoon or dinner, but not after."
    c.   "I suggest you drink warm milk instead to help you sleep."
    d.   "Let me refer you to the Group Alcoholic Anonymous to help you with your problem."

46. An 80-year old man comes to the clinic for his annual check-up. The nurse understands that expected pulmonary changes in an elderly include
    a.   Decreased residual volume
    b.   Increase in functional alveoli
    c.   Increased ciliary action in the bronchi
    d.   Decreased lung elasticity

47. An elderly male client asks for some salt during one of his meals. He states that the foods are not tasty as before. What is the most probable cause of this?

a. The body seeks out more sodium to balance water loss
b. It is a compensatory mechanism to cause fluid retention that will increase much needed intravascular fluids
c. A declining number of taste buds
d. A sign of confusion

48. Which assessment finding in the elderly population is caused by increased peripheral vascular resistance and decreased vessel elasticity?
a. Dementia
b. Irregular heart rhythm
c. Hypertension
d. Tachycardia

49. A 69-year old widower has been admitted for correction of his chronic constipation. In his initial interview, the nurse noted that he repeatedly states he wishes he was as strong as when he was younger. What is the correct nursing action?
a. Encourage reminiscence
b. Explain the expected changes in aging
c. Change to a more humorous topic
d. Confront the client on his mood

50. A nurse is caring for an elderly client with a hearing deficit. Which of the following actions of the nurse needs further improvement?
a. Facing the client, speaking slowly and clearly
b. Cleaning the ears of cerumen
c. Assisting with the use of hearing aid
d. Speaking loudly and overemphasizing each word

51. A 75-year old male client is admitted for a routine colonoscopy. In the interview, he tells the nurse that he is feeling depressed. What story does the nurse expect the client to tell?
a. Plans for an upcoming trip
b. Decreased desire to attend an annual home care event
c. Being angry at losing a chess game
d. A fight with a good friend over the TV remote

52. The nurse is reviewing the expected physiologic changes in aging. Which of the following findings does the nurse consider as pathologic in an 80-year old client?
a. Increased residual volume
b. Decreased sphincter control of the bladder
c. Significant increase in diastolic pressure
d. Decreased response to touch, heat and pain

53. A 60-year old elderly admits to being sexually active and confides to the nurse that she experiences dyspareunia during intercourse and that she has vaginal dryness. Which of the following should be included in the nurse's care plan?
    a. Provide health teachings on the importance of increasing fluid intake to prevent vaginal dryness
    b. Review all medications that the client is taking and identify those that can cause the dryness
    c. Advise the client to use water based lubricant to ease discomfort during intercourse
    d. Refer the client to the physician for a diagnostic work-up

54. An 86-year old with Alzheimer's disease has recently moved in to live with his son. He has increasing episodes of forgetfulness and tends to wander. Which of the following response by the son alerts the nurse to a possible problem?
    a. "I need help sorting out all his medications"
    b. "He got the bruises from bumping into things all the time. He just couldn't remember."
    c. "I'm not sure if I can handle all these by myself."
    d. "I am thinking that maybe the facility for the aged is the best place for him right now."

55. An 85-year old elderly male suspected of having hyperthyroidism complains of fatigue, weight loss, and tachycardia. Which finding further supports the nurse's suspicion?
    a. Chronic constipation that has been resolved
    b. Cold clammy skin
    c. Decreased respiratory rate
    d. Increased urinary dribbling

56. A nurse is caring for an elderly lady in a hospice care. She appoints her eldest daughter as her health care proxy. The nurse understands that a health care proxy is someone
    a. Appointed by the client to make health decisions for the client in case she becomes incapacitated by disability or disease
    b. The client trusts to execute all her wishes with regards to her wealth
    c. A lawyer who will take care of all legal matters for the client upon her death
    d. Of nearest kin who will be informed in case of her demise

57. A 79-year old client with mild dementia has been encouraged by the nurse to make legal arrangements for her health care. In the course of these legalities, the nurse helps the client make a list of treatments and procedures which she will allow and refuse in case she becomes incapacitated. This list is called
    a. Durable power of attorney
    b. Do-not-resuscitate order
    c. Living will
    d. Health care proxy

58. An elderly patient was brought in by authorities who found him confused and bleeding in one

hand. After the nurse tends to his wound, the nurse interviews the client to determine if the cause of his confusion is delirium or dementia. Which of the following is accurate in distinguishing between the two?

a.   Dementia is acute. Confusion is noted in a span of days or weeks. Confusion in delirium is slow and progresses over the years

b.   Orientation to place in dementia is impaired while in the early stages of delirium it may not be apparent yet.

c.   A demented client has labile mood while a delirious client has a flat affect

d.   Dementia is caused by diminishing functioning brain cells while delirium is a sequala of infections, hospitalizations and medications

59. A nurse is doing her rounds in a health care facility. What signs when exhibited by older elderly clients indicate the possibility of pneumonia?

a.   Fever and chills

b.   Purulent rhinorrhea

c.   Tachypnea and confusion

d.   Diarrhea

60. A client is brought in by concerned neighbors after being seen wandering wearing only light clothes on a chilly night. The client is a widow and lives alone. Upon interview, the client insists that the nurse calls her husband at work. When asked of the present date, she became irritated but did not reply. Going through her medical records, she had been recently hospitalized for upper airway infection. Based on these findings, what condition is the client most likely suffering from?

a.   Mild cognitive impairment

b.   Delirium

c.   Dementia

d.   Normal forgetfulness

61. An elderly client has just turned 60 years of age. Which vaccine should the nurse administer in the immediate future to prevent herpetic lesions and neuralgia?

a.   MMR

b.   DT

c.   Zoster

d.   Pneumococcal

62. The nurse is performing a fall risk assessment on several clients. Who among the following is at greatest risk for falls?

a.   An 89-year old client recently hospitalized and taking pain meds for cancer

b.   An active 70-year old client who has friends called "bandits"

c.   A 63-year old retired principal obsessed about cleanliness

d.   A 68-year old gardener still tending the facility's yard.

63. A nurse conducts home visitation on several clients to conduct fall risk assessment. She identifies which client as someone needing further teaching?
    a.   A 76-year old widower bragging about his new walker and showing the nurse his 'garage'
    b.   A 67-year old living in a house with four adults
    c.   A retired school teacher having his house renovated and having grab bars installed.
    d.   A 67-year old female recently been visited by grandchildren and whose house has toys on the ground.

64. A nurse is conducting health teaching about safety in polypharmacy (taking multiple medications at the same time). Which of the following is an important parameter to be assessed by the nurse?
    a.   Smoking habits
    b.   Alcohol consumption
    c.   Duration of treatment
    d.   Age of client

65. A nurse working in a health facility is caring for an elderly client. Which of the following nursing action encourages autonomy in the client?
    a.   Giving him his oral medications on time
    b.   Decorating his room
    c.   Scheduling his dental appointment
    d.   Allowing him to choose leisure activities

ANSWERS

1. B
   Aging causes the aorta and other arteries to become stiff and atherosclerotic which cause systolic hypertension. The diastolic pressure stops increasing by 60 years of age. With increasing systolic hypertension and stable diastolic pressure, the pulse pressure widens.

2. A
   Actinic purpura are patches of unraised macular lesions on the skin of older people. It is caused by the rupture of frail capillaries.

3. D
   Due to fewer lacrimal production, older people often experience dry eyes.

4. C
   As a person ages, the chest wall becomes stiffer and respiratory muscles weaken. The chest will have increased AP (anteroposterior) diameter. Lung recoil and lung capacity decrease, so small alveoli are prone to atelectasis.

5. C
   S1 and S2 are normal heart sounds in all individuals. S4 can be heard in otherwise healthy older adults. The S3 sound is normal in children and young adults but is pathologic in the older adults. It signifies heart failure and valvular disease.

6. A
   Aging does not affect sexual desire and interest. In older men, erections happen mostly because of tactile stimulation. The penis also decreases in size and the scrotum appears more pendulous.

7. A
   Mucopurulent vaginal discharge is a sign of infection and is always abnormal. In older women, the vagina is atrophied, and the ovaries become non-palpable. The pubic hairs also turn gray.

8. A
   Older patients who have impaired hearing related to aging will have difficulty hearing high-frequency tones, so it is important to speak clearly in an audible voice and turn off distracting noises such as the television when conversing with them.

9. B
   In older patients, hyperthyroidism would have manifestations of fatigue, weight loss, and tachycardia. Heat intolerance, diaphoresis, and hyperreflexia which are commonly exhibited by younger patients may not be apparent in older people.

10. D

The SPICES mnemonic that describes geriatric syndromes refers to Sleep disorders, Problems with eating or feeding, Incontinence, Confusion, Evidence of Falls, and Skin Breakdown.

11. A

Instrumental Activities of Daily Living or IADLs are those activities necessary for independent living beyond self-care. Examples of AIDLs are using a phone, driving, using public transportation, and shopping, among others.

12. B

Hospitalized older adults are prone to adverse drug reactions if they have more than four co-morbid conditions, if they have heart or kidney failure or liver disease, those aged 80 and above, those with a history of having adverse drug reactions, and those who have stayed in the hospital for 12 days or longer, among others.

13. C

Acute pain has a distinct onset and is of short duration. Common causes of acute pain are post-surgical wound, trauma, and headache. Cancer, arthritic, and neuropathic pain are usually persistent pains.

14. B

The DIAPERS mnemonic refers to Delirium, Infection-urinary, Atrophic vaginitis, Pharmaceuticals, Psychological disorders, Excess urine output, Restricted mobility and Stool impaction.

15. C

A score of 3 or more in a female older patient or 4 or more in an older female, is positive for risky behaviors in using alcohol or alcohol abuse.

16. A

Orthostatic hypotension in common in older patients. Manifestations of orthostatic hypotension include feeling faint and lightheaded, unsteady and having blurry vision. Sometimes, the patient loses consciousness called syncope.

17. A

Melanoma is a type of skin cancer presenting as a raised lesion with varying dark colors and irregular borders.

18. B

Smoking, UV light exposure, high alcohol consumption, smoking, steroids, and trauma can cause cataract formation.

19. A

Mitral regurgitation is the most common cause of murmurs in older patients. The nurse will note a harsh holosystolic murmur at the apex radiating to the axilla.

20. A

The Ankle-Brachial Index is 70% sensitive and 90% specific to peripheral arterial disease. When the nurse finds diminished or absent peripheral pulses, they may take the Ankle-Brachial Index.

21. C

Parkinson disease is manifested by Tremors, Rigidity, Akinesia, Postural instability (TRAP).

22. A

The current recommendations for exercise in the older adults are 2.5 hours of moderate-intensity or 1.25 of vigorous-intensity aerobic activity as well as muscle strengthening activities on at least two days every week.

23. B

Heavy tools or supplies that an older patient may need must not be stored in high places. It will be difficult for them to reach those things, and attempting to reach them might cause the tools to fall on the patient and cause injury.

24. C

Delirium is usually caused by stress, and in this situation, the physiologic stress is the urinary tract infection. In both delirium and dementia, there is disorientation and altered speech.

25. D

Palliative and end-of-life care deals with the alleviation of pain and improving the quality of life of the patient when they have a few more months to live. The care plan would not include treatments that would attempt to save the patient's life.

26. B

A functional assessment assesses three parameter namely activities of daily living, instrumental activities of daily living, and mobility.

27. D

ADLs are activities for self-care. Examples are grooming, changing clothes, toileting, walking and eating.

28. A

The Katz Index of ADL assesses the independence of clients in bathing, dressing, using the toilet, transferring oneself from bed to chair and vice versa, urinary and bowel control and feeding. The client is given a score of 1 for every parameter where he is completely independent, and a score of 0 for any signs of dependence. A score of 1 indicates that of the 6 parameters, the client is independent in only one parameter.

29. D

The Rapid Disability Rating Scale-2 is completed by a member of the client's family or a caregiver who ideally should be living with the client. This is because familiarity of the client's ADL is necessary. It measures what the client actually does, and not what he could possibly perform.

30. C

IADLs are abilities that enable a client to be independent in community living. Examples of IADLs are grocery shopping, meal preparation, self-administration of medication and use of transport.

31. C, D, E

The Lawton IADL assesses 8 parameters namely: telephone use, marketing and grocery shopping, preparation of meals, home maintenance or housekeeping, doing the laundry, transportation, self-medication and financial management.

32. B

The Older Americans Resources and Services Multidimensional Functional Assessment Questionnaire-IADL (OARS-IADL) assesses functioning of the client in social, economic, physical and mental health areas of his life, and his capacity for self-care.

33. D

The Get Up and Go test assesses the client's functional mobility to give a quantifiable indication of the client's safety when going outdoors. The nurse instructs to and observes how the client sits on a chair, stands up from a sitting position, walks and returns to seat.

34. A

The HARP assessment instrument is used to assess loss of ADL functions after hospitalization due to a medical reason. It assesses three parameters: age, mental state and IADL status before hospitalization.

35. B

Delirium is a type of altered cognition wherein signs and symptoms usually develop during or after acute illness. The person may exhibit confusion, disorientation, varying levels of consciousness and even hallucinations.

36. C, E

The main focus of measures to prevent depression in the elderly is to lengthen the duration by which a client maintains independence and to preserve functional abilities.

37. D

Elder mistreatment is a likely result of caregiver burnout, which the nurse should prevent and prioritize.

38. A, B, E

Services of home care include skilled nursing care, primary care, physical, occupational, and speech therapies, social work, nutrition, case management, assistance in activities of daily living, and some durable medical equipment.

39. A

Assisted living facilities are becoming popular because they offer more choices and independence than home health. They do not feel too committed and dependent as in long-term facilities. The facilities are homelike with opportunities for socialization. They also offer assistance in ADLs.

40. A

Advantages of exercise in the elderly include decreased in body fat, improved muscle tone and strength, promotes flexibility, range of motion and psychological well-being.

41. C

The recommended type of and duration of exercise in the elderly is 2 ½ hours of moderate intensity aerobic exercise, or 75 minutes of vigorous aerobic exercise.

42. A

Throw rugs should have rubber bases without loose edges. They should be made of anti-slip materials to prevent falls in the elderly or they can be avoided altogether.

43. C

Certain factors cause falls and injuries. These are syncope, poor vision, problems in gait and equilibrium, nerve problems, dementia and use of psychotropic medications that cause drowsiness and dizziness.

44. C

Worsening dementia is an indication that driving privileges of the client should be withheld for safety purposes.

45. B

Alcohol intake is allowed to only one standard drink in a day taken before dinner.

46. D

As people age, the chest wall becomes stiffer and harder to move (decreased chest compliance), respiratory muscles weaken, and the lungs lose some of their elastic recoil. Lung mass declines, and residual volume increases.

47. C

Taste buds begin to diminish in number starting at the 4th decade of life. At age 60, the older adult becomes more insensitive to taste qualities.

48. C
Blood pressure increases as a result of thickening and decreased elasticity of blood vessels. Because of this, there is impedance and resistance in distributing blood to different parts of the body causing hypertension.

49. A
Engaging in a "life review" process or reminiscence is one method of assisting the client reach development milestones for this age group. The task of adjusting to declining physical strength needs to be done to preserve ego integrity.

50. D
Raising the voice emits high frequency sounds that an elderly client with presbycussis will have more difficulty hearing. All other options are correct nursing actions.

51. B
There are many psychosocial symptoms that a client with depression may exhibit, including feelings of hopelessness, helplessness, increased anxiety and decreased desire for socialization. These feelings contribute to despair rather than ego integrity.

52. C
A modest increase in systolic blood pressure and not the diastolic pressure is expected in the elderly due to increased vascular resistance and decreased vessel elasticity. The significant change in diastolic pressure needs to be evaluated.

53. C
Vaginal dryness or decreased secretions is caused by a decrease in estrogen. The decline in estrogen is caused by the atrophy of the ovaries. To preserve ego integrity in this client, the nurse advises the client to use a water-based lubricant to help ease discomfort during sexual intercourse.

54. B
It is the nurse's role to screen all older patients for possible mistreatment, which includes abuse, neglect, exploitation, and abandonment. Depression, dementia, and malnutrition are independent risk factors to mistreatment. Bruises should be a cause for suspicion of abuse.

55. A
In elderly clients, the most common presentations of hyperthyroidism are fatigue, weight loss, and tachycardia. Older patients are more likely to have anorexia and atrial fibrillation; heat intolerance, increased sweating, and hyperreflexia are rarer. An atypical sign of hyperthyroidism is a chronic constipation that has 'resolved' by itself (instead of diarrhea).

56. A

A health care proxy is a relative or friend whom the client appoints to make health decisions for her in case she becomes incapacitated by disability or disease. This person is also responsible for carrying out the clients wishes with regards to her health and hospital stay in the same circumstances. The durable power of attorney makes this appointment legally binding.

57. C

A living will is a category of an advanced directive recognized by the law that lists treatments and medical procedures that the patient will allow or refuse in case the client becomes incapacitated by disease or disability. Usually the physician and the nurse help the client make this list.

58. D

Dementia is a slow progressive condition of confusion and forgetfulness that happens in a span of years. It is caused by diminishing number of functioning neurons. In its early stages, orientation to place is not yet apparent, although in later stages disorientation happens, too. Patients with dementia usually exhibit a flat or depressed affect. On the other hand, delirium is a sequela of infections, medications or hospitalization. The onset of confusion is acute and noted from the time trigger factors happened. Delirious clients are oftentimes disoriented to time, place and person, and they have labile fluctuating mood.

59. C

Due to physiologic changes in aging, typical signs of pneumonia that are apparent in younger clients may not be observed in the very elderly clients. They have impaired thermoregulation and decreased ciliary action within airways that makes fever and secretions not readily observable. Rather, they exhibit signs like tachypnea and confusion. The nurse should be alert to further assess the client for pneumonia.

60. B

Delirium is condition of confusion that is oftentimes a sequela of infections, medications or hospitalization. The onset of confusion is acute, noted from the time trigger factors happened. Delirious clients are oftentimes disoriented to time, place and person, and they have labile and fluctuating mood.

61. C

Zoster vaccine is recommended at age 60 years, regardless of whether the patient reports a history of herpes zoster. Studies show that vaccination reduces incidence of herpes zoster by approximately 50% and incidence of postherpetic neuralgia by more than 65%.

62. A

This client has 3 risk parameters for falls: advanced age, possibility of delirium due to hospitalization, and the intake of narcotics for pain.

63. D

Clutter in an elderly's home can cause falls. This client needs to be reminded to clear all passageways, and exits of clutter like cords, toys, plants and jars.

64. B

The nurse should assess alcohol consumption when dealing with polypharmacy because alcohol interacts with a lot of medications.

65. D

Autonomy is the right to direct one's life without disregarding the rights of others. It is encouraged in the elderly to promote ego integrity. Loss of autonomy is a real fear among the elderly.

Putting It All Together

Questions

1. A novice nurse is to perform physical assessment and history. Which of the following should NOT be characteristic of the nurse's assessments?
    a. Do repeated rehearsals
    b. Arrange separate steps to create fluidity of assessment
    c. Minimize the number of position changes
    d. When time is pressing, there is no need for introduction

2. Put the following in the recommended sequence:
    > A. Measurements
    > B. Introduction
    > C. Health history and general appearance
    > D. Skin
    a. B, C, A, D
    b. C, B, A, D
    c. B, A, C, D
    d. B, D, C, A

3. A nurse assesses the radial pulse, counts respirations and measures blood pressure and temperature. Which of the following parameters is the nurse assessing?
    a. Measurements
    b. General status
    c. Vital signs
    d. Circulatory system

4. A nurse is assessing the function of cranial nerves III, IV and VI. Which of the following organ is the nurse examining?
    a. Eyes
    b. Ears
    c. Tongue
    d. Throat

5. The nurse is moving the auricle and moving the tragus to check for tenderness. Which of the following organs is the nurse assessing?
    a. Eyes
    b. Ears
    c. Nose
    d. Mouth

6. Put the following in the recommended sequence:
    > A. Neck
    > B. Heart

    C. Chest- anterior
    D. Chest- posterior
a. B, A, D, C
b. C, D, A, B
c. A, D, C, B
d. A, B, C, D

7. The nurse is seen testing ROM and muscle strength of a group of joints and muscles. She is also checking for epitrochlear nodes, temperature, capillary refill and radial and brachial pulses. Which of the following is the nurse currently assessing?
    a. Vital signs
    b. Upper extremities
    c. Lower extremities
    d. Abdomen

8. The nurse prepares a female client for a clinical breast examination. How should the client be positioned?
    a. Supine, no pillow, head of bed elevated 30 degrees
    b. Semi-fowlers
    c. Left lateral
    d. Flat on bed, no elevation

9. A nurse is conducting a clinical breast examination. Put the following in the correct sequence:
    A. Palpate lymph nodes
    B. Lift one arm up and palpate the breast of the same side
    C. Drape the client appropriately
    D. Teach breast examination
    E. Palpate tail Spence, areolae, nipples after each breast
    a. D, C, B, E, A
    b. D, B, E, A, C
    c. C, B, E, A, D
    d. C, B, A, E, D

10. A nurse is to assess the breasts, the neck vessels, the heart, the inguinal area and the abdomen. Which of these sites should the nurse assess first?
    a. Neck vessels
    b. Breasts
    c. Heart
    d. Inguinal area

11. The physician instructs the nurse to monitor for jugular vein distention. Which of the following anatomical location should the nurse particularly assess?

a. The back of the knee
b. The neck
c. The nape
d. The upper arm

12. The physician instructs the nurse to note any heaves and thrills, and to count the apical pulse. Which of the following should the nurse pay particular attention to?
    a. Upper extremities
    b. Heart
    c. Lower extremities
    d. Abdomen

13. The nurse wants to assess the liver for enlargement and tenderness. Which of the following should the nurse percuss and palpate ?
    a. Upper left quadrant of the abdomen, below the costal margin
    b. Upper right quadrant of the abdomen, below the costal margin
    c. Costovertebral angle
    d. 9th to 12th right intercostal space

14. The nurse tests the client for stereognosis, and asks the client to distinguish superficial pain, light touch and vibration. Which of the following functions is the nurse assessing?
    a. Cardiac
    b. Neurologic
    c. ROM
    d. Gastrointestinal

15. A novice nurse is to perform an examination of the male genitalia. The experienced nurse reminds her of the correct sequence which is:
    A.   Teach testicular self-examination
    B.   Check for hernia
    C.   Inspect the penis and the scrotum
    D.   Inspect the contents of the scrotum
    a. D, C, B, A
    b. C, D, B, A
    c. A, D, C, B
    d. D, A, B, C

16. The nurse is to examine several areas of the client's anatomy and physiology. Which of the following is a correct grouping of activities?
    a. Checking for heaves and thrills, and checking for pulsations in the inguinal area
    b. Palpating rectal walls, assessing the prostate and saving a specimen for hemoccult test
    c. Palpating the breast, checking for jugular vein distention and palpating costovertebral angle

for tenderness

    d.   Inspecting the pinna, checking for occulomotor function and assessing for tingling sensation in the hands

17. The nurse is now documenting her findings. Which of the following statements is true regarding proper documentation?
    a.   It is important to be specific and redundancies are encouraged
    b.   In a legal view, examinations and procedures that are not documented are not done
    c.   Describe in great detail every finding even if normal
    d.   Omit patient subjective complaints

18. A nurse is to check the client's family history. Which of the following should be included in the nurse's documentation?
    a.   Illnesses of the client in the past
    b.   Vaccination record of family members including parents
    c.   Genogram
    d.   A stickman

19. The nurse wants to indicate results of deep tendon reflexes. Which of the following should the nurse utilize to clearly indicate findings?
    a.   Stickman
    b.   Genogram
    c.   Simple drawing
    d.   Detailed description

20. Which of the following tests will necessitate the client to stand up?
    a.   Jugular vein pressure
    b.   Romberg test
    c.   Test for heaves and thrills
    d.   Deep tendon reflexes

21. The nurse is drying a newborn who has just been delivered. Which of the following assessment parameter is the best indicator of adjustment to extrauterine life?
    a.   1-minute Apgar score
    b.   5-minute Apgar score
    c.   Respiratory pattern
    d.   Heart rate

22. Which of the following is a correct technique of examining a neonate?
    a.   Having a heat source over the examination table
    b.   Putting a male neonate on the examination table without diapers
    c.   Putting a female neonate on the examination table with a baby shirt that opens in front

d. Putting a male neonate on the examination table with a baby shirt that opens in front

23. A nurse conducting a physical examination of a neonate is competent to put the following activities in which proper sequence?
    A. General appearance
    B. Chest
    C. Vital signs
    D. Measurement
    a. A, C, D, B
    b. C, A, D, B
    c. C, D, A, B
    d. A, B, C, D

24. A nurse is plotting data on growth curves for a 4-month old infant. Which of the following parameters should be plotted on the growth curves? Select all that apply.
    a. Weight
    b. Length
    c. Waist circumference
    d. Head circumference
    e. Age

25. A nurse is observing a neonate on the examination table. She notes that the client is alert and responsive, with acrocyanosis, with symmetrical limbs and with no deformities. Which of the following parameters is the nurse assessing?
    a. Measurement
    b. Upper extremities
    c. Lower extremities
    d. General appearance

26. A nurse is assessing several pediatric clients. Who of the following patients would need a follow-up evaluation?
    a. A newborn whose head circumference equals chest circumference
    b. A newborn with irregular respirations
    c. A newborn with a soft spot above the forehead
    d. A 6-month old sitting up without support

27. A nurse is assessing a 4-month old baby. Which of the following findings necessitates a physician's immediate attention?
    a. Absent startle reflex
    b. Positive Babinski reflex
    c. Chest retractions
    d. Increased heart rate when crying

28. A nurse is assessing a newborn. Which of the following is NOT a normal finding?
    a. Umbilical cord has two veins and one artery
    b. The abdomen is globular
    c. All four extremities are slightly flexed
    d. Both hands form a fist

29. A nurse wants to assess a 4-month old infant's eyes. Which of the following technique is best to use to facilitate her examination? Select all that apply.
    a. Put the baby in a supine position, support the baby's head and shoulders and slightly hyperextend the neck
    b. Use an ophthalmoscope to elicit blink reflex
    c. Use a penlight to assess for any nystagmus
    d. Use a penlight to assess for pupillary reflex
    e. Have the parent hold her baby with the baby's face above her shoulder

30. A nurse taps her fist on the table, creating a loud noise in the process. Which of the following is the nurse assessing for in a newborn when she does this? Select all that apply.
    a. General appearance
    b. Skin tone
    c. Startle reflex
    d. Babinski reflex
    e. Hearing

31. A competent nurse caring for a 3-month old infant is sure to reserve which test at the last of the examination procedure?
    a. ROM
    b. Ophthalmoscopic exam
    c. Otoscopic exam
    d. Reflexes

32. A nurse wants to assess a 4-month old infant for any head lag. Which technique is best to use when assessing for head lag?
    a. Position the baby prone
    b. Wrap hands around the infant's hand, and pull the infant to a sitting position
    c. Gently shake the baby back and forth
    d. Carry the baby upright over the shoulder

33. A nurse is drying a female newborn with clean towels. As she puts on her diapers, she notes a waxy cheese-like substance in between her labia. Which of the following is best for the nurse to do?
    a. Clean the perineum with betadine solution
    b. Continue putting on the diaper, wrap the infant warmly and document findings

c. Request for an anti-fungal cream
d. Inform the physician

34. A nurse is inspecting the genitalia of a male newborn. Which of the following indicates that the nurse needs further teaching?
a. Checks for rugae of the scrotum
b. Observes for strength of the urine stream
c. Retracts the foreskin to check for obstruction
d. Palpates the testes

35. A nurse is conducting a physical examination on a preschool child. Which of the following procedures would most likely cause the most anxiety in a child?
a. Rinne test
b. Test for Range of motion
c. Assessing the throat with a tongue blade
d. Test for pupillary reflex

36. A nurse wants to assess the lung sounds of a female preschool child. Which of the following technique would most likely elicit the child's cooperation?
a. Demonstrate how to inhale and exhale first before having the client perform it
b. Ask the child to inhale and blow into a pinwheel
c. Get a doll and point to the chest as the area to be examined
d. Use direct and precise instructions

37. A nurse is to perform a thorough physical assessment in a young child. Which of the following sequence is most effective to use?
   A. Head, face and neck
   B. Upper extremities
   C. Eyes
   D. Nose
a. B, A, C, D
b. A, C, D, B
c. C, D, A, B
d. A, B, C, D

38. A nurse is assessing the length of the spinous processes. To which of the following group of examination procedures does assessment of the spinous processes belong?
a. Abdomen
b. Head
c. Lower extremities
d. Thorax

39. A nurse is to perform a transillumination test. The test would detect an abnormality is which client?
    a. A three-year old girl with murmur
    b. A 2-year old girl with fever due to gastroenteritis
    c. A male newborn with undescended testis
    d. A 7-month old female infant with talipes equinovarus

40. Which of the following technique of physical examination is applicable to adolescent clients?
    a. Keeping street clothes on during examination
    b. Preparing a reward to take home after the assessment
    c. Using an anatomical replica of the body parts to be examined
    d. Asking them to change into a hospital gown without underpants

41. The competent nurse is caring for several patients. Which of the following assessment parameters entails continuous monitoring? Select all that apply.
    a. Central venous pressure
    b. Pulse oximetry
    c. Urinalysis results
    d. Intracranial pressure
    e. Deep tendon reflexes

42. A nurse is to conduct a health history on a client. Which of the following is NOT appropriate to do before or during the interview?
    a. Note any flags or markers on the client's door that indicate special needs or precautions
    b. Introduce oneself as their nurse while quickly assessing the client's pulse oximeter
    c. Assess if the client is having any pain or discomfort
    d. Validate significant client symptoms that were assessed during the previous shift

43. A nurse reads in the documentation of the nurse from an earlier shift that the client is 'alert, oriented to time and place, and responds appropriately'. Which of the following assessment parameters was the nurse referring to?
    a. Facial expression
    b. Level of consciousness
    c. Articulation
    d. Cranial nerve function

44. A nurse is taking the vital signs of a client. Which of the following is NOT a correct technique?
    a. Counting the apical pulse when the radial pulse is barely palpable
    b. Taking the blood pressure on the arm with a fistula
    c. Taking the oral temperature when the tympanic thermometer is not available
    d. Counting the respirations while the client is reading a book

45. A nurse just administered morphine to treat the client's pain. Which of the following is the nurse's main responsibility after administration of this medication?
    a. Assess pain level after 1 hour
    b. Check for adverse effect after 72 hours
    c. Promptly endorse assessment of pain levels to the nurse of the incoming shift
    d. Assess pain level after 15 minutes

46. A competent nurse should use which proper sequence when conducting assessment of an adult client?
    A. Health history
    B. Neurologic assessment
    C. Measurement
    D. General appearance
    a. A, B, C, D
    b. D, C, A, B
    c. A, D, C, B
    d. D, A, B, C

47. A client's pulse oximeter reading has been decreasing for the past 24 hours. He had an abdominal surgery 2 days ago. The last reading was 94%. Which of the following equipment should the nurse have a client use to improve his oxygenation?
    a. Brown paper bag
    b. Treadmill
    c. Incentive spirometer
    d. Ventilator

48. A nurse is assessing the cardiovascular system of a client. Which of the following actions by the nurse indicates a need for further teaching?
    a. Checking the apical pulse and the radial pulse at the same time
    b. Assessing the heart sounds over a gown of a client who complains of chills
    c. Assessing for heart rhythm at the apex
    d. Checking capillary refill at both upper and lower extremities

49. A nurse is having difficulty assessing the peripheral pulses of an obese client. Which of the following equipment would help her in her assessment?
    a. Otoscope
    b. A hand-held Doppler ultrasound
    c. Stethoscope
    d. MRI

50. Which of the following sequence of adult physical assessment reflects competence in a nurse?

A. Respiratory system
B. Cardiovascular system
C. Abdomen
D. Skin

a.   A, B, C, D
b.   A, B, D, C
c.   B, A, C, D
d.   A, C, D, B

51. After abdominal surgery, a client has been allowed to eat soft foods as tolerated. Which of the following should be included in the nurse's findings before resumption of eating is allowed?
    a.   No reports of pain
    b.   Wound is approximated with no signs of infection
    c.   Reports of passing of flatus
    d.   Client can stand up

52. A client has just undergone abdominal surgery. The client has an IV, is receiving oxygen, and still with a Foley catheter. After 6 hours, which of the following findings may need to be reported to the physician?
    a.   Urine bag has a content of 50ml
    b.   Heart rate is 100 per minute
    c.   Client is drowsy
    d.   Oxygen saturation 96%

53. A post-surgical client has been encouraged to ambulate. His Foley catheter has been removed. The nurse understands that the client should have voided at least once in how many hours?
    a.   1-2 hours
    b.   4-6 hours
    c.   30 minutes to 1hour
    d.   8-10 hours

54. A nurse has assisted a client in putting on an antiembolic hose. Which of the following should the nurse advise the client regarding its use? Select all that apply.
    a.   Apply talcum powder inside the hose prior to use
    b.   Wear for 22 hours
    c.   Remove only for bathing
    d.   Put on while the foot is dangling on the bed for at least five minutes
    e.   It is best to put it on before bed

55. The nurse makes several findings on different clients. Which of the following findings requires immediate attention?
    a.   Pupils - PERLA

b. Oxygen saturation 90%
c. Nausea and vomiting after chemotherapy
d. Pain at the surgical site, level 4, eight hours after surgery

56. A nurse is to access important medical information of a client. Which of the following is the digitalized medical record?
    a. Chart
    b. EHR
    c. Billing
    d. Patient satisfaction survey

57. The EHR contains which of the following information?
    a. Billing
    b. Schedule of future visits
    c. Transfer details
    d. Patient information

58. Digitalization of patient health data has numerous benefits. Which of the following is the benefit of computer physician order entry (CPOE)?
    a. It allows redundancies in medication
    b. It allows only one physician to prescribe medications
    c. It decreases errors in prescribing and transcription of medications
    d. It allows the nurse to view initial physician assessment findings via a computer

59. A novice nurse is having difficulty using the EHR. She has to be reminded that there are numerous advantages of using an electronic medical record. Select all advantages.
    a. Helps detect healthcare associated infections
    b. Requires expertise in the use of current technology
    c. Increases patient safety
    d. Helps identify medications
    e. Helps prevent prescription errors

60. The nurse uses the SBAR to organize assessment data for verbal communication. Which of the following is NOT part of SBAR?
    a. S- Situation
    b. B- Background
    c. A- Assessment
    d. R- Recognition

61. The nurse wants to take measurements of the range of motions of a patient's joints. Which instrument should the nurse obtain?
    a. Reflex hammer

   b. Pulse oximeter
   c. Doppler
   d. Goniometer

62. A novice nurse asks a senior nurse what a stadiometer is. Which of the following is an accurate description of a stadiometer?
   a. It measures height
   b. It measures weight
   c. It measures pulse quality
   d. It measures the maximum volume of air in the lungs

63. A nurse is obtaining an obese patient's blood pressure measurements but is having difficulty hearing the Korotkoff sounds. Which of the following instruments should the nurse obtain to better hear the pulse beats?
   a. A pulse oximeter
   b. A scoliometer
   c. A Doppler
   d. An extra large BP cuff

64. The nurse is about to begin a head-to-toe assessment of the patient. Which of the following set of tasks should the nurse perform first?
   a. Perform handwashing, make an introduction, explain the procedure
   b. Prepare the patient's charts and inform the supervisor
   c. Put on gloves and other personal protective equipment
   d. Prepare equipment and supplies on a table just outside the examination room

65. Which of the following parameters will the nurse be UNABLE to assess by just observing the patient and the environment?
   a. Presence of background noise
   b. Safety of the immediate surrounding
   c. The patient's thought processes
   d. The patient's grooming

66. The nurse is to obtain a patient's vital signs, but the patient's clothing makes it difficult for the nurse to make the assessments. Which of the following is best for the nurse to do to successfully obtain vital signs?
   a. Have the patient lie down
   b. Roll the sleeves up
   c. Remove all upper garments
   d. Ask the patient to change into a hospital gown

67. After taking the vital signs, which of the following assessments should the nurse do next?

a. Inspection of the integument
b. Mental status examination
c. Inspection of the head and face
d. Body measurements

68. How should the patient be positioned before starting to assess the integument?
   a. Sitting up in bed and slightly leaning forward on an overbed table
   b. Sitting on the edge of the bed or examining table, with the feet dangling
   c. Supine in bed
   d. Semi-fowler's

69. When examining the eyes, which test should be done first?
   a. Test for acuity
   b. Inspection of the outer structures
   c. Inspection of the inner eye
   d. Test for visual fields

70. The nurse is to examine the patient's ear. Which of the following instruments or supplies will the nurse need?
   a. A Snellen chart
   b. Cotton balls
   c. An ophthalmoscope
   d. A tuning fork

71. The nurse is evaluating the patient's nose and sinuses next. Which cranial nerve is needed to be tested at this time?
   a. CN I
   b. CN II
   c. CN III
   d. CN IV

72. The nurse needs to palpate for the patient's thyroid gland and examine the posterior chest. What is the best position for the nurse to be in to perform these assessments?
   a. Sitting down so that the nurse is lower than the patient
   b. Standing behind the seated patient
   c. Facing the patient's left side
   d. Facing the patient's right side

73. In which area of assessment will the nurse determine costovertebral angle tenderness?
   a. Abdomen
   b. Anterior thorax
   c. Posterior thorax

d.   Upper extremities

74. The nurse is to perform a cardiac assessment to listen to signs of aortic stenosis or murmur. How should the patient be positioned for this examination?
   a.   Sitting
   b.   Supine
   c.   Side-lying
   d.   Semi-fowler's

75. The nurse is to assess both the carotid artery and the jugular vein. How should the patient be positioned for this examination?
   a.   Supine with the bed flat
   b.   Semi-fowlers with HOB 30°
   c.   Side-lying
   d.   Sitting up

76. Which should follow cardiovascular assessments while the patient is still lying down?
   a.   Examination of the musculoskeletal system (upper body)
   b.   Examination of the musculoskeletal system (lower body)
   c.   Breast examination
   d.   Abdomen

77. The nurse is to perform an examination of the patient's abdomen. How should the nurse proceed with the assessment?
   a.   Inspection, auscultation, percussion, palpation
   b.   Inspection, percussion, palpation, auscultation,
   c.   Inspection, palpation, auscultation, percussion,
   d.   auscultation, inspection, palpation, percussion,

78. Which body parts should the nurse examine to assess for peripheral vascular status?
   a.   Anterior chest
   b.   Posterior chest
   c.   Arms and legs
   d.   Head and neck

79. The nurse is to assess the musculoskeletal system of the patient next while the patient is still lying down. Which body part should the nurse start examining first?
   a.   The upper body
   b.   The lower body
   c.   The anterior chest
   d.   The posterior chest

80. The nurse is to perform neurologic assessments. Which of the following will elicit a neurologic motor response?
    a. Stereognosis
    b. Position sense
    c. Deep tendon reflexes
    d. Vibration

81. The nurse is to perform neurologic assessments, particularly the Romberg test. How should the patient be positioned during this test?
    a. Sitting up leaning forward
    b. Sitting by the side of the bed
    c. Standing up
    d. Sitting up on a chair

82. A nurse is to assist in the pelvic examination of a female patient. How should the nurse prepare the speculum?
    a. Put a disposable probe on the tips
    b. Soak it in warm water
    c. Put petroleum jelly on the tips
    d. Cover the tips with gauze

83. A physician orders oxygen saturation measurements for a patient. Which of the following supplies/equipment should the nurse obtain to comply with the physician's order?
    a. A venipuncture set
    b. A Doppler
    c. A BP apparatus
    d. A pulse oximeter

84. Which of the following does NOT reflect respect for the patient's privacy?
    a. Closing the door before the examination
    b. Closing the curtain before the examination
    c. Asking the patient to undress and put on a gown while equipment and supplies are prepared in front of them
    d. Exposing only the body part to be examined

85. Which of the following tool should the nurse use to assess for the patient's cognitive functions?
    a. The Mini-Mental Status Examination (MMSE) tool
    b. The CAGE questionnaire
    c. The Glasgow Coma Scale
    d. Beck Depression Inventory

ANSWERS

1. D

    To ensure that the client trusts the nurse, there should be formal introduction even if time is pressing. During emergencies, however, introduction can be skipped.

2. A

    The recommended sequence for assessment procedures should start with proper introduction, followed by history taking together with general appearance and then assessment of the skin.

3. C

    The vital signs include radial pulse, temperature, blood pressure and respiration.

4. A

    Cranial nerves III, IV, and VI are responsible for the sensory and motor functions of the eyes.

5. B

    The tragus and the auricle are parts of the external ear.

6. C

    The recommended sequence is neck, posterior chest, anterior chest and then the heart.

7. B

    When assessing the upper extremities, the nurse performs ROM exercises and checks muscle strength. She also checks for epitrochlear nodes, temperature, capillary refill and radial and brachial pulses.

8. A

    Before a clinical breast examination in a female client, the nurse positions the client supine with the head flat and the head of the bed elevated to 30 degrees.

9. C

    The correct sequence is to first drape the client appropriately, lift the arm of the side to be palpated, palpate the breast tissue and then the tail of Spence, the areola and nipple of the same breast and then the lymph nodes up to the axilla. The health teaching comes last.

10. B

    The proper sequence of the above is: Breasts, neck vessels, heart, abdomen and then the inguinal area.

11. B

    Jugular vein distention can be assessed by looking at the client's neck.

12. B

    Heaves are observable pulsations of the heart and thrills are palpable pulsations. The apical pulse is to be assessed on the 5th intercostal space, left midclavicular line in a non-enlarged heart.

13. B

    The liver is located at the right upper quadrant of the abdomen, below the costal margin.

14. B

    Tests for stereognosis and distinguishing superficial pain, light touch and vibrations are part of a neurologic assessment.

15. B

    The correct sequence in examining the male genitalia is to first to inspect the penis and scrotum and then to assess for scrotal content. The nurse checks the surrounding areas and palpates for presence of inguinal hernias. Teaching testicular self-examination is the last.

16. B

    The correct grouping of activities is: assessment rectal walls, assessing the prostate and saving a specimen for hemoccult test. They all involve entry to the anal canal.

17. B

    It is important to know that while it is important for the nurse to use clear and concise phrases, and to include relevant normal and abnormal findings, any findings not documented are considered not done at all.

18. C

    A genogram will show health histories from both the mother's side and the father's side.

19. A

    A stickman will best depict findings of deep tendon reflexes.

20. B

    For the Romberg test, the client needs to be standing up. He will then be asked to close his eyes and maintain the position for at least 20 minutes.

21. B

    The best indicator of adjustment to extrauterine life is the 5-minute Apgar score. The 1-minute Apgar score determines how the baby tolerated labor and birthing. Both test for breathing effort, heart rate, muscle tone, reflexes and skin color.

22. A

    A heat source should be placed over the examination table because neonates are prone to cold stress. A male neonate should wear diapers that should be removed only when inspecting the genitalia and the buttocks. The baby should have no other clothing.

23. C
The correct sequence when conducting physical assessment of a neonate is to first take vital signs and measurements, and then assess the general appearance followed by the chest and the heart.

24. A, B, D, E

25. D
Assessment of general appearance includes parameters such as, alertness, skin color, symmetry, cry, movement and deformities if present.

26. A
A newborn whose head circumference is equal to the chest circumference has microcephaly. The client needs to undergo further evaluation.

27. C
Chest retractions in an infant indicate respiratory distress. This warrants immediate medical attention. The startle reflex is gone at four months. Babinski reflex persists until the 12th month. When crying, the heart rate increases.

28. A
The umbilical cord of a newborn should have two arteries and one vein.

29. A, C, E
When assessing the baby's eyes, the nurse may opt to slightly hyperextending the neck while supporting the head and shoulders or have the parent carry the baby upright with the face above the parent's shoulder. The nurse uses the penlight to assess for pupillary, blink and corneal reflexes, and the ophthalmoscope to check for the red reflex.

30. D, E
The nurse produces a loud sound to both assess for startle reflex and hearing in a newborn.

31. C
The nurse should conduct the otoscopic examination last because this creates the most anxiety in a young infant because of the probing nature of the procedure.

32. B
When assessing for head lag in a very young infant, the nurse wraps her hands around the infant's hand and pulls the infant to a sitting position.

33. B

The waxy cheese-like substance found in between the labia of a newborn is vernix caseosa. It is a normal finding.

34. C

Retracting the foreskin can traumatize the thin skin, which will cause pain.

35. C

Preschoolers are very cooperative, but they fear bodily injury. Probing examinations such as inserting a tongue blade in the mouth creates undue anxiety in the child.

36. B

The nurse can best elicit a preschool child's cooperation when assessing for lung sounds by having the child blow on a pinwheel. It can also be used as a positive reinforcement for cooperation by telling her she can have it after the examination.

37. A

The best sequence of assessment activities is: examination of the upper extremities, of the head face and neck, followed by the eyes and then the nose.

38. D

The spinous processes of the spine belong to the group of activities in the assessment of the thorax.

39. C

The transillumination test is usually used to check presence of testis in the scrotum. The room is dimmed and a flashlight is lit over the scrotum. The outline of the testis should normally be visible.

40. A

The adolescent is self-conscious and will not be comfortable undressing. The examination should proceed with the street clothes on. Anatomical replicas to explain a procedure are usually used when the client is for a medical or surgical procedure.

41. A, B, D

Assessment parameters that need continuous monitoring are central venous pressure, intracranial pressure, pulse oximetry, adventitious breath sounds, abnormal blood pressure, and deteriorating level of consciousness among others.

42. B

When introducing oneself as a nurse, use direct eye contact.

43. B

Checking for alertness, orientation to place, person and time, responsiveness and attentiveness is assessing for level of consciousness.

44. B
The client should refrain from taking blood pressure measurements on the arm with fistulas, recent arterial access or IV access.

45. D
After administering pain medications, assess the level of the client's pain 1 hour after oral medications, and after 15 minutes if given IV. IV medications take effect faster.

46. C
The proper sequence at the beginning of assessment is: health history, assessment of general appearance, performing measurements followed by neurologic assessments.

47. C
An incentive spirometer is a device that encourages lung expansion and improve oxygenation. The client puts the mouthpiece in the mouth, and forms a seal with the lips. He then inhales as deep as possible and holds his breath for 2-6 seconds.

48. B
Auscultating heart and lung sounds over a gown will interfere with hearing significant heart and lung sounds, and should be avoided.

49. B
A hand-held Doppler ultrasound will detect blood flow in the arteries and veins of the extremities when assessment of the pulse through palpation is difficult.

50. B
The nurse should ideally follow this sequence when conducting an adult physical examination: Assessment of the respiratory and then the cardiovascular system, of the skin and then of the abdomen.

51. C
A client's bowels should have resumed motility before the client can eat. If not, he may experience bloating, nausea and vomiting. Indications that bowel activities have resumed are passing flatus or stool, or hearing bowel sounds through auscultation.

52. A
A post-operative client with a Foley catheter should be continuously draining urine. The normal output is 30ml/hr. An urinary output of 50ml for the last 6 hours may indicate a stricture or obstruction in the urinary tract.

53. B

   Post-surgical clients, whose Foley catheter has been removed, should at least have 1 voiding within 4-6 hours after the surgery.

54. B, C

   Thromboembolic disease hose should be worn before getting up from bed in the morning, worn for 22 hours, and removed only for bathing and cleaning purposes.

55. B

   An SaO2 of 90% is a red flag, meaning the client has poor oxygenation and therefore requires immediate medical attention.

56. B

   The electronic health record (EHR) is the digitalized form of client's health data that has replaced paper documentation or charts.

57. D

   The electronic health record contains all known health information on a client.

58. C

   The primary benefit of computer physician order entry (CPOE) is that it decreases errors in prescribing and transcription of medications.

59. A, C, D, E

   The advantages of an EHR are: it helps detect healthcare-associated infections, helps identify medications and prevent prescription errors. Overall, it increases patient safety.

60. D

   SBAR stands for Situation, Background, Assessment, and Recommendation. It is used to organize assessment data for verbal communication.

61. D

   A goniometer is an instrument that measures angles, and it is used to determine a patient's range of motion.

62. A

   A stadiometer is an instrument that is used to measure height. It is either mounted on the wall or portable. It has a horizontal headpiece that is rested on the patient's head.

63. C

   A Doppler amplifies sounds. When Korotkoff sounds are difficult to hear using a stethoscope, the nurse may obtain a Doppler to listen to the beats better.

64. A

Before beginning a thorough assessment, the nurse must perform handwashing to prevent the spread of microorganisms that cause infections. It is also important to introduce oneself as part of building rapport. The nurse also needs to explain the procedure so that the patient will know what to expect out of the nurse-patient encounter.

65. C

To assess the patient's thought processes, the nurse needs to interview the patient. Observation will not explore the patient's thoughts.

66. D

When a patient's clothing is getting in the way of the nurse's assessments, the nurse may assist the patient to change into a hospital gown. A gown will expose the arms for blood pressure measurements and make the rest of the examination convenient for both the nurse and the patient.

67. D

To ensure that the examination proceeds in a logical flow, the nurse should take the patient's body measurements after taking the vital signs. Body measurements include the height, weight, and Body Mass Index (BMI).

68. B

The best patient position for integument assessment is to have the patient sitting at the edge of the bed with the feet dangling. Before doing so, ensure that the patient is able to sit up without support. This position enables the nurse to see them and inspect the skin up close.

69. A

To ensure that the examination of the eye proceeds in a logical flow, the nurse must begin testing the patient's visual acuity first. This test should be followed in correct sequence by the inspection of the outer structures, testing of the visual field, eye muscle tests, and finally an ophthalmoscopic examination.

70. D

A tuning fork is needed to conduct the Weber and Rinne tests. These tests assess for conductive and sensorineural hearing losses.

71. A

The Cranial Nerve I or the olfactory nerve functions will need to be tested during the examination of the patient's nose and sinuses. The nurse has to prepare objects with different scents to evaluate the olfactory nerve function.

72. B

To be able to palpate for the patient's thyroid gland efficiently and also to start the examination of the posterior chest, the nurse should stand behind the seated patient.

73. C

The assessment for costovertebral angle tenderness involves percussion of the back at the angle formed by the spine and the costal margin. Tapping this area elicits pain in patients with inflamed kidneys.

74. A

To efficiently auscultate for murmurs, the patient should be sitting up. The nurse should also use the bell of the stethoscope in auscultation.

75. B

To start assessing the carotid pulse and the jugular vein, the patient must be lying supine with the head of the bed elevated 30°.

76. C

Breast examination should follow cardiovascular assessments while the patient is still lying in bed. The abdomen should be assessed next after doing breast exams.

77. A

In the examination of the abdomen, auscultation should follow inspection because palpation and percussion may alter bowel sounds and render the result of the examination inaccurate.

78. C

The patient's peripheral vascular status is assessed by examining the patient's arms and legs. The nurse checks the patient's radial, brachial, femoral, popliteal, posterior tibia, and dorsalis pedis pulses. This is also the time to check for color changes, symmetry, and for the presence of edema and lesions.

79. B

While the patient is still lying down after the examination of the abdomen, the nurse should proceed to examine the musculoskeletal system of the lower body next, starting with the hips. After the lower body is examined, the musculoskeletal structures of the upper body are assessed next.

80. C

Deep tendon reflexes are a neurologic motor response. Stereognosis, position sense, vibration, pain and light touch are all neurologic sensory functions.

81. C

To perform the Romberg test, the patient should be standing up. The nurse can also check for gait and balance problems while the patient is walking.

82. B

Before the speculum is to be used for pelvic examination, it is the nurse's responsibility to warm the speculum by putting it in a clean container with warm water. Using a cold metal speculum can make the patient uncomfortable, and tense the perineal muscles, making the examination difficult.

83. D

A pulse oximeter is a non-invasive equipment that monitors a patient's oxygen saturation. It is clipped on a finger with good perfusion.

84. C

During a physical examination, the nurse must ensure the patient's privacy by closing doors, windows, and curtains as appropriate. They must also adequately cover the patient, and expose only the body parts that are to be examined.

85. A

The Mini-Mental Status Examination tool (MMSE) is used to test the patient's cognitive functions and mental status.